NEURO-NUTRACEUTICALS AND DRUG DISCOVERY AND DELIVERY IN ALZHEIMER'S DISEASE

Volume 1

Targeting Key Pathological Pathways

Neuro-Nutraceuticals and Drug Discovery and Delivery in Alzheimer's Disease, 2-volume set:
ISBN: 978-1-77491-844-9 (hbk)

Volume 1: Targeting Key Pathological Pathways
ISBN: 978-1-77491-942-2 (hbk)
ISBN: 978-1-00357-035-6 (ebk)

Volume 2: Strategies to Unlock the Brain's Fortress
ISBN: 978-1-77491-944-6 (hbk)
ISBN: 978-1-00357-058-5 (ebk)

NEURO-NUTRACEUTICALS AND DRUG DISCOVERY AND DELIVERY IN ALZHEIMER'S DISEASE

Volume 1

Targeting Key Pathological Pathways

Varinder Singh, PhD
Amit Kumar, PhD
Parul Sood, PhD
Editors

AAP | APPLE ACADEMIC PRESS

First edition published 2025

Apple Academic Press Inc.
1265 Goldenrod Circle, NE,
Palm Bay, FL 32905 USA

760 Laurentian Drive, Unit 19,
Burlington, ON L7N 0A4, CANADA

CRC Press
2385 NW Executive Center Drive,
Suite 320, Boca Raton FL 33431

4 Park Square, Milton Park,
Abingdon, Oxon, OX14 4RN UK

Library and Archives Canada Cataloguing in Publication

CIP data on file with Canada Library and Archives

Library of Congress Cataloging-in-Publication Data

CIP data on file with US Library of Congress

ISBN: 978-1-77491-942-2 (hbk)
ISBN: 978-1-77491-943-9 (pbk)
ISBN: 978-1-00357-035-6 (ebk)

Dedication

This book is dedicated to
God Almighty and our parents.

About the Editors

Varinder Singh, PhD
Assistant Professor, Department of Pharmaceutical Sciences & Technology, Maharaja Ranjit Singh Punjab Technical University, Bathinda, Punjab, India

Varinder Singh, PhD, is working as an Assistant Professor in the Department of Pharmaceutical Sciences and Technology at Maharaja Ranjit Singh Punjab Technical University, Bathinda, Punjab, India. His research interests primarily lie in the discovery and development of natural products for therapeutic use. He is well-versed in the fields of natural product chemistry (isolation and characterization of bioactive natural compounds), drug discovery, and pharmacology. He has a strong record of publications in high-impact peer-reviewed journals (39 peer-reviewed publications), with many of his papers cited extensively in the field of natural products. He has one patent granted. He has been awarded with numerous travel grants from government and non-government organizations, including the Alzheimer's Association International, the Indian Department of Science and Technology, Indian Council of Medical Research, and International Brain Research Organization. He earned his PhD (Pharmaceutical Sciences) at Punjabi University, Patiala, Punjab, India.

Amit Kumar, PhD
Associate Professor, Chitkara College of Pharmacy, Chitkara University, Punjab, India

Amit Kumar, PhD, is working as an Associate Professor at Chitkara College of Pharmacy, Chitkara University, Punjab, India. He has 12 years of teaching and research experience and has published more than 20 research articles in international journals. He has to date 371 citations and an h-index of 11. He has filed three patents. His area of research includes neuroprotective drug development and elucidating pathological features of diseases. He has received various awards and grants from the International Brain Research Organization, the Indian Department of Science and Technology

(DST)-Science and Engineering Research Board, and the Indian Council of Medical Research. He is a certified trainer of Scientific Medical Writing approved from the Life Sciences Sector Skill Development Council and DST (Govt. of India). He received his graduate, postgraduate, and PhD degrees in Pharmaceutical Sciences from Punjabi University Patiala, Punjab, India.

Parul Sood, PhD
Associate Professor, Chitkara School of Pharmacy, Chitkara University, Himachal Pradesh, India

Parul Sood, PhD, is working as an Associate Professor at Chitkara School of Pharmacy, Chitkara University, Himachal Pradesh, India. She has more than 14 years of professional experience in teaching and research. Her area of specialization and research is exploring herbal plants for the treatment of various neurological disorders including, Alzheimer's disease, as well as pharmacognostical and phytochemical evaluation, and standardization of herbal drugs and herbal drug formulation development. She is a gold medalist in MPharm and GATE as well as GPAT qualified. She has total of 12 publications in reputed journals and has presented a total of 15 oral/poster presentations at national and international conferences and was awarded third position at two national conferences. She completed her PhD at the Department of Pharmaceutical Sciences, Punjabi University Patiala, Punjab, India.

Contents

Contributors

K. Anitha
Department of Pharmacology, Amity Institute of Pharmacy, Amity University Madhya Pradesh, Gwalior, Madhya Pradesh, India

Shiveena Bhatia
Department of Pharmacology and Toxicology, Department of Pharmacy, Birla Institute of Technology and Science Pilani, Pilani Campus, Rajasthan, India

Shvetank Bhatt
School of Pharmacy, Dr. Vishwanath Karad MIT World Peace University, Pune, Maharashtra, India

Shilpi Chauhan
Lloyd Institute of Management and Technology, Greater Noida, Uttar Pradesh, India

Dimple Sethi Chopra
Department of Pharmaceutical Sciences and Drug Research, Punjabi University, Patiala, Punjab, India

Sunayna Choudhary
Department of Pharmacognosy, M.M. College of Pharmacy, Maharishi Markandeshwar (Deemed to be University), Mullana, Ambala, Haryana, India

Kamal Dua
Discipline of Pharmacy, Graduate School of Health, University of Technology Sydney, NSW, Australia; Faculty of Health, Australian Research Center in Complementary and Integrative Medicine, University of Technology Sydney, Ultimo, NSW, Australia

Vinod Kumar Gauttam
Department of Pharmacognosy, Shiva Institute of Pharmacy, Bilaspur, Himachal Pradesh, India

Parveen Kumar Goyal
Department of Pharmacy, Panipat Institute of Engineering and Technology (PIET), Samalkha, Panipat, Haryana, India

Nisha Gupta
Lloyd Institute of Management and Technology, Greater Noida, Uttar Pradesh, India

Sumeet Gupta
Department of Pharmacy, M.M. College of Pharmacy, M.M. (Deemed to be University), Mullana, Ambala, Haryana, India

Amteshwar Singh Jaggi
Department of Pharmaceutical Sciences and Drug Research, Punjabi University, Patiala, Punjab, India

Manish Kumar Jeengar
Department of Pharmacology, School of Pharmacy, Amrita Vishwa Vidyapeetham, AIMS Health Sciences Campus, AIMS Ponekkara, Ernakulam, Kochi, Kerala, India

Ayush Kandpal
Department of Pharmaceutical Sciences and Drug Research, Punjabi University, Patiala, Punjab, India

Shreya Kaul
Amity Institute of Pharmacy, Amity University, Noida, Uttar Pradesh, India

Simrat Kaur
Department of Pharmaceutical Sciences and Drug Research, Punjabi University, Patiala, Punjab, India

Monika Kaushik
Department of Pharmacology, Amity Institute of Pharmacy, Amity University Madhya Pradesh, Gwalior, Madhya Pradesh, India

Suman Khurana
Amity Institute of Pharmacy, Amity University Haryana, Amity Education Valley, Manesar, Gurugram, Haryana, India; Department of Pharmacy, Panipat Institute of Engineering and Technology (PIET), Samalkha, Panipat, Haryana, India

Amit Kumar
Chitkara College of Pharmacy, Chitkara University, Punjab, India

Kuldeep Kumar
Department of Pharmaceutical Sciences and Drug Research, Punjabi University, Patiala, Punjab, India

Mohit Kumar
Department of Pharmaceutical Sciences and Technology, Maharaja Ranjit Singh Punjab Technical University, Bathinda, Punjab, India

Rahul Kumar
Department of Biological Science, National Institute of Pharmaceutical Education and Research (NIPER), Hyderabad, Telangana, India

Preeti Maan
Lloyd Institute of Management and Technology, Greater Noida, Uttar Pradesh, India

Indrani Maji
Department of Pharmaceutics, National Institute of Pharmaceutical Education and Research (NIPER), Hyderabad, Telangana, India

Vasudevan Mani
Department of Pharmacology and Toxicology, College of Pharmacy, Qassim University, Buraydah, Kingdom of Saudi Arabia

Mintu Mathew
Department of Pharmacology, Amrita School of Pharmacy, Amrita Vishwa Vidyapeetham, AIMS Health Sciences Campus, Kochi, Ernakulam, Kerala, India

Anuradha Mishra
Department of Food Technology, M.M.I.C.T. & B.M., Maharishi Markandeshwar (Deemed to be University), Mullana, Ambala, Haryana, India

Arun Mittal
Amity Institute of Pharmacy, Amity University Haryana, Amity Education Valley, Manesar, Gurugram, Haryana, India

Kavita Munjal
Assistant Professor, Department of Pharmacy, Amity Institute of Pharmacy, Amity University, Noida, Uttar Pradesh, India

Nikita Nain
Department of Pharmacy, M.M. College of Pharmacy, M.M. (Deemed to be University), Mullana, Ambala, Haryana, India

Prachi Parvatikar
Department of Biotechnology, Allied Health Sciences BLDE (DU), Vijayapura, Karnataka, India

Rohini Pujari
School of Pharmacy, Dr. Vishwanath Karad MIT World Peace University, Pune, Maharashtra, India

Satish Sardana
Amity Institute of Pharmacy, Amity University Haryana, Amity Education Valley, Manesar, Gurugram, Haryana, India

Shreya Sharma
School of Pharmacy, Dr. Vishwanath Karad MIT World Peace University, Pune, Maharashtra, India

Satish Shilpi
Faculty of Pharmacy, DIT University, Dehradun, Uttarakhand, India

Dhandeep Singh
Department of Pharmaceutical Sciences and Drug Research, Punjabi University, Patiala, Punjab, India

Hasandeep Singh
Department of Pharmaceutical Sciences, Guru Nanak Dev University, Amritsar, Punjab, India

Manjinder Singh
Chitkara College of Pharmacy, Chitkara University, Punjab, India

Nirmal Singh
Professor and Former Head, Department of Pharmaceutical Sciences and Drug Research, Punjabi University, Patiala, Punjab, India

Pankaj Kumar Singh
Department of Pharmaceutics, National Institute of Pharmaceutical Education and Research (NIPER), Hyderabad, Telangana, India

Shashi Bala Singh
Department of Biological Science, National Institute of Pharmaceutical Education and Research (NIPER), Hyderabad, Telangana, India

Tanveer Singh
Department of Neuroscience and Experimental Therapeutics, College of Medicine, Texas A&M Health Science Center, TX, USA

Varinder Singh
Department of Pharmaceutical Sciences and Technology, Maharaja Ranjit Singh Punjab Technical University, Bathinda, Punjab, India

Rajan Swami
Chitkara Collage of Pharmacy, Chitkara University, Punjab, India

Jaya Thomas
Department of Pharmacology, Amrita School of Pharmacy, Amrita Vishwa Vidyapeetham, AIMS Health Sciences Campus, Kochi, Ernakulam, Kerala, India

Vaishnavi R. Unnithan
Department of Pharmacology, Amrita School of Pharmacy, Amrita Vishwa Vidyapeetham, AIMS Health Sciences Campus, Kochi, Ernakulam, Kerala, India

S. Vijayaraj
Department of Pharmaceutical Analysis and Chemistry, Dr. Kalam College of Pharmacy, Avanam, Thanjavur, Tamil Nadu, India

Harlokesh Narayan Yadav
Department of Pharmacology, All India Institute of Medical Sciences, New Delhi, India

Kamica Yadav
Department of Pharmacy, Starex University, Gurugram, Haryana, India; Amity Institute of Pharmacy, Amity University Haryana, Amity Education Valley, Manesar, Gurugram, Haryana, India

Preface

Within the enigmatic realm of the human brain lies the devastating impact of Alzheimer's disease—an affliction that robs individuals of their memories, their identities, and their very essence. As our global population ages, the urgency to combat this formidable adversary grows exponentially. The search for effective treatments and potential cures has become a paramount quest, one that demands unwavering dedication, relentless research, and a multifaceted approach. This book, titled *Neuro-Nutraceuticals and Drug Discovery in Alzheimer's Disease, Volume 1: Targeting Key Pathological Pathways,* represents a collective effort to delve into the potential of nature's pharmacopeia in our battle against Alzheimer's disease.

As we delve into the depths of Alzheimer's disease, we uncover the key pathological pathways that fuel its progression—amyloid-beta aggregation, tau hyperphosphorylation, neuroinflammation, oxidative stress, and synaptic dysfunction. Each of these pathways holds crucial clues to potential therapeutic targets, offering a glimmer of hope in the fight against this relentless ailment. Conventional drugs, while providing symptomatic relief, have often fallen short of halting the relentless progression of this neurodegenerative disorder. In the face of such challenges, the exploration of nutraceuticals derived from medicinal plants emerges as a promising frontier. Nature, with its bountiful offerings, holds the potential to provide safer and more effective therapeutic candidates, while also addressing concerns about undesirable side effects and soaring costs associated with existing treatments.

In this book, we embark on a profound exploration of the world of neuropsychopharmacology, drug discovery, and the emerging field of nutraceutical interventions for Alzheimer's disease. Our journey takes us into the intricate pathways of this debilitating condition, where we unravel the underlying mechanisms and complexities of the disease's pathology.

The purpose of this book is to consolidate the latest research and advancements in the field of natural product drug discovery and Alzheimer's disease. Our esteemed team of editors, Dr. Varinder Singh, Dr. Amit Kumar, and Dr. Parul Sood, have meticulously curated two comprehensive sections to cover diverse aspects of this subject.

Section I lays the foundation by unveiling the underlying pathological, biochemical, molecular, and genetic aspects of Alzheimer's disease. These chapters provide essential insights into the intricacies of the disease and serve as a springboard for the subsequent discussions on potential therapeutic interventions. Section II forms the heart of the book, shining a spotlight on the vast potential of nutraceuticals in managing Alzheimer's disease. This section explores a plethora of medicinal plants and their secondary metabolites that show promise in treating this devastating condition. From preclinical findings to clinical studies, these chapters present a wealth of knowledge on memory improvement effects and the mechanisms underlying the actions of these neuronutraceuticals.

As we journey through the pages of this book, it is our hope that readers, whether seasoned researchers, practitioners, or aspiring students, will find themselves enlightened by the wealth of scientific knowledge presented herein. The compilation of cutting-edge research and in-depth exploration of the therapeutic potential of nature's offerings shall contribute to the ongoing efforts in managing dementia and cognitive disorders.

While the journey to discovering effective treatments and preventive measures for Alzheimer's disease is a complex and challenging one, it is not devoid of hope. This book is a testament to the indomitable spirit of the scientific community, whose collective efforts strive to unravel the mysteries of this disease and bring forth solutions that can transform lives.

We extend our heartfelt gratitude to all the contributors who have lent their expertise and insights to this compilation. Their dedication and commitment have been instrumental in shaping this book into a valuable resource for the scientific community.

Finally, we express our deepest appreciation to you, the reader, for embarking on this intellectual expedition with us. It is our sincere belief that this volume will inspire continued exploration, spark innovative ideas, and pave the way for advancements in the treatment of Alzheimer's disease.

—***Editors***

PART I

Molecular and Genetic Pathways in Alzheimer's Disease

CHAPTER 1

Pathophysiology and Diagnosis of Alzheimer's Disease: Past and Recent Developments

NIRMAL SINGH,[1*] KULDEEP KUMAR,[1] SIMRAT KAUR,[1]
AYUSH KANDPAL,[1] HARLOKESH NARAYAN YADAV,[2]
DHANDEEP SINGH,[1] DIMPLE SETHI CHOPRA,[1]
AMTESHWAR SINGH JAGGI,[1] AMIT KUMAR,[3] and VASUDEVAN MANI[4]

[1]*Department of Pharmaceutical Sciences and Drug Research, Punjabi University, Patiala, Punjab, India*

[2]*Department of Pharmacology, All India Institute of Medical Sciences, New Delhi, India*

[3]*Chitkara College of Pharmacy, Chitkara University, Punjab, India*

[4]*Department of Pharmacology and Toxicology, College of Pharmacy, Qassim University, Buraydah, Kingdom of Saudi Arabia*

[*]Corresponding author.

ABSTRACT

Alzheimer's disease (AD) is an irreversible, progressive neurodegenerative disorder and is one of the primary causes of dementia. It is typically characterized by the formation of extra neuronal deposits of amyloid beta (Aβ) plaques and intra-neuronal neurofibrillary tangles (NFTs) in the brain. Additionally, it is accompanied by the development of oxidative stress and neuroinflammation contributing significantly to extreme cognitive decline, neurodegeneration, and mortality. Various hypotheses such as the β-amyloid plaque hypothesis, tau hypothesis, neurotransmitter imbalance, gut microbiome disruption, autophagy, genetic variations, etc., are suggested to

Neuro-Nutraceuticals and Drug Discovery and Delivery in Alzheimer's Disease, Volume 1: Targeting Key Pathological Pathways. Varinder Singh, Amit Kumar, Parul Sood (Eds.)

intricately express the pathophysiology of AD. Due to the progressive nature of AD, early diagnosis is in heavy demand at the time. Several neuroimaging techniques and novel biomarkers are employed to assess the patient's mental capacity. These neuroimaging techniques for evaluating the biomarkers are focused on the early detection of AD because various therapeutic interventions for preventing or postponing the onset of symptoms are highly effective in the early stages of AD. The current book chapter provides insights into the fundamental pathophysiology of AD and recent developments in AD pathology. The focus is also to highlight the differential imaging techniques and biomarkers for early diagnosis and detection of AD patients. This chapter will be of great information to the researchers working in the relevant area.

1.1 INTRODUCTION

Alzheimer's disease (AD), a progressive neurodegenerative disorder, contributes to 50–60% of the cases of dementia and is one of the significant healthcare challenges of the 21st century [1, 2]. Dementia is characterized by memory loss, aphasia, apraxia, agnosia, and mood changes [3]. The Centers for Disease Control and Prevention (CDC) published a report on the epidemiology of AD, stating that around 5.8 million Americans were suffering from AD in 2020, projected to triple to 14 million people by 2060 [4]. The high prevalence of AD in older people indicates its association with aging [5]. The incidences of men suffering from AD were found to be 19–29% lower than women [6]. AD begins with a progressive decline in cognitive function. It differs from age-related degeneration in cognitive function because it has more gradations and is not associated with severe disability. Severe brain damage is the last checkpoint in AD pathology [1].

The pathology of AD encompasses the injury and death of neurons, which initiates in the brain's hippocampal region and spreads to other areas in the brain, eventually leading to atrophy of the whole brain [7]. Since the discovery of AD in 1906, many neurologists have detected amyloid plaques and neurofibrillary tangles (NFTs) in brain samples of AD patients, indicating their role in AD pathology [8]. Amyloid plaques are formed by the extracellular deposition of β-amyloid peptide (Aβ) in the parenchyma and blood vessels of the brain. NFTs comprise paired helical filaments with hyperphosphorylated tau proteins [9]. These proteinaceous complexes act as precursors for neuronal cell damage [10]. Apart from the role of amyloid plaques and NFTs in the pathophysiology of AD, the irregular release of some neurotransmitters, such as glutamate, results in inflammation and neuronal cell death. Neuroinflammation and specific immunological changes, such as increased proinflammatory cytokine levels in the cerebrospinal fluid (CSF), have also been found to play an intricate role in developing AD [11].

In the last two decades, there has been marked progress in the development and accessibility of *in-vivo* AD biomarkers, in identifying the nature and cause of the disease, and application of this development in diagnosing AD [12]. The most precise diagnosis of AD involves post-mortem examination of the brain tissue. However, diagnostic tests, including examination of CSF and positron emission tomography (PET) biomarkers, combined with novel clinical criteria, can help diagnose AD in living patients [13]. The current treatment strategies for patients with any stage of mild to moderate AD dementia are acetylcholinesterase inhibitor drugs (donepezil, rivastigmine, and galantamine), whereas, for patients with moderate to severe AD dementia, the United States Food and Drug Administration (USFDA) has approved memantine (an N-methyl-D-aspartic acid (NMDA) receptor antagonist) as a practical therapeutic approach [14, 15].

The current chapter provides insights into the basic pathophysiology of AD and its recent developments. We also highlighted the differential diagnostic techniques and new detection approaches for AD patients. This chapter will certainly help researchers/scientists find new therapeutic strategies for managing AD at the clinical level.

1.2 PATHOPHYSIOLOGY

Since the detection of amyloid plaques and hyperphosphorylated NFTs in AD patients in 1907, scientists and clinicians have hypothesized various causal factors (such as the cholinergic hypothesis, infectious diseases hypothesis, gut microbiome disruption, autophagy, etc.) that explain this multifactorial disorder [6, 16].

1.2.1 AB PLAQUES HYPOTHESIS

According to the Aβ plaques hypothesis, the plaques of Aβ are formed and accumulated in different areas of the brain [17]. The brain recognizes these depositions as foreign entities that lead to the activation of microglial cells and the release of cytokines that further initiate an inflammatory [18] and immune response [19] responsible for neurodegeneration. The amyloid precursor protein (APP) is cleaved by the various secretase enzymes, i.e., α, β, and γ into Aβ peptides which develop into amyloid plaques and get deposited in the brain [20]. The formation of Aβ plaque begins with the enzymatic cleavage of APP by β-secretase or β-site APP cleaving enzyme (BACE 1), also known as aspartyl protease 2 (Asp2) or memapsin-2, at sites Asp1 and Glu11 to form a C-terminal membrane with 89–99 amino acids (C_{99}) bound to it [21]. Then, the γ-secretase with presenilin 1 (PS1) or presenilin 2 (PS2) as its main components cleaves the C_{99} into Aβ1–40 and Aβ1–42 isoforms. Among these isoforms, $A\beta_{1-40}$ is soluble, whereas $A\beta_{1-42}$ is insoluble. $A\beta_{1-42}$ consists of two different amino acids, i.e., alanine and leucine, rendering it vulnerable to aggregation and forming plaque [22]. This alteration in the cleavage pattern occurs due to a genetic mutation in the APP gene, PS1/PS2 gene, and apolipoprotein E (APOE4) gene [23]. Besides hereditary factors, several neuropeptides are speculated to be involved in forming plaques. Decreased levels of corticotropin-releasing hormone (CRH), somatostatin, neuropeptide Y, and increased angiotensin II levels are probably involved in either impaired cleavage of the APP or improper removal of $A\beta_{1-42}$ fragments [24–26]. However, the Aβ hypothesis has been contentious, as a recent report has suggested that amyloid plaque formation inhibitory drugs have failed in reversing or arresting cognitive decline. This indicates that either the hypothesis is inaccurate, or the brain develops resistance to the anti-amyloid therapy after a certain period (Figure 1.1) [27].

1.2.2 TAU HYPOTHESIS

In the late 20th century, many research laboratories determined that NFTs are composed of microtubule-associated proteins, tau [28]. The NFTs are the complex of tau filaments that play a crucial role in the pathology of AD [29]. The microtubule-binding domain of tau proteins is involved in the microtubule assembly's polymerization and stabilization, which further play a vital role in maintaining the integrity of the cytoskeleton [30]. Several kinases, such as Fyn kinase, glycogen synthase kinase-3β (GSK3β), cyclin-dependent kinase-5 (CDK5), etc., are found to regulate the binding of tau proteins with microtubules by phosphorylating serine/threonine residues. Among these kinases, CDK5 plays a prominent role in generating NFTs.

Additionally, the activation of calpain and deregulation of p35 by Aβ leads to cytosolic calcium overload and splitting of p35 into p25, respectively, which in turn hyperactivates the CDK5 [31]. The hyperactivation of CDK5 triggers the hyperphosphorylation of tau [32] resulting in decreased affinity of tau proteins to microtubules [33], eventually leading to the generation of NFTs. These NFTs accumulate in the cytosol and cannot perform normal functions such as maintaining the integrity of the cell, synaptic transmission, axonal transport, etc. (Figure 1.1) [6].

1.2.3 NEUROTRANSMITTER IMBALANCE

The role of the cholinergic system in cognitive neuroscience is well-established [34]. Cholinergic dysregulation is one of the major causes of various kinds of dementia, including AD [35]. The amyloid plaques and NFTs also get deposited in the cholinergic regions in the nucleus basalis of Meynert, leading to the deterioration of cognitive function due to the induction of inflammatory response. In addition, the cholinergic deficit results in altered blood-brain-barrier (BBB) permeability that hampers the removal of the amyloid plaques, thus exaggerating the disease [36]. The decreased activity of choline acetyltransferase and the increased expression of acetylcholinesterase (AChE) contribute to the decline in acetylcholine (Ach) levels and worsening dementia.

Moreover, AChE promotes plaque formation by interacting with the Aβ peptide [37]. Besides the cholinergic system, the noradrenergic system is also involved in cognitive functioning [38]. It has been reported that noradrenergic receptors are abundantly present in the astrocytes in the locus coeruleus, which on activation, improves synaptic plasticity and learning and memory as well [39]. Therefore, degeneration of the noradrenergic neurons in the locus coeruleus region of the brain contributes to cognitive impairment [40].

Furthermore, the loss of serotonergic neurons from the brainstem and decreased brain serotonin levels in AD patients have been reported to be involved in AD pathology [41]. The serotonergic dysfunction in the midbrain raphe nuclei leads to memory loss as they regulate cortical plasticity and memory formation [42]. Glutamate is another neurotransmitter involved in maintaining synaptic plasticity. It modulates synaptic function by acting on N-Methyl-D-aspartate (NMDA) and α-amino-3-hydroxy-5-methyl-4-isoxazole propionic acid (AMPA) receptors [43]. An imbalance in the glutamate/glutamine metabolism leads to constant depolarization of the neurons, causing excitotoxicity that eventually results in synaptic injury. Besides this, the Aβ peptide interacts with NMDA receptors causing a loss of hypersensitization of NMDA receptors resulting in neuronal excitotoxicity [44]. In the dorsal raphe nuclei (a region of the brain stem), an association between serotonin and gamma-aminobutyric acid (GABA) regulates the brain's cognitive function. A study has reported that 5HT6R antagonists improved cognitive decline by increasing serotonin levels through the modulation of GABAergic neurons. It also decreases the formation of amyloid plaques due to its inhibitory effect on γ-secretase activity [45]. Therefore, several neurotransmitters working in conjunction are necessary for the normal cognitive functioning of the brain. Hence, altering the levels of any of the neurotransmitters mentioned above may exaggerate the AD symptoms (Figure 1.1).

1.2.4 NEUROINFLAMMATION HYPOTHESIS

Acute neuroinflammation protects the brain against harmful stimuli such as amyloid plaques, NFTs, etc. However, prolonged activation of microglial cells decreases their ability to remove plaques. On the contrary, there is no effect on their proinflammatory cytokine-releasing ability that eventually leads to an imbalance between pro- and anti-inflammatory cytokines [46]. Aβ deposition leads to the activation of various Toll-like receptors (TLR) such as TLR2, TLR4, TLR6, etc., and their co-receptors (CD36, CD14, and CD47 expressed by microglia) [47]. The principal proinflammatory cytokines involved in the neuroinflammatory pathway are interleukin-1β (IL-1β) and interleukin-18 (IL-18), expressed by activated caspase-1 or caspase-8. It is also well-documented that the Nod-like Receptor family pyrin domain containing 3 (NLRP3) inflammasome promotes the activation of caspase-1 and can also sense Aβ deposition [48]. The rise in these proinflammatory cytokines further causes damage to the dendrites and interferes with the removal of Aβ. They also interact with neurons and microglia and increase the synthesis of nitric oxide (NO) by expressing inducible nitric oxide synthase (iNOS) that further enhances the peptide's ability to aggregate and suppress synaptic functions [46]. These cytokines activate the CDKs, resulting in the hyperphosphorylation of tau and enhancing the formation of amyloid plaques. Additionally, GABAergic dysregulation leads to the loss of inhibitory action of GABA on activated microglia, which releases proinflammatory cytokines (Figure 1.1) [49].

1.2.5 GENETIC VARIATIONS

The role of genetic variations in the pathophysiology of AD might be crucial, but genetic inheritance is not the only factor behind the majority of cases of AD. Genetic variations have been identified to cause AD in patients below the age of 65 and account for 0.1% of the total cases of AD [1]. AD may be categorized as familial and sporadic based on the types of genes involved [50]. The familial type of AD is characterized as an autosomal dominant disorder usually affecting individuals before the age of 65. The APP gene on chromosome 21 was identified as the first genetic mutation leading to familial-type AD [51]. The APP gene mutation is found to be the causal factor behind only a few cases of familial-type AD. Other mutations, such as PS1 and PS2, which are highly homologous genes, are responsible for most familial-type AD cases [52, 53]. Another type of genetic factor associated with AD, the APOE4 ε4 allele, was reported by two independent groups in 1993 [54, 55]. The APOE4 ε4 allele was found to modify the age of onset of the disease, with each copy of the allele decreasing the age of onset by 10 years (Figure 1.1) [50, 56].

1.2.6 OXIDATIVE STRESS

The role of mitochondrial dysfunction and oxidative stress has been well-defined in the pathobiology of early AD. Mitochondrial dysfunction is associated with decreased levels of cytochrome C oxidase. The oxidative stress leads to the overactivation of GSK3β, which alters the permeability of mitochondria and eventually contributes to the increased production of reactive oxygen species (ROS) [57]. Metal ions such as zinc and copper tend to bind with Aβ plaque and increase ROS production, leading to oxidative changes in the Aβ peptide, hampering its excretion. The accumulation of Aβ peptide leads to lipid and protein oxidation of the cellular membrane and increases its permeability, making it susceptible to degeneration [58, 59]. Another major factor responsible for the increase in oxidative stress is calcium ions. Aβ plaques disrupt the storage of calcium ions in the endoplasmic reticulum. This impairment results in the depletion of glutathione as well as the accumulation of ROS in the cell [60]. Moreover, excessive stimulation of NMDA receptors alters the cell permeability and contributes to the increased calcium influx, further producing reactive nitrogen species (RNS) and ROS. Besides, Aβ peptides can initiate the production of free radicals by activating nicotinamide adenine dinucleotide phosphate hydrogen (NADPH) oxidase enzyme (Figure 1.1) [61, 62].

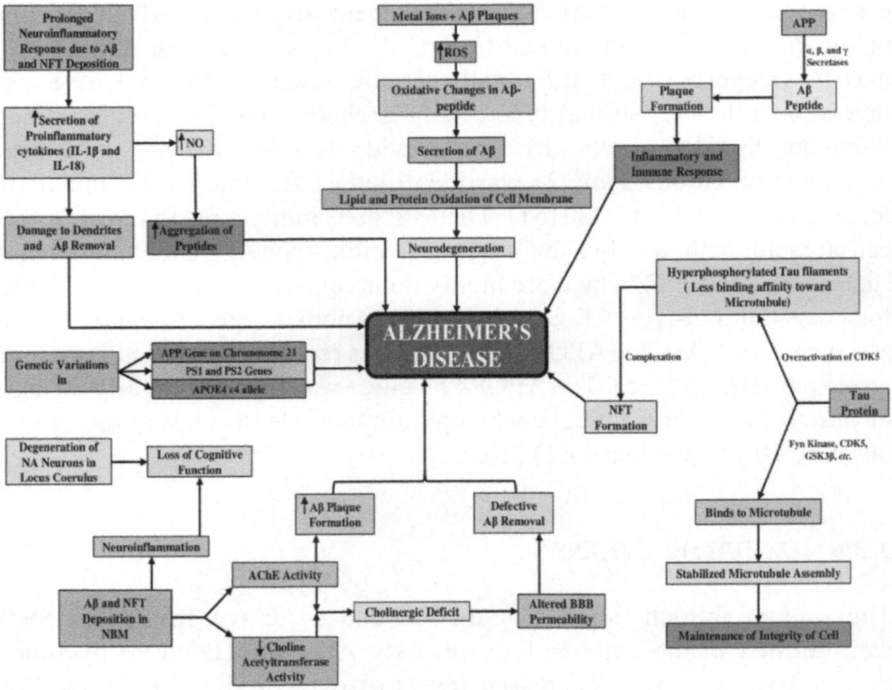

FIGURE 1.1 Various pathophysiological hypotheses of Alzheimer's disease.

Abbreviations: Aβ: Amyloid beta; AChE: acetylcholinesterase; APP: amyloid precursor protein; APOE: apolipoprotein-E; BBB: blood-brain barrier; CDK-5: cycline dependent kinase-5; GSK-3β: glycogen synthase kinase-β; IL: interleukin; NA: noradrenaline; NBM: nucleus basalis of Meynert; NFT: neurofibrillary tangles; NO: nitric oxide; PS-1: presenilin-1; PS-2: presenilin-2; and ROS: reactive oxygen species.

1.3 RECENT DEVELOPMENTS IN AD PATHOLOGY

1.3.1 GUT MICROBIOME DISRUPTION

The brain-gut metabolic axis provides an excellent platform for the bidirectional communication between the brain and the gut [63]. A good number of studies have established a positive link between AD and microbiome disruption in the gut. Trouble in the gut microflora increases the production of secondary cytotoxic bile acid, which tends to cross the BBB and accumulate in the brain leading to cell death, ROS production, inflammatory response, etc. [64, 65]. It is speculated that gut microbiota affects the brain's synthesis, absorption, and transportation of serotonin and GABA. Furthermore, a few bacterial species are involved in the formation of amyloid plaque, which is responsible for initiating the inflammatory response and, therefore, increasing the vulnerability to AD [66].

NO is another culprit behind various neurodegenerative disorders, including AD. Different gut microbes such as *Bifidobacteria* and *Lactobacilli* are found to convert nitrate and nitrite to NO, whereas microflora like gut bacilli and Streptomyces are capable of producing NO by their NO synthetase (NOS) [67, 68]. Alterations in any of these microbes' activities might result in excessive NO production, which further causes axonal degeneration and neuroinflammation [57]. Additionally, disruption in microbiota can contribute to AD progression by enhancing the secretion of immunogenic lipopolysaccharides (LPSs) and amyloids which readily diffuse into the brain and worsen AD symptoms [69]. The gut bacteria-derived amyloids may diffuse into the gastrointestinal tract (g.i.t.) and increase the levels of specific proinflammatory cytokines (TNFα, IL10, IL6, IL22, etc.) further increasing ROS concentration and activating nuclear factor kappa-B (NF-kB) signaling [70]. It was also reported that patients infected with certain bacteria, such as *Chlamydia pneumonia, Borrelia burgdorferi*, and *Helicobacter pylori*, showed a significant increase in levels of Aβ-40, Aβ-42, and inflammatory mediators associated with AD [71].

1.3.2 AUTOPHAGY

Autophagy, also known as the cell's housekeeping or waste management system, comprises engulfing the damaged proteins and cell constituents. It initiates with the formation of a phagophore which encloses all the damaged proteins or dysfunctional cellular organelles resulting in the formation of closed vacuolar structures called autophagosomes. Eventually, the fusion of autophagosomes with lysosomes leads to the formation of autolysosomes which are responsible for the degradation of all its contents [72]. Several factors, such as PS1 proteins, oxidative stress, NFTs, etc., disrupt the autophagosome's normal functioning, thus contributing to AD pathology [73].

1.3.3 INFECTIOUS DISEASE HYPOTHESIS

The amyloid proteins tend to possess antimicrobial activity. It has been speculated that an infection in the brain (neurons) with Spirochetes and some other microbes, such as Chlamydia and herpes simplex virus 1 (HSV-1), has been associated with the deposition of Aβ and NFTs in the infection regions of the brain. Therefore, any untreated infection might play a crucial role in the pathogenesis of AD [74]. Moreover, the condition leads to the activation of the immune system, which activates a specific component of the innate immune system, viz., toll-like proteins that further play a role in the pathogenesis of AD [75].

1.4 DIAGNOSIS

As the population ages and the number of AD patients rises, great emphasis is being given to diagnosing the disease as early as possible. The diagnosis of AD mainly focuses on identifying and scanning biomarkers that can accurately depict specific pathophysiological processes of AD. Currently, cerebrospinal fluid (CSF) protein analysis and positron emission tomography (PET) of tracer compounds are the main methods being used to diagnose AD [76]. It is possible to employ phosphorylated tau 181 (P-tau181) as a predictive and confirmatory diagnostic biomarker for AD. It is released in the CSF and deposited in the brain, then further crosses the BBB to reach into the blood, where it can be utilized as a biomarker for AD [77, 78]. A particular PET scan demonstrates 100% specificity and 96% sensitivity in AD and for individuals with milder illnesses. However, due to the very high cost, $_{18}$F-based tracers are not frequently utilized as PET ligands for diagnosis.

Further, assessing p-tau, Aβ-42, and total tau levels in CSF is less expensive. Due to the invasive nature of the procedure (lumbar puncture) and the lack of laboratory facilities available for fluid analysis, this approach takes considerable time to complete. However, the accuracy of both the PET imaging and CSF analysis is comparable, indicating that the best diagnostic test will rely on the patient's preferences, cost, and accessibility of facilities [6, 79]. The results of both PET imaging and CSF analysis showed that the pathological alterations begin twenty years before the manifestation of symptoms [80]. Therefore, diagnosing AD at this point would not be particularly helpful for managing AD. Hence, it is proposed to use the biomarkers, which can aid in early AD detection, for better diagnosis and therapy.

1.4.1 VARIOUS TECHNIQUES FOR DETECTION OF AD

1.4.1.1 BRAIN IMAGING

Aging and AD cause significant changes in the brain's structure and functions. The pathology of AD spreads through the brain in a usual pattern, with some regions being impacted first and others being damaged in the advanced stages of AD [81]. The medial temporal lobe components, the entorhinal and perirhinal cortex, and the hippocampus showed the earliest abnormalities in the topographic pattern distinguishing AD [82]. A significant loss of cortical neurons and loss of connections between brain systems leads to the development of AD. Recent developments in brain imaging have confirmed unique disruptions in functional neural networks [83]. MRI techniques can distinguish AD from other brain disorders by identifying brain damage patterns associated with the risk of AD from Mild Cognitive Impairment (MCI) and other behavioral disorders [84]. Both structural and functional MRIs are performed to assess the brain and amyloid metabolisms [6]. Some other diagnostic techniques such as diffusion tensor imaging (DTI) and related tractography technologies, arterial spin labeling assessments of cerebral blood flow and magnetic resonance spectroscopy (MRS), and functional magnetic resonance imaging (fMRI) are the additional MRI techniques under development that are also improving the understanding of AD (Figure 1.2) [84].

1.4.1.2 POSITRON EMISSION TOMOGRAPHY (PET)

The primary method of diagnosing AD is positron emission tomography (PET) using tracer molecules. PET has emerged as a crucial clinical tool for non-invasive *in-vivo* characterization, imaging, and quantifying physiological processes [85]. The success of PET imaging is based on the introduction of radiolabeled compounds (tracers) in sub-pharmacological doses for carrying out nuclear imaging procedures [86–88]. The fundamental principle of tracer-based tomography is that the concentration and distribution of the tracer serve as a measure for the regionalized abundances of the tracers. Fluorodeoxyglucose (FDG), amyloid-binding tracers, and tau-binding tracers are the three major categories of PET tracers essential for the *in-vivo* detection of AD. Although there are numerous other PET tracers (such as cholinergic tracers, inflammatory tracers, and [15] O-based imaging) that can be used to study AD pathology, the use of only FDG is found to be clinically relevant at this moment [89, 90]. However, the use of amyloid as well as tau tracers is steadily increasing (Figure 1.2) [91].

1.4.1.3 FLUORODEOXYGLUCOSE POSITRON EMISSION TOMOGRAPHY (FDG-PET)

FDG (2-[18F]-fluoro-2-deoxy-D-glucose) is a glucose analog that does not undergo glycolysis and accumulates in the brain at the same rate as glucose is digested. Moreover, FDG has been used for decades to measure brain glucose metabolism [92, 93]. Fluorodeoxyglucose positron emission tomography (FDG-PET) allows for measuring cerebral glucose metabolism in the resting state, which is a substitute for cognitive activity and a detective measure of neuronal activity [94]. It is well-documented that AD patients, compared to healthy individuals, have progressive and typically bilateral glucose hypometabolism, revealing patterns of metabolic abnormalities that further produce a so-called FDG-PET endophenotype [83]. This endophenotype is an aspect of AD affecting specific brain areas or regions [95]. It is also depicted that hypometabolism of glucose occurs in the frontal, posterior, and cingulate cortices, as well as in the parietal and temporal cortices [96]. FDG-PET has been used to examine changes in the primary visual cortex (regionalized or global) which becomes the basis for treating AD. FDG-PET has also been used to track the extent of the hypometabolism distribution area, which is related to the severity of AD dementia [97].

Currently, single photon emission computed tomography and 18F-fluorodeoxyglucose-positron emission tomography (18F FDG PET) are being used in clinical settings [98, 99]. Recently, Lohith and colleagues reported the usefulness of 18F-MK-6240 as a neurofibrillary tangle (NFT) imaging PET tracer [100]. They noted that 18F-MK-6240 displays regional accumulation in a way that is consistent with AD NFT pathology. Indeed, there was no indication of off-target binding in healthy participants, and the signal magnitude in terms of semi-quantitative Standardized Uptake Value Ratio (SUVR) or fully quantitative total volume of distribution (VT) values was higher in AD/MCI subjects compared to healthy subjects in NFT depositing regions (Figure 1.2) [100].

1.4.1.4 AMYLOID-POSITRON EMISSION TOMOGRAPHY (AMYLOID-PET)

AD patients exhibit cortical amyloid retention in the orbitofrontal, inferior parietal/posterior cingulate, and precuneus cortices more than healthy senior individuals [101]. The first amyloid tracer was Pittsburgh compound B or PIB (N-methyl-[11C]-2-(4-methylaminophenyl)-6-hydroxy benzothiazole), a thioflavin-T derivative [102]. It has been demonstrated that PIB is sensitive to soluble and insoluble types of amyloid protein, and the accumulation of PIB *in vivo* matches exceptionally well with amyloid identified in the AD patient's brain after autopsy. Additionally, the retention of PIB is linked with the hypometabolism of glucose in the parietal-temporal areas in AD patients but not among those with MCI [103]. On the other hand, the short half-life of the $_{11}$C atom (approx. 20 min) has posed the biggest challenge to the clinical acceptance of PIB and significantly restricted its use. This has led to the adoption of $_{18}$F-based tracers for amyloid imaging because its half-life is substantially longer (over two hours). Three fluorine-based tracers such as florbetapir, florbetaben, and flutemetamol have shown satisfactory results and coincide well with the findings of PIB investigations and post-mortem autopsies and, therefore, have been approved for use in various clinical settings [104, 105]. However, the major limitation of the Aβ-PET is the lack of any standard method for quantifying Aβ plaques (Figure 1.1) [106].

1.4.1.5 TAU-POSITRON EMISSION TOMOGRAPHY (TAU-PET)

In contrast to the usual pattern associated with amyloid accumulation, tau NFTs follow a well-defined sequential spreading pattern, which is a significant benefit of tau-PET over Aβ-PET. The growth of tau tangles might be a sign of *in-vivo* disease development [107]. It has been speculated that tau-PET is better than amyloid-PET and volumetric MR investigations in predicting and assessing cognitive decline [108]. Further, the ultrastructural paired helical fragments (PHF) type of tau aggregates is the most prevalent in AD; therefore, most researchers focus on tracking these PHFs in terms of the production of tau-PET tracers [109]. The currently available tau tracers are categorized based on their structural similarities, including nonselective tracer $_{18}$F-FDDNP, quinoline derivatives, pyrido-indole derivatives, and PBB3 [110]. Four high-affinity binding sites for tau tracers have been found by computational modeling of tau fibrils using cryo-EM structures of PHFs and straight filaments. One binding site is located on the surface, whereas the other three are hidden deep within the fibril's core (Figure 1.2) [111, 112].

1.5 BIOMARKERS

The term "biomarker" refers to an indicator used to evaluate both pathogenic and normal physiological processes and the pharmacological effects of any intervention. Biomarkers are generally used to check the disease status of aged AD patients [113]. AD's two primary pathogenic features are an extracellular Aβ protein deposition and aggregated forms of hyperphosphorylated tau protein in the brain [114]. Recently, Lashley et al. thoroughly evaluated the current status and future of all the significant molecular biomarkers of AD [115].

1.5.1 CSF BIOMARKERS

Nowadays, CSF measurements of $A\beta_{1-42}$, t-tau, and p-tau have gained immense popularity as AD-specific markers due to the availability of better assay methods. Previous *in-vitro* studies and human trials have suggested that the non-essential heavy metals such as cadmium (Cd), mercury (Hg), lead (Pb), and arsenic (As) have a role in the aggregation of the Aβ protein as well as in the high levels of tau hyperphosphorylation [116, 117]. A unique "Alzheimer's CSF profile" is produced by an ELISA test called INNOTEST that has been employed for two decades to quantify t-tau, p-tau, and Aβ42 in CSF. This Alzheimer's CSF profile revealed an increasing t-tau and p-tau with a lower level of Aβ42 in AD patients [118]. C-reactive protein (CRP) levels are strongly linked with the CSF amyloid levels and the ApoE genotype [119]. A previous study by O'Bryant and colleagues found that mean CRP levels considerably declined in AD patients [120].

Numerous other markers, including soluble vascular endothelial growth factor receptor-1 (sVEGFR-1), soluble vascular cell adhesion molecule-1 (sVCAM-1), interferon gamma-induced protein 10 (IP-10), macrophage migration inhibitory factor (MIF), and complement component 1q (C1q), have been strongly linked to the pathological tau levels regardless of the patient's age. Therefore, each of these molecules has a different impact on aging on CSF marker levels. In the late stages of AD, events, including neuronal death caused by inflammatory signaling in response to tissue damage, are present, and the CSF tau level also rises. It has been revealed that CSF biomarkers only coincide with abnormal brain activity in AD's later stages [121].

The assessment of biomarkers in CSF samples has some drawbacks due to the invasive technique, high cost, and limited availability of PET investigations. Additionally, in elderly patients, lumbar puncture CSF fluid collection results in nausea, back pain, and weakness [6]. These drawbacks lead to its limited usage for the diagnosis of AD (Figure 1.2).

1.5.2 BLOOD AND URINE BIOMARKERS

The technological advancements in very sensitive immunoassays and mass spectrometry-based techniques showed convincing evidence for blood biomarkers that can be used to screen for amyloid deposition in the brain and neurodegeneration [122]. Assessment of Aβ42 and Aβ40 plasma levels has become recognized biomarkers for AD. Preclinical reports have depicted that plasma and CSF levels of Aβ42 and Aβ40 in AD transgenic mice rise with age but eventually fall when Aβ42 starts accumulating in the brain, initiating the process of cognitive impairment. In 2008, Schupf and colleagues investigated the alteration in these biomarkers throughout the onset of cognitive impairment or AD. They also determined the prognostic value of Aβ levels in aged individuals, reporting that those with rising Aβ42 levels over the follow-up period had a three-fold greater risk of developing AD [123]. In another investigation, the total Aβ percentage was calculated from plasma samples using an immuno-infrared sensor. The biomarker amide I band was considerably lower in AD patients. Amide I is a biomarker that can identify AD in people even before the manifestation of clinical symptoms of dementia. According to the test's positive probability ratio of 7.9, it is strongly evidenced that this biomarker can promisingly detect AD [124].

Brain lipids are crucial molecules because they play a pivotal role in various biological and physiological processes in the central nervous system, including impulse transmission and cell signaling. The most prevalent types of brain lipids include cholesterol, ceramides, glucosyl ceramides, phosphatidylcholine, sphingomyelin, and sulfatides [125]. In addition, long-chain fatty acid derivatives like prostaglandins, leukotrienes, and neuroprotectants are also found in the brain [126]. It is documented that sphingolipid levels are decreased in AD patients [127]. The discovery of the lipid mentioned above biomarkers may be considered a less intrusive diagnostic approach for the predictions of the progression of AD. Although histological and cytological approaches are also feasible for lipid identification and measurement. In these techniques, many dyes are used in tissues and cells to detect and trace different lipids (Figure 1.2) [128].

1.5.3 GENETIC BIOMARKERS

AD is complicated and diverse and can also be inherited. Numerous genes and environmental factors have been identified that affect the risk and rate of disease progression in late-onset AD [26]. Three significant genes that encode for PS1, PS2, and the amyloid precursor have been shown to have more than 160 mutations. The other important risk factor for developing AD is the Epsilon 4 (ε4) allele of the APOE gene, which has a frequency of 14% but rises to 40% in AD patients. Additionally, it is associated with increased Aβ pathology and the onset of AD dementia at an earlier age. It is documented that amyloid plaques are highly prevalent in ε4 allele carriers, with lower levels of Aβ1–42 and higher levels of PiB in the CSF that are witnessed to be coupled to Aβ aggregates on PET imaging [130]. Parental inheritance causes familial AD, which accounts for less than 1% of the burden of AD [121]. Studies suggest that the ε4 allele at the ApoE locus is associated with an elevated risk of late-onset AD in a more precise and reliable genetic manner [131, 132]. The ApoE gene encodes the carriers of the ε4 allele that have increased amyloid deposition and harmful impacts on memory and executive functioning [133]. The studies have well-established that the individuals with the presence of the ApoE ε4 allele have a lower age than average AD manifestation. Therefore, the focus is to increase the accuracy of a comprehensive biomarker panel for AD (Figure 1.2) [128].

1.5.4 BRAIN-DERIVED NEUROTROPHIC FACTOR (BDNF)

Hippocampal volume (HV) loss and memory deterioration associated with high Aβ levels have been previously documented in healthy individuals; however, Lim and colleagues demonstrated that BDNF Val66Met exacerbates these conditions in the preclinical stage of AD [134]. It was reported that the rate of HV reduction in individuals with high levels of Aβ and the Met allele was significantly high. Moreover, a higher decline rate in HV was also reported in Val/Val homozygotes with high Aβ levels irrespective of the BDNF Val66Met polymorphism over 36 months. Although hippocampal atrophy and increased memory loss in adults with MCI and high Aβ have previously been reported, Lim and coworkers provided a preliminary report. They established a link between high Aβ and BDNF Val66Met polymorphism in MCI due to AD, suggesting they are important prognostic markers of increased hippocampal atrophy and memory loss (Figure 1.2) [135].

1.5.5 KIDNEY/BRAIN (KIBRA) PROTEIN – A MEMORY-ASSOCIATED PROTEIN

The KIBRA protein is distributed throughout the brain but is primarily abundant in the hippocampal postsynaptic density. It interacts with several postsynaptic proteins, such as dendrin and synaptopodin, and these interactions have a pivotal role in memory-related processes [136]. Tracy and colleagues reported aberrant K274 and K281 acetylation on tau in AD brains, which exacerbated memory loss and impaired synaptic plasticity by lowering the postsynaptic KIBRA protein [137]. Memory problems and a reduced hippocampal long-term potentiation (LTP) were seen in transgenic mice that could acetylate K274 and K281. It is speculated that by increasing the expression of the KIBRA protein or stimulating actin polymerization, the LTP deficit may be prevented. The loss of KIBRA protein in dementia-related AD patients has been linked to a rise in tau acetylation. This finding showed a novel mechanism by which pathogenic tau contributes to AD's synapse disruption and cognitive loss. Many genes such as APOE, BDNF, KIBRA, klotho (KL), Spondin-1 (SPON1), CUB, and Sushi multiple domains 1 (CSMD1) are documented to be significant indicators of cognitive change. Porter and colleagues strongly emphasized identifying gene risk profiling to evaluate the therapeutic efficacy of any drug in preclinical trials for AD with cognition (Figure 1.2) [138].

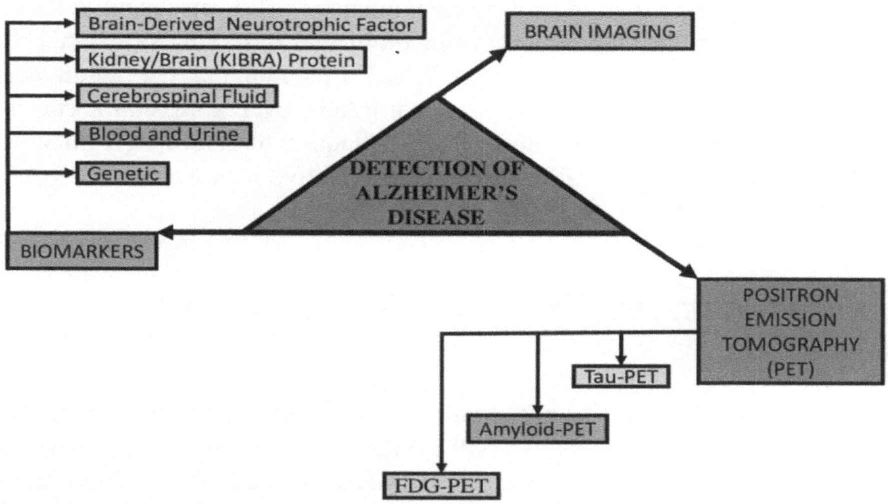

FIGURE 1.2 Various diagnostic techniques of Alzheimer's disease.

Abbreviations: FDG-PET: Fluorodeoxyglucose positron emission tomography; KIBRA: kidney/brain protein; and PET: positron emission tomography.

1.5.6 SYNAPTIC VESICLE GLYCOPROTEIN 2A

The synaptic density is reflected by synaptic vesicle glycoprotein 2A (SV2A), a measure proposed to have therapeutic significance in AD [139]. Lower levels of SV2A may be a promising biomarker of synaptic loss in AD because this protein is found in the cell membrane of secretory vesicles and is widely expressed throughout the brain. A PET radiotracer called 18F-UCBJ is speculated to be sensitive to synapse loss because variations in its uptake in the grey matter were linked to alterations in SV2A expression and reduced synaptic density [140, 141]. Although these results are encouraging, extensive validation of this and additional radiotracers is required to fully utilize the clinical potential of SV2A in AD [142].

1.5.7 RECEPTOR FOR ADVANCED GLYCATION END PRODUCTS

There is convincing evidence that the Receptor for Advanced Glycation End Products (RAGE) regulates the toxicity of Aβ in AD [143]. ROS mediates the development of senile plaques and NFTs that are released as a result of RAGE binding with Aβ. Additionally, RAGE levels in AD patients are significantly higher than in healthy individuals [144]. Consequently, it has been proposed that RAGE is a promising biomarker of AD in its early stages. It has been documented that for brain RAGE PET imaging, the radiotracer, i.e., 11C-FPS-ZM1, is used [144]. Indeed, RAGE overexpression is speculated to occur before the development of Aβ plaques; therefore, PET imaging of RAGE using 11C-FPS-ZM1 may be an effective technique in the early detection of AD [143].

1.5.8 PLATELET-DERIVED GROWTH FACTOR RECEPTOR-B (SPDGFRB)

Recent studies have intricately explored a new shredded form of platelet-derived growth factor receptor-b (sPDGFRb), a protein highly expressed in brain capillary pericytes and detected in CSF, as a potential early biomarker for BBB disruption in the early stages of AD [145]. Further, in clinical practice, another technique, i.e., CSF sPDGFR and dynamic contrast-enhanced magnetic resonance imaging (DCE-MRI), may detect early BBB damage to help identify individuals at early stages [146].

1.5.9 IRON

Excessive iron deposition in particular brain regions is reported to be associated with AD [147]. Although iron is essential for preserving homeostasis and is vital for many biological functions, AD has been linked to aberrant iron accumulation in subcortical and deep grey matter nuclei. Quantitative susceptibility mapping (QSM) has been employed in numerous investigations to assess the local magnetic susceptibility resulting from MRI images induced by deposits containing both Aβ and iron [147, 148]. Furthermore, it has been documented that employing QSM to detect iron has a clinical benefit for determining the correlation between Aβ accumulation and iron loads [147]. Therefore, early AD detection by imaging Aβ may benefit from assessing iron using QSM [149].

1.6 NOVEL IMPLICATIONS OF IMAGING TECHNIQUES IN THE DETECTION OF AD

1.6.1 DIFFUSION TENSOR IMAGING

Diffusion tensor imaging (DTI) is a more sophisticated diffusion MRI. This method detects the migration of water molecules in three dimensions to assess the structural integrity of living tissues [84]. By measuring the mean diffusivity, DTI has been utilized to evaluate the structural integrity of different brain areas in AD [150]. Studies have established a correlation between white matter integrity and disease severity, demonstrating the importance of DTI in evaluating white matter architecture [151]. Moreover, Hoy and coworkers reported white matter degeneration as a pathological biomarker for the early diagnosis of AD [152]. The specific link connecting disease severity and white fiber tracts needs to be investigated to fully utilize DTI as a diagnostic tool for AD [151].

1.6.2 OPTICAL COHERENCE TOMOGRAPHY

Optical coherence tomography (OCT) is another intriguing imaging method that could be used in AD research. Recently, pathological alterations in the retina have already been linked to AD [153]. These alterations include the development of Aβ plaques, RNFL thinness, ganglion cell degeneration, and diminished vessel density. According to a research study conducted by Song and colleagues, OCT data indicates that individuals with AD frequently have thinner choroidal, macular, and retinal tissue than healthy people [154]. However, the authenticity and integrity of these indicators are still contentious due to the possibility of other underlying disorders, such as glaucoma, which might lead to similar pathological changes, such as Aβ accumulation in the lens, RNFL thickness analysis, and ganglion cell loss. Nevertheless, OCT is a feasible and cost-effective imaging method that needs to be explored in depth to translate its clinical applicability in diagnosing AD [97].

1.7 NOVEL APPROACHES FOR AD'S DIAGNOSIS

These days, various trials are using newer approaches for the detection of AD. These approaches include detection of AD using blood-based biomarkers, and characterization of AD based on some biomarkers from CSF [36, 118]; some physiological parameters that help in the evaluation of Aβ/amyloid-based markers such as tau/neurofibrillary pathology and other neurodegenerative/neuronal injury markers [50]; neuroimaging techniques like fMRI and PET scan for the assessment of the integrity of neural networks [155]; magnetic stimulation to stimulate nerve cells to assess cholinergic, GABAergic, and/or glutamatergic circuit impairment [156, 157]; electroencephalography: recording of electrical activity of cortical neurons; [129] electrovestibulography: measurement of field potential activity in the external ear canal (Table 1.1).

TABLE 1.1 Novel Approaches for AD's Diagnosis

SL. No.	Method	Principle	References
1.	Biomarkers	Detection of blood- and CSF-based hallmarks of AD.	[36, 118]
2.	A/T/N system (A: Aβ/amyloid-based markers; T: tau/neurofibrillary pathology; and N: neurodegenerative/neuronal injury markers)	Categorizing as either positive or negative based on the presence or absence of the specified markers (A/T/N).	[50]
3.	Neuroimaging	Utilizing techniques such as fMRI and PET for the assessment of the integrity of neural networks.	[155]
4.	Transcranial magnetic stimulation.	Based on using changing magnetic field to stimulate nerve cells to assess cholinergic, GABAergic, and/or glutamatergic circuits.	[156, 157]
5.	Electroencephalography	Based on recording the electrical activity of cortical neurons.	[129]
6.	Electrovestibulography	Measurement of field potential activity in the external ear canal in the presence of a vestibular stimulus.	[157]

1.8 CONCLUSION

Clinical management of AD is still a massive challenge due to the complex and unknown pathophysiology and the lack of early diagnosis of AD patients. Delineating the recent developments in the pathophysiology and early diagnosis of AD will certainly open new avenues for the timely beginning of AD treatment. Recent developments in the pathophysiology and diagnosis of AD described exhaustively in this chapter will be of great help and importance for the persons involved in research pertaining to AD.

KEYWORDS

- **Alzheimer's disease**
- **amyloid beta**
- **biomarkers**
- **neurofibrillary tangles**
- **neuroimaging**
- **neuroinflammation**

REFERENCES

1. Duthey, B. (2013). Background Paper 6.11: Alzheimer Disease and Other Dementias. A Public Health Approach to Innovation (pp. 1–74).
2. World Health Organization. (2022). Dementia. Retrieved from: https://www.who.int/news-room/fact-sheets/detail/dementia (accessed on 22 July 2024).
3. Dementia UK. (2019). What is Dementia. Dementia UK. Retrieved from: https://www.dementiauk.org/about-dementia/dementia-information/what-is-dementia (accessed on 22 July 2024).
4. Centers for Disease Control and Prevention. (2020). Alzheimer's disease and related dementias. Retrieved from: https://www.cdc.gov/aging/aginginfo/alzheimers.htm (accessed on 22 July 2024).
5. Trevisan, K., Cristina-Pereira, R., Silva-Amaral, D., & Aversi-Ferreira, T. A. (2019). Theories of aging and the prevalence of Alzheimer's disease. BioMed Research International, 2019, Article 9171424. https://doi.org/10.1155/2019/9171424.
6. Khan, S., Barve, K. H., & Kumar, M. S. (2020). Recent advancements in pathogenesis, diagnostics, and treatment of Alzheimer's disease. Current Neuropharmacology, 18(11), 1106–1125. https://doi.org/10.2174/1570159X18666200528142429.
7. Shaffer, J. L. (2013). Alzheimer's Disease Neuroimaging Initiative: Predicting cognitive decline in subjects at risk for Alzheimer disease by using combined cerebrospinal fluid, MR imaging, and PET biomarkers. Radiology, 266(2), 583–591.

8. Ramirez-Bermudez, J. (2012). Alzheimer's disease: Critical notes on the history of a medical concept. Archives of Medical Research, 43(8), 595–599. https://doi.org/10.1016/j.arcmed.2012.11.008.
9. Anand, R., Gill, K. D., & Mahdi, A. A. (2014). Therapeutics of Alzheimer's disease: Past, present and future. Neuropharmacology, 76, 27–50. https://doi.org/10.1016/j.neuropharm.2013.07.004.
10. Barage, S. H., & Sonawane, K. D. (2015). Amyloid cascade hypothesis: Pathogenesis and therapeutic strategies in Alzheimer's disease. Neuropeptides, 52, 1–8. https://doi.org/10.1016/j.npep.2015.06.008.
11. Revett, T. J., Baker, G. B., Jhamandas, J., & Kar, S. (2013). Glutamate system, amyloid β peptides and tau protein: Functional interrelationships and relevance to Alzheimer disease pathology. Journal of Psychiatry and Neuroscience, 38(1), 6–23. https://doi.org/10.1503/jpn.110190.
12. Dubois, B., Villain, N., Frisoni, G. B., Rabinovici, G. D., Sabbagh, M., Cappa, S., Bejanin, A., Bombois, S., Epelbaum, S., Teichmann, M., & Habert, M. O. (2021). Clinical diagnosis of Alzheimer's disease: Recommendations of the International Working Group. Lancet Neurology, 20(6), 484–496. https://doi.org/10.1016/S1474-4422(21)00066-1.
13. Budson, A. E., & Solomon, P. R. (2012). New criteria for Alzheimer's disease and mild cognitive impairment: Implications for the practicing clinician. The Neurologist, 18(6), 356. https://doi.org/10.1097/NRL.0b013e31826a998d.
14. Mossello, E., & Ballini, E. (2012). Management of patients with Alzheimer's disease: Pharmacological treatment and quality of life. Therapeutic Advances in Chronic Disease, 3(4), 183–193. https://doi.org/10.1177/2040622312452387.
15. Fish, P. V., Steadman, D., Bayle, E. D., & Whiting, P. (2019). New approaches for the treatment of Alzheimer's disease. Bioorganic & Medicinal Chemistry Letters, 29(2), 125–133. https://doi.org/10.1016/j.bmcl.2018.11.034.
16. Kumar, A., & Dogra, S. (2008). Neuropathology and therapeutic management of Alzheimer's disease–An update. Drugs of the Future, 33(5), 433–446.
17. Thapa, K., Khan, H., Sharma, U., Grewal, A. K., & Singh, T. G. (2021). Poly (ADP-ribose) polymerase-1 as a promising drug target for neurodegenerative diseases. Life Sciences, 267, Article 118975. https://doi.org/10.1016/j.lfs.2020.118975.
18. Wang, W. Y., Tan, M. S., Yu, J. T., & Tan, L. (2015). Role of pro-inflammatory cytokines released from microglia in Alzheimer's disease. Annals of Translational Medicine, 3(10), 136. https://doi.org/10.3978%2Fj.issn.2305-5839.2015.03.49.
19. Blasko, I., & Grubeck-Loebenstein, B. (2003). Role of the immune system in the pathogenesis, prevention and treatment of Alzheimer's disease. Drugs & Aging, 20(2), 101–113. https://doi.org/10.2165/00002512-200320020-00002.
20. De Strooper, B., Vassar, R., & Golde, T. (2010). The secretases: Enzymes with therapeutic potential in Alzheimer disease. Nature Reviews Neurology, 6(2), 99–107. https://doi.org/10.1038/nrneurol.2009.218.
21. Grimm, M. O., & Hartmann, T. (2012). Recent understanding of the molecular mechanisms of Alzheimer's disease. *Journal of Addiction Research & Therapy*, *5*, 1–27.
22. Lundkvist, J., & Näslund, J. (2007). Gamma-secretase: A complex target for Alzheimer's disease. *Current Opinion in Pharmacology*, *7*(1), 112–118. https://doi.org/10.1016/j.coph.2006.10.002.
23. Cacabelos, R. (2008). Pharmacogenomics in Alzheimer's disease. *Mini Reviews in Medicinal Chemistry*, *8*(2), 213–357. https://doi.org/10.2174/1389557023406458.

24. Pedersen, W. A., McCullers, D., Culmsee, C., Haughey, N. J., Herman, J. P., & Mattson, M. P. (2001). Corticotropin-releasing hormone protects neurons against insults relevant to the pathogenesis of Alzheimer's disease. *Neurobiology of Disease*, *8*(3), 492–503. https://doi.org/10.1006/nbdi.2001.0395.
25. Iwata, N., Higuchi, M., & Saido, T. C. (2005). Metabolism of amyloid-β peptide and Alzheimer's disease. *Pharmacology & Therapeutics*, *108*(2), 129–148. https://doi.org/10.1016/j.pharmthera.2005.03.010.
26. Begcevic, I., Brinc, D., Brown, M., Martinez-Morillo, E., Goldhardt, O., Grimmer, T., Magdolen, V., Batruch, I., & Diamandis, E. P. (2018). Brain-related proteins as potential CSF biomarkers of Alzheimer's disease: A targeted mass spectrometry approach. *Journal of Proteomics*, *182*, 12–20. https://doi.org/10.1016/j.jprot.2018.04.027.
27. Mullane, K., & Williams, M. (2018). Alzheimer's disease (AD) therapeutics-1: Repeated clinical failures continue to question the amyloid hypothesis of AD and the current understanding of AD causality. *Biochemical Pharmacology*, *159*, 359–375. https://doi.org/10.1016/j.bcp.2018.09.026.
28. Binder, L. I., Guillozet-Bongaarts, A. L., Garcia-Sierra, F., & Berry, R. W. (2005). Tau, tangles, and Alzheimer's disease. *Biochimica et Biophysica Acta (BBA)–Molecular Basis of Disease*, *1739*(2–3), 216–223. https://doi.org/10.1016/j.bbadis.2004.08.014.
29. Goedert, M., Spillantini, M. G., & Davies, S. W. (1998). Filamentous nerve cell inclusions in neurodegenerative diseases. *Current Opinion in Neurobiology*, *8*(5), 619–632. https://doi.org/10.1016/S0959-4388(98)80090-1.
30. Shahani, N., & Brandt, R. (2002). Functions and malfunctions of the tau proteins. *Cellular and Molecular Life Sciences (CMLS)*, *59*(10), 1668–1680.
31. Pao, P. C., & Tsai, L. H. (2021). Three decades of Cdk5. *Journal of Biomedical Science*, *28*(1), 1–7.
32. Shah, K., & Lahiri, D. K. (2017). A tale of the good and bad: Remodeling of the microtubule network in the brain by Cdk5. *Molecular Neurobiology*, *54*(3), 2255–2268. https://doi.org/10.1007/s12035-016-9792-7.
33. Huang, F., Wang, M., Liu, R., Wang, J. Z., Schadt, E., Haroutunian, V., Katsel, P., Zhang, B., & Wang, X. (2019). CDT2-controlled cell cycle reentry regulates the pathogenesis of Alzheimer's disease. *Alzheimer's & Dementia: The Journal of the Alzheimer's Association*, *15*(2), 217–231. https://doi.org/10.1016/j.jalz.2018.08.013.
34. Haense, C., Kalbe, E., Herholz, K., Hohmann, C., Neumaier, B., Krais, R., & Heiss, W. D. (2012). Cholinergic system function and cognition in mild cognitive impairment. *Neurobiology of Aging*, *33*(5), 867–877. https://doi.org/10.1016/j.neurobiolaging.2010.08.015.
35. Bekdash, R. A. (2021). The cholinergic system, the adrenergic system and the neuropathology of Alzheimer's disease. *International Journal of Molecular Sciences*, *22*(3), Article 1273. https://doi.org/10.3390/ijms22031273.
36. Hampel, H., Mesulam, M. M., Cuello, A. C., Farlow, M. R., Giacobini, E., Grossberg, G. T., Khachaturian, A. S., Vergallo, A., Cavedo, E., Snyder, P. J., & Khachaturian, Z. S. (2018). The cholinergic system in the pathophysiology and treatment of Alzheimer's disease. *Brain*, *141*(7), 1917–1933. https://doi.org/10.1093/brain/awy132.
37. Ferreira-Vieira, T. H., Guimaraes, I. M., Silva, F. R., & Ribeiro, F. M. (2016). Alzheimer's disease: Targeting the cholinergic system. *Current Neuropharmacology*, *14*(1), 101–115. https://doi.org/10.2174/1570159x13666150716165726.

38. Robertson, I. H. (2013). A noradrenergic theory of cognitive reserve: Implications for Alzheimer's disease. *Neurobiology of Aging*, *34*(1), 298–308. https://doi.org/10.1016/j.neurobiolaging.2012.05.019.
39. Bekar, L. K., He, W., & Nedergaard, M. (2008). Locus coeruleus α-adrenergic–mediated activation of cortical astrocytes in vivo. *Cerebral Cortex*, *18*(12), 2789–2795. https://doi.org/10.1093/cercor/bhn040.
40. Matchett, B. J., Grinberg, L. T., Theofilas, P., & Murray, M. E. (2021). The mechanistic link between selective vulnerability of the locus coeruleus and neurodegeneration in Alzheimer's disease. *Acta Neuropathologica*, *141*(5), 631–650. https://doi.org/10.1007/s00401-020-02248-1.
41. Vakalopoulos, C. (2017). Alzheimer's disease: The alternative serotonergic hypothesis of cognitive decline. *American Journal of Alzheimer's Disease*, *60*(3), 859–866. https://doi.org/10.3233/JAD-170364.
42. Kuhn, M., Popovic, A., & Pezawas, L. (2014). Neuroplasticity and memory formation in major depressive disorder: An imaging genetics perspective on serotonin and BDNF. *Restorative Neurology and Neuroscience*, *32*(1), 25–49. https://doi.org/10.3233/RNN-139005.
43. Lutzu, S., & Castillo, P. E. (2021). Modulation of NMDA receptors by G-protein-coupled receptors: Role in synaptic transmission, plasticity and beyond. *Neuroscience*, *456*, 27–42. https://doi.org/10.1016/j.neuroscience.2020.02.019.
44. Guo, J. L., Narasimhan, S., Changolkar, L., He, Z., Stieber, A., Zhang, B., Gathagan, R. J., Iba, M., McBride, J. D., Trojanowski, J. Q., & Lee, V. M. (2016). Unique pathological tau conformers from Alzheimer's brains transmit tau pathology in nontransgenic mice. *Journal of Experimental Medicine*, *213*(12), 2635–2654. https://doi.org/10.1084/jem.20160833.
45. Yun, H. M., Park, K. R., Kim, E. C., Kim, S., & Hong, J. T. (2015). Serotonin 6 receptor controls Alzheimer's disease and depression. *Oncotarget*, *6*(29), 26716. https://doi.org/10.18632/oncotarget.5777.
46. Heneka, M. T., Golenbock, D. T., & Latz, E. (2015). Innate immunity in Alzheimer's disease. *Nature Immunology*, *16*(3), 229–236. https://doi.org/10.1038/ni.3102.
47. Yu, Y., & Ye, R. D. (2015). Microglial Aβ receptors in Alzheimer's disease. *Cellular and Molecular Neurobiology*, *35*(1), 71–83. https://doi.org/10.1007/s10571-014-0101-6.
48. Barczuk, J., Siwecka, N., Lusa, W., Rozpędek-Kamińska, W., Kucharska, E., & Majsterek, I. (2022). Targeting NLRP3-mediated neuroinflammation in Alzheimer's disease treatment. *International Journal of Molecular Sciences*, *23*(16), Article 8979. https://doi.org/10.3390/ijms23168979.
49. Kinney, J. W., Bemiller, S. M., Murtishaw, A. S., Leisgang, A. M., Salazar, A. M., & Lamb, B. T. (2018). Inflammation as a central mechanism in Alzheimer's disease. *Alzheimer's & Dementia: Translational Research & Clinical Interventions*, *4*, 575–590. https://doi.org/10.1016/j.trci.2018.06.014.
50. Jack, C. R., Bennett, D. A., Blennow, K., Carrillo, M. C., Feldman, H. H., Frisoni, G. B., Hampel, H., Jagust, W. J., Johnson, K. A., Knopman, D. S., & Petersen, R. C. (2016). A/T/N: An unbiased descriptive classification scheme for Alzheimer disease biomarkers. *Neurology*, *87*(5), 539–547. https://doi.org/10.1212/WNL.0000000000002923.
51. Goate, A., Chartier-Harlin, M. C., Mullan, M., Brown, J., Crawford, F., Fidani, L., Giuffra, L., Haynes, A., Irving, N., James, L., & Mant, R. (1991). Segregation of a

missense mutation in the amyloid precursor protein gene with familial Alzheimer's disease. *Nature*, *349*(6311), 704–706. https://doi.org/10.1038/349704a0.
52. Sherrington, R., Rogaev, E. I., Liang, Y. A., Rogaeva, E. A., Levesque, G., Ikeda, M., Chi, H., Lin, C., Li, G., Holman, K., & Tsuda, T. (1995). Cloning of a gene bearing missense mutations in early-onset familial Alzheimer's disease. *Nature*, *375*(6534), 754–760. https://doi.org/10.1038/375754a0.
53. Levy-Lahad, E., Wasco, W., Poorkaj, P., Romano, D. M., Oshima, J., Pettingell, W. H., Yu, C. E., Jondro, P. D., Schmidt, S. D., & Wang, K. (1995). Candidate gene for the chromosome 1 familial Alzheimer's disease locus. *Science*, *269*(5226), 973–977. https://doi.org/10.1126/science.7638622.
54. Corder, E. H., Saunders, A. M., Strittmatter, W. J., Schmechel, D. E., Gaskell, P. C., Small, G., Roses, A. D., Haines, J. L., & Pericak-Vance, M. A. (1993). Gene dose of apolipoprotein E type 4 allele and the risk of Alzheimer's disease in late onset families. *Science*, *261*(5123), 921–923. https://doi.org/10.1126/science.8346443.
55. Poirier, J., Bertrand, P., Kogan, S., Gauthier, S., Davignon, J., & Bouthillier, D. (1993). Apolipoprotein E polymorphism and Alzheimer's disease. *The Lancet*, *342*(8873), 697–699. https://doi.org/10.1016/0140-6736(93)91705-5.
56. Meyer, M. R., Tschanz, J. T., Norton, M. C., Welsh-Bohmer, K. A., Steffens, D. C., Wyse, B. W., & Breitner, J. C. (1998). APOE genotype predicts when—not whether—one is predisposed to develop Alzheimer disease. *Nature Genetics*, *19*(4), 321–322. https://doi.org/10.1038/ng0898_321.
57. Luca, M., Di Mauro, M., Di Mauro, M., & Luca, A. (2019). Gut microbiota in Alzheimer's disease, depression, and type 2 diabetes mellitus: The role of oxidative stress. *Oxidative Medicine and Cellular Longevity*, *2019*, Article 4730539. https://doi.org/10.1155/2019/4730539.
58. Pithadia, A. S., & Lim, M. H. (2012). Metal-associated amyloid-β species in Alzheimer's disease. *Current Opinion in Chemical Biology*, *16*(1–2), 67–73. https://doi.org/10.1016/j.cbpa.2012.01.016.
59. Cheignon, C., Tomas, M., Bonnefont-Rousselot, D., Faller, P., Hureau, C., & Collin, F. (2018). Oxidative stress and the amyloid beta peptide in Alzheimer's disease. *Redox Biology*, *14*, 450–464. https://doi.org/10.1016/j.redox.2017.10.014.
60. Wang, Y., Shi, Y., & Wei, H. (2017). Calcium dysregulation in Alzheimer's disease: A target for new drug development. *Journal of Alzheimer's Disease & Parkinsonism*, *7*(5). https://doi.org/10.4172/2161-0460.1000374.
61. Nakamura, T., & Lipton, S. A. (2010). Preventing Ca2+-mediated nitrosative stress in neurodegenerative diseases: Possible pharmacological strategies. *Cell Calcium*, *47*(2), 190–197. https://doi.org/10.1016/j.ceca.2009.12.009.
62. Fragoso-Morales, L. G., Correa-Basurto, J., & Rosales-Hernández, M. C. (2021). Implication of nicotinamide adenine dinucleotide phosphate (NADPH) oxidase and its inhibitors in Alzheimer's disease murine models. *Antioxidants*, *10*(2), 218. https://doi.org/10.3390/antiox10020218.
63. Osadchiy, V., Martin, C. R., & Mayer, E. A. (2019). The Gut-Brain Axis and the Microbiome: Mechanisms and Clinical Implications. *Clinical Gastroenterology and Hepatology*, *17*(2), 322–332. https://doi.org/10.1016/j.cgh.2018.10.002.
64. Hu, X., Wang, T., & Jin, F. (2016). Alzheimer's disease and gut microbiota. *Science China Life Sciences*, *59*(10), 1006–1023. https://doi.org/10.1007/s11427-016-5083-9.

65. Mahmoudian Dehkordi, S., Arnold, M., Nho, K., Ahmad, S., Jia, W., Xie, G., Louie, G., Kueider-Paisley, A., Moseley, M. A., Thompson, J. W., Alzheimer's Disease Neuroimaging Initiative, & Alzheimer's Disease Metabolomics Consortium. (2019). Altered bile acid profile associates with cognitive impairment in Alzheimer's disease—An emerging role for gut microbiome. *Alzheimer's & Dementia*, *15*(1), 76–92.
66. de J. R. De-Paula, V., Forlenza, A. S., & Forlenza, O. V. (2018). Relevance of gut microbiota in cognition, behaviour and Alzheimer's disease. *Pharmacological Research*, *136*, 29–34. https://doi.org/10.1016/j.phrs.2018.07.007.
67. Calabrese, V., Boyd-Kimball, D., Scapagnini, G., & Butterfield, D. A. (2004). Nitric oxide and cellular stress response in brain aging and neurodegenerative disorders: The role of vitagenes. *In Vivo*, *18*(3), 245–268.
68. Tiso, M., & Schechter, A. N. (2015). Nitrate reduction to nitrite, nitric oxide and ammonia by gut bacteria under physiological conditions. *PLoS One*, *10*(3), e0119712. https://doi.org/10.1371/journal.pone.0119712.
69. Dehhaghi, M., Kazemi Shariat Panahi, H., & Guillemin, G. J. (2018). Microorganisms' footprint in neurodegenerative diseases. *Frontiers in Cellular Neuroscience*, *12*, 466. https://doi.org/10.3389/fncel.2018.00466.
70. Pistollato, F., Sumalla Cano, S., Elio, I., Masías Vergara, M., Giampieri, F., & Battino, M. (2016). Role of gut microbiota and nutrients in amyloid formation and pathogenesis of Alzheimer disease. *Nutrition Reviews*, *74*(10), 624–634. https://doi.org/10.1093/nutrit/nuw023.
71. Angelucci, F., Cechova, K., Amlerova, J., & Hort, J. (2019). Antibiotics, gut microbiota, and Alzheimer's disease. *Journal of Neuroinflammation*, *16*(1), 1–0. https://doi.org/10.1186/s12974-019-1494-4.
72. Funderburk, S. F., Marcellino, B. K., & Yue, Z. (2010). Cell "self-eating" (autophagy) mechanism in Alzheimer's disease. *Mount Sinai Journal of Medicine: A Journal of Translational and Personalized Medicine*, *77*(1), 59–68. https://doi.org/10.1002/msj.20161.
73. Cai, Z., Zhao, B., Li, K., Zhang, L., Li, C., Quazi, S. H., & Tan, Y. (2012). Mammalian target of rapamycin: A valid therapeutic target through the autophagy pathway for Alzheimer's disease? *Journal of Neuroscience Research*, *90*(6), 1105–1118. https://doi.org/10.1002/jnr.23011.
74. Ashraf, G. M., Tarasov, V. V., Makhmutova, A., Chubarev, V. N., Avila-Rodriguez, M., Bachurin, S. O., & Aliev, G. (2019). The possibility of an infectious etiology of Alzheimer disease. *Molecular Neurobiology*, *56*(6), 4479–4491. https://doi.org/10.1007/s12035-018-1388-y.
75. Bir, S. C., Chernyshev, O. Y., & Minagar, A. (2018). Roles of toll-like receptors in pathophysiology of Alzheimer's Disease and multiple sclerosis. *Journal of Neuroinflammation, 2018*, 541–562. https://doi.org/10.1016/B978-0-12-811709-5.00033-8.
76. Bateman, R. J., Barthelemy, N. R., & Horie, K. (2020). Another step forward in blood-based diagnostics for Alzheimer's disease. *Nature Medicine*, *26*(3), 314–316. https://doi.org/10.1038/s41591-020-0797-4.
77. Janelidze, S., Mattsson, N., Palmqvist, S., Smith, R., Beach, T. G., Serrano, G. E., Chai, X., Proctor, N. K., Eichenlaub, U., Zetterberg, H., & Blennow, K. (2020). Plasma P-tau181 in Alzheimer's disease: Relationship to other biomarkers, differential

diagnosis, neuropathology and longitudinal progression to Alzheimer's dementia. *Nature Medicine*, *26*(3), 379–386. https://doi.org/10.1038/s41591-020-0755-1.

78. Thijssen, E. H., La Joie, R., Wolf, A., Strom, A., Wang, P., Iaccarino, L., Bourakova, V., Cobigo, Y., Heuer, H., Spina, S., VandeVrede, L., & Rabinovici, G. D. (2020). Diagnostic value of plasma phosphorylated tau181 in Alzheimer's disease and frontotemporal lobar degeneration. *Nature Medicine*, *26*(3), 387–397. https://doi.org/10.1038/s41591-020-0762-2.
79. Weller, J., & Budson, A. (2018). Current understanding of Alzheimer's disease diagnosis and treatment. *F1000Research*, *7*. https://doi.org/10.12688/f1000research.14506.1.
80. Fagan, A. M., Xiong, C., Jasielec, M. S., Bateman, R. J., Goate, A. M., Benzinger, T. L., Ghetti, B., Martins, R. N., Masters, C. L., Mayeux, R., & Ringman, J. M. (2014). Longitudinal change in CSF biomarkers in autosomal-dominant Alzheimer's disease. *Science Translational Medicine*, *6*(226), 226ra30. https://doi.org/10.1126/scitranslmed.3007901.
81. Jagust, W. (2018). Imaging the evolution and pathophysiology of Alzheimer disease. *Nature Reviews Neuroscience, 19*(11), 687–700. https://doi.org/10.1038/s41583-018-0067-3.
82. Mosconi, L. (2013). Glucose metabolism in normal aging and Alzheimer's disease: Methodological and physiological considerations for PET studies. *Clinical Translational Imaging, 1*(4–5), 217–233. https://doi.org/10.1007/s40336-013-0026-y.
83. Johnson, K. A., Fox, N. C., Sperling, R. A., & Klunk, W. E. (2012). Brain imaging in Alzheimer disease. *Cold Spring Harbor Perspectives in Medicine, 2*(4), a006213. https://doi.org/10.1101/cshperspect.a006213.
84. Chandra, A., Dervenoulas, G., Politis, M., & Alzheimer's Disease Neuroimaging Initiative. (2019). Magnetic resonance imaging in Alzheimer's disease and mild cognitive impairment. *Journal of Neurology, 266*(6), 1293–1302. https://doi.org/10.1007/s00415-018-9016-3.
85. Acosta, C., Anderson, H. D., & Anderson, C. M. (2017). Astrocyte dysfunction in Alzheimer disease. *Journal of Neuroscience Research, 95*(12), 2430–2447. https://doi.org/10.1002/jnr.24075.
86. Higashi, T., Nishii, R., Kagawa, S., Kishibe, Y., Takahashi, M., Okina, T., Suzuki, N., Hasegawa, H., Nagahama, Y., Ishizu, K., & Oishi, N. (2018). 18F-FPYBF-2, a new F-18-labelled amyloid imaging PET tracer: First experience in 61 volunteers and 55 patients with dementia. *Annals of Nuclear Medicine, 32*(3), 206–216. https://doi.org/10.1007/s12149-018-1236-1.
87. Villa, A., Klein, B., Janssen, B., Pedragosa, J., Pepe, G., Zinnhardt, B., Vugts, D. J., Gelosa, P., Sironi, L., Beaino, W., & Damont, A. (2018). Identification of new molecular targets for PET imaging of the microglial anti-inflammatory activation state. *Theranostics, 8*(19), 5400–5418. https://doi.org/10.7150/thno.25572.
88. Bao, W., Xie, F., Zuo, C., Guan, Y., & Huang, Y. H. (2021). PET neuroimaging of Alzheimer's disease: Radiotracers and their utility in clinical research. *Frontiers in Aging Neuroscience, 13*, 624330. https://doi.org/10.3389/fnagi.2021.624330.
89. Herscovitch, P. (2015). Regulatory approval and insurance reimbursement: The final steps in clinical translation of amyloid brain imaging. *Clinical and Translational Imaging, 3*(2), 75–77. https://doi.org/10.1007/s40336-015-0101-7.
90. Schmidt, M. E., Janssens, L., Moechars, D., Rombouts, F. J., Timmers, M., Barret, O., Constantinescu, C. C., Madonia, J., Russell, D. S., Sandiego, C. M., & Kolb, H.

(2020). Clinical evaluation of [18 F] JNJ-64326067, a novel candidate PET tracer for the detection of tau pathology in Alzheimer's disease. *European Journal of Nuclear Medicine and Molecular Imaging, 47*(12), 3176–3185. https://doi.org/10.1007/s00259-020-04880-1.

91. Chetelat, G., Arbizu, J., Barthel, H., Garibotto, V., Law, I., Morbelli, S., van de Giessen, E., Agosta, F., Barkhof, F., Brooks, D. J., & Carrillo, M. C. (2020). Amyloid-PET and 18F-FDG-PET in the diagnostic investigation of Alzheimer's disease and other dementias. *The Lancet Neurology, 19*(11), 951–962. https://doi.org/10.1016/S1474-4422(20)30314-8.
92. Hampel, H., Frank, R., Broich, K., Teipel, S. J., Katz, R. G., Hardy, J., Herholz, K., Bokde, A. L., Jessen, F., Hoessler, Y. C., & Sanhai, W. R. (2010). Biomarkers for Alzheimer's disease: Academic, industry and regulatory perspectives. *Nature Reviews Drug Discovery, 9*(7), 560–574. https://doi.org/10.1038/nrd3115.
93. Ou, Y. N., Xu, W., Li, J. Q., Guo, Y., Cui, M., Chen, K. L., Huang, Y. Y., Dong, Q., Tan, L., & Yu, J. T. (2019). FDG-PET as an independent biomarker for Alzheimer's biological diagnosis: A longitudinal study. *Alzheimer's Research & Therapy, 11*(1), 57. https://doi.org/10.1186/s13195-019-0512-1.
94. Marcus, C., Mena, E., & Subramaniam, R. M. (2014). Brain PET in the diagnosis of Alzheimer's disease. *Clinical Nuclear Medicine, 39*(10), 413. https://doi.org/10.1097/RLU.0000000000000547.
95. Liu, X., Chen, K., Wu, T., Weidman, D., Lure, F., & Li, J. (2018). Use of multimodality imaging and artificial intelligence for diagnosis and prognosis of early stages of Alzheimer's disease. *Translational Research, 194*, 56–67. https://doi.org/10.1016/j.trsl.2018.01.001.
96. Henry, M. S., Passmore, A. P., Todd, S., McGuinness, B., Craig, D., & Johnston, J. A. (2013). The development of effective biomarkers for Alzheimer's disease: A review. *International Journal of Geriatric Psychiatry, 28*(4), 331–340. https://doi.org/10.1002/gps.3829.
97. Van Oostveen, W. M., & De Lange, E. C. (2021). Imaging techniques in Alzheimer's disease: A review of applications in early diagnosis and longitudinal monitoring. *International Journal of Molecular Sciences, 22*(4), 2110. https://doi.org/10.3390/ijms22042110.
98. Ma, D., Yee, E., Stocks, J. K., Jenkins, L. M., Popuri, K., Chausse, G., Wang, L., Probst, S., & Beg, M. F. (2021). Blinded clinical evaluation for dementia of Alzheimer's type classification using FDG-PET: A comparison between feature-engineered and non-feature-engineered machine learning methods. *American Journal of Alzheimer's Disease and Other Dementias, 80*(2), 715–726. https://doi.org/10.3233/JAD-201591.
99. Hanyu, H., Koyama, Y., Horita, H., Aoki, T., Sato, T., Takenoshita, N., Kanetaka, H., Shimizu, S., Hirao, K., & Watanabe, S. (2022). Characterization of Alzheimer's Disease Subtypes Based on Magnetic Resonance Imaging and Perfusion Single-Photon Emission Computed Tomography. *Journal of Alzheimer's Disease, 87*(2), 781–789. https://doi.org/10.3233/JAD-215674.
100. Lohith, T. G., Bennacef, I., Vandenberghe, R., Vandenbulcke, M., Salinas, C. A., Declercq, R., Reynders, T., Telan-Choing, N. F., Riffel, K., Celen, S., & Serdons, K. (2019). Brain imaging of Alzheimer dementia patients and elderly controls with 18F-MK-6240, a PET tracer targeting neurofibrillary tangles. *Journal of Nuclear Medicine, 60*(1), 107–114. https://doi.org/10.2967/jnumed.118.208215.

101. Villemagne, V. L., Ong, K., Mulligan, R. S., Holl, G., Pejoska, S., Jones, G., O'Keefe, G., Ackerman, U., Tochon-Danguy, H., Chan, J. G., & Reininger, C. B. (2011). Amyloid imaging with 18F-florbetaben in Alzheimer disease and other dementias. *Journal of Nuclear Medicine, 52*(8), 1210–1217. https://doi.org/10.2967/jnumed.111.089730.
102. Yeo, S. K., Shepelytskyi, Y., Grynko, V., & Albert, M. S. (2020). Molecular imaging of fluorinated probes for tau protein and amyloid-β detection. *Molecules, 25*(15), 3413. https://doi.org/10.3390/molecules25153413
103. Carneiro, C. D., Faria, D. D., Coutinho, A. M., Ono, C. R., Duran, F. L., da Costa, N. A., Garcez, A. T., da Silveira, P. S., Forlenza, O. V., Brucki, S. M., & Nitrini, R. (2022). Evaluation of 10-minute post-injection 11C-PiB PET and its correlation with 18F-FDG PET in older adults who are cognitively healthy, mildly impaired, or with probable Alzheimer's disease. *Brazilian Journal of Psychiatry, 44*, 495–506. https://doi.org/10.47626/1516-4446-2021-2374.
104. Clark, C. M., Schneider, J. A., Bedell, B. J., Beach, T. G., Bilker, W. B., Mintun, M. A., Pontecorvo, M. J., Hefti, F., Carpenter, A. P., Flitter, M. L., & Krautkramer, M. J. (2011). Use of florbetapir-PET for imaging β-amyloid pathology. *JAMA, 305*(3), 275–283. https://doi.org/10.1001/jama.2010.2008.
105. Meyer, P. F., McSweeney, M., Gonneaud, J., & Villeneuve, S. (2019). PET amyloid imaging across the Alzheimer's disease spectrum: From disease mechanisms to prevention. *Progress in Molecular Biology and Translational Science, 165, 63–106.* https://doi.org/10.1016/bs.pmbts.2019.05.001.
106. Ricci, M., Cimini, A., Camedda, R., Chiaravalloti, A., & Schillaci, O. (2021). Tau biomarkers in dementia: Positron emission tomography radiopharmaceuticals in tauopathy assessment and future perspective. *International Journal of Molecular Sciences, 22*(23), 1–23. https://doi.org/10.3390/ijms222313002.
107. Bucci, M., Chiotis, K., & Nordberg, A. (2021). Alzheimer's disease profiled by fluid and imaging markers: Tau PET best predicts cognitive decline. *Molecular Psychiatry, 26*(10), 5888–5898. https://doi.org/10.1038/s41380-021-01263-2.
108. Jouanne, M., Rault, S., & Voisin-Chiret, A. S. (2017). Tau protein aggregation in Alzheimer's disease: An attractive target for the development of novel therapeutic agents. *European Journal of Medicinal Chemistry, 139*, 153–167. https://doi.org/10.1016/j.ejmech.2017.07.070.
109. Okamura, N., Harada, R., Ishiki, A., Kikuchi, A., Nakamura, T., & Kudo, Y. (2018). The development and validation of tau PET tracers: Current status and future directions. *Clinical and Translational Imaging, 6*, 305–316. https://doi.org/10.1007/s40336-018-0290-y.
110. Damasceno, P. F., La Joie, R., Maia, P. D., Visani, A., Iaccarino, L., Strom, A., Edwards, L., Tempini, M. L., Jagust, W. J., Miller, B. L., & Rabinovici, G. D. (2020). Colocalization of atrophy and tau improves AI classification of Alzheimer phenotypical variants: Tau imaging. *Alzheimer's & Dementia, 16*, e046258. https://doi.org/10.1002/alz.046258.
111. Hammes, J., Bischof, G. N., Bohn, K. P., Onur, Ö., Schneider, A., Fliessbach, K., Hönig, M. C., Jessen, F., Neumaier, B., Drzezga, A., & van Eimeren, T. (2021). One-stop shop: 18F-flortaucipir PET differentiates amyloid-positive and-negative forms of neurodegenerative diseases. *Journal of Nuclear Medicine, 62*(2), 240–246. https://doi.org/10.2967/jnumed.120.244061.

112. Humpel, C. (2011). Identifying and validating biomarkers for Alzheimer's disease. *Trends in Biotechnology, 29*(1), 26–32. https://doi.org/10.1016/j.tibtech.2010.09.007.
113. Hansson, O., Seibyl, J., Stomrud, E., Zetterberg, H., Trojanowski, J. Q., Bittner, T., Lifke, V., Corradini, V., Eichenlaub, U., Batrla, R., & Buck, K. (2018). CSF biomarkers of Alzheimer's disease concord with amyloid-β PET and predict clinical progression: A study of fully automated immunoassays in BioFINDER and ADNI cohorts. *Alzheimer's & Dementia, 14*(11), 1470–1481. https://doi.org/10.1016/j.jalz.2018.01.010.
114. Lashley, T., Schott, J. M., Weston, P., Murray, C. E., Wellington, H., Keshavan, A., Foti, S. C., Foiani, M., Toombs, J., Rohrer, J. D., & Heslegrave, A. (2018). Molecular biomarkers of Alzheimer's disease: Progress and prospects. *Disease Models & Mechanisms, 11*(5), dmm031781. https://doi.org/10.1242/dmm.031781.
115. Yang, Y. W., Liou, S. H., Hsueh, Y. M., Lyu, W. S., Liu, C. S., Liu, H. J., Chung, M. C., Hung, P. H., & Chung, C. J. (2018). Risk of Alzheimer's disease with metal concentrations in whole blood and urine: A case–control study using propensity score matching. *Toxicology and Applied Pharmacology, 356*, 8–14. https://doi.org/10.1016/j.taap.2018.07.015.
116. Huat, T. J., Camats-Perna, J., Newcombe, E. A., Valmas, N., Kitazawa, M., & Medeiros, R. (2019). Metal toxicity links to Alzheimer's disease and neuroinflammation. *Journal of Molecular Biology, 431*(9), 1843–1868. https://doi.org/10.1016/j.jmb.2019.01.018.
117. Blennow, K., & Zetterberg, H. (2018). Biomarkers for Alzheimer's disease: Current status and prospects for the future. *Journal of Internal Medicine, 284*(6), 643–663. https://doi.org/10.1111/joim.12816.
118. Kok, E. H., Alanne-Kinnunen, M., Isotalo, K., Luoto, T., Haikonen, S., Goebeler, S., Perola, M., Hurme, M. A., Haapasalo, H., & Karhunen, P. J. (2011). CRP gene variation affects early development of Alzheimer's disease-related plaques. *Journal of Neuroinflammation, 8*(1), 1–9. https://doi.org/10.1186/1742-2094-8-96.
119. O'Bryant, S. E., Waring, S. C., Hobson, V., Hall, J. R., Moore, C. B., Bottiglieri, T., Massman, P., & Diaz-Arrastia, R. (2010). Decreased C-reactive protein levels in Alzheimer disease. *Journal of Geriatric Psychiatry and Neurology, 23*(1), 49–53. https://doi.org/10.1177/0891988709351832.
120. Brosseron, F., Traschütz, A., Widmann, C. N., Kummer, M. P., Tacik, P., Santarelli, F., Jessen, F., & Heneka, M. T. (2018). Characterization and clinical use of inflammatory cerebrospinal fluid protein markers in Alzheimer's disease. *Alzheimer's Research & Therapy, 10*, 1–4. https://doi.org/10.1186/s13195-018-0353-3.
121. Bateman, R. J., Blennow, K., Doody, R., Hendrix, S., Lovestone, S., Salloway, S., Schindler, R., Weiner, M., Zetterberg, H., Aisen, P., & Vellas, B. (2019). Plasma biomarkers of AD emerging as essential tools for drug development: An EU/US CTAD task force report. *Journal of Prevention of Alzheimer's Disease, 6*, 169–173. http://dx.doi.org/10.14283/jpad.2019.21.
122. Schupf, N., Tang, M. X., Fukuyama, H., Manly, J., Andrews, H., Mehta, P., Ravetch, J., & Mayeux, R. (2008). Peripheral Aβ subspecies as risk biomarkers of Alzheimer's disease. *Proceedings of the National Academy of Sciences, 105*(37), 14052–14057. https://doi.org/10.1073/pnas.0805902105.
123. Nabers, A., Perna, L., Lange, J., Mons, U., Schartner, J., Güldenhaupt, J., Saum, K. U., Janelidze, S., Holleczek, B., Rujescu, D., & Hansson, O. (2018). Amyloid blood biomarker detects Alzheimer's disease. *EMBO Molecular Medicine, 10*(5), 1–11. https://doi.org/10.15252/emmm.201708763.

124. Cermenati, G., Mitro, N., Audano, M., Melcangi, R. C., Crestani, M., De Fabiani, E., & Caruso, D. (2015). Lipids in the nervous system: From biochemistry and molecular biology to patho-physiology. *Biochimica et Biophysica Acta (BBA)–Molecular and Cell Biology of Lipids, 1851*(1), 51–60. https://doi.org/10.1016/j.bbalip.2014.08.011.
125. Kumar, A., Behl, T., Jamwal, S., Kaur, I., Sood, A., & Kumar, P. (2020). Exploring the molecular approach of COX and LOX in Alzheimer's and Parkinson's disorder. *Molecular Biology Reports, 47*, 9895–9912. https://doi.org/10.1007/s11033-020-06033-x.
126. Beal, E. (2011). Plasma lipid biomarkers for early-stage Alzheimer disease. *Nature Reviews Neurology, 7*(9), 474. http://www.nature.com/doifinder/10.1038/nrneurol.2011.125.
127. Zarrouk, A., Debbabi, M., Bezine, M., Karym, E. M., Badreddine, A., Rouaud, O., Moreau, T., Cherkaoui-Malki, M., El Ayeb, M., Nasser, B., & Hammami, M. (2018). Lipid biomarkers in Alzheimer's disease. *Current Alzheimer Research, 15*(4), 303–312. https://doi.org/10.2174/1567205014666170505101426.
128. Knopman, D. S., Amieva, H., Petersen, R. C., Chételat, G., Holtzman, D. M., Hyman, B. T., Nixon, R. A., & Jones, D. T. (2021). Alzheimer disease. *Nature Reviews Disease Primers, 7*(1), 33. https://doi.org/10.1038/s41572-021-00269-y.
129. Dastgheib, Z. A., Lithgow, B. J., & Moussavi, Z. K. (2022). An unbiased algorithm for objective separation of Alzheimer's, Alzheimer's mixed with cerebrovascular symptomology, and healthy controls from one another using electrovestibulography (EVestG). *Medical & Biological Engineering & Computing, 60*(3), 797–810. https://doi.org/10.1007/s11517-022-02507-1.
130. Sharma, V., Kaur, A., & Singh, T. G. (2020). Counteracting role of nuclear factor erythroid 2-related factor 2 pathway in Alzheimer's disease. *Biomedicine & Pharmacotherapy, 129*, 110373. https://doi.org/10.1016/j.biopha.2020.110373.
131. Sims, R., Hill, M., & Williams, J. (2020). The multiplex model of the genetics of Alzheimer's disease. *Nature Neuroscience, 23*(3), 311–322. https://doi.org/10.1038/s41593-020-0599-5.
132. Raulin, A. C., Doss, S. V., Trottier, Z. A., Ikezu, T. C., Bu, G., & Liu, C. C. (2022). ApoE in Alzheimer's disease: Pathophysiology and therapeutic strategies. *Molecular Neurodegeneration, 17*(1), 1–26. https://doi.org/10.1186/s13024-022-00574-4.
133. Lim, Y. Y., Villemagne, V. L., Laws, S. M., Ames, D., Pietrzak, R. H., Ellis, K. A., Harrington, K. D., Bourgeat, P., Salvado, O., Darby, D., & Snyder, P. J. (2013). BDNF Val66Met, Aβ amyloid, and cognitive decline in preclinical Alzheimer's disease. *Neurobiology of Aging, 34*(11), 2457–2464. https://doi.org/10.1016/j.neurobiolaging.2013.05.006.
134. Lim, Y. Y., Villemagne, V. L., Laws, S. M., Ames, D., Pietrzak, R. H., Ellis, K. A., Harrington, K., Bourgeat, P., Bush, A. I., Martins, R. N., & Masters, C. L. (2014). Effect of BDNF Val66Met on memory decline and hippocampal atrophy in prodromal Alzheimer's disease: A preliminary study. *PLoS ONE, 9*(1), e86498. https://doi.org/10.1371/journal.pone.0086498.
135. Kauppi, K., Nilsson, L. G., Adolfsson, R., Eriksson, E., & Nyberg, L. (2011). KIBRA polymorphism is related to enhanced memory and elevated hippocampal processing. *Journal of Neuroscience, 31*(40), 14218–14222. https://doi.org/10.1523/JNEUROSCI.3292-11.2011.
136. Tracy, T. E., Sohn, P. D., Minami, S. S., Wang, C., Min, S. W., Li, Y., Zhou, Y., Le, D., Lo, I., Ponnusamy, R., & Cong, X. (2016). Acetylated tau obstructs KIBRA-mediated

signaling in synaptic plasticity and promotes tauopathy-related memory loss. *Neuron, 90*(2), 245–260. https://doi.org/10.1016/j.neuron.2016.03.005.

137. Porter, T., Villemagne, V. L., Savage, G., Milicic, L., Lim, Y. Y., Maruff, P., Masters, C. L., Ames, D., Bush, A. I., Martins, R. N., & Rainey-Smith, S. (2018). Cognitive gene risk profile for the prediction of cognitive decline in presymptomatic Alzheimer's disease. *Personalized Medicine in Psychiatry, 7*, 14–20. https://doi.org/10.1016/j.pmip.2018.03.001.
138. Bao, W., Jia, H., Finnema, S., Cai, Z., Carson, R. E., & Huang, Y. H. (2017). PET imaging for early detection of Alzheimer's disease: From pathologic to physiologic biomarkers. *PET Clinics, 12*(3), 329–350. https://doi.org/10.1016/j.cpet.2017.03.001.
139. Finnema, S. J., Nabulsi, N. B., Eid, T., Detyniecki, K., Lin, S. F., Chen, M. K., Dhaher, M., Matuskey, D., Baum, E., Holden, D., & Spencer, D. D. (2016). Imaging synaptic density in the living human brain. *Science Translational Medicine, 8*(348), 348ra96. https://doi.org/10.1126/scitranslmed.aaf6667.
140. Mercier, J., Provins, L., & Valade, A. (2017). Discovery and development of SV2A PET tracers: Potential for imaging synaptic density and clinical applications. *Drug Discovery Today: Technologies, 25*, 45–52. https://doi.org/10.1016/j.ddtec.2017.11.003.
141. Cai, Z., Li, S., Matuskey, D., Nabulsi, N., & Huang, Y. (2019). PET imaging of synaptic density: A new tool for investigation of neuropsychiatric diseases. *Neuroscience Letters, 691*, 44–50. https://doi.org/10.1016/j.neulet.2018.07.038.
142. Kong, Y., Liu, C., Zhou, Y. Q., Zhang, C., Sun, B., Wang, J., & Guan, Y. (2020). Progress of RAGE molecular imaging in Alzheimer's disease. *Frontiers in Aging Neuroscience, 12*, 227. https://doi.org/10.3389/fnagi.2020.00227.
143. Luzi, F., Savickas, V., Taddei, C., Hader, S., Singh, N., Gee, A. D., & Bongarzone, S. (2020). Radiolabeling of [11C] FPS-ZM1, a receptor for advanced glycation end products-targeting positron emission tomography radiotracer, using a [11C] CO2-to-[11C] CO chemical conversion. *Future Medicinal Chemistry, 12*(6), 511–521. https://doi.org/10.4155/fmc-2019-0329.
144. Nation, D. A., Sweeney, M. D., Montagne, A., Sagare, A. P., D'Orazio, L. M., Pachicano, M., Sepehrband, F., Nelson, A. R., Buennagel, D. P., Harrington, M. G., & Benzinger, T. L. (2019). Blood–brain barrier breakdown is an early biomarker of human cognitive dysfunction. *Nature Medicine, 25*(2), 270–276.
145. Zhang, Q., & Xie, C. (2021). Apolipoprotein E drives early blood–brain barrier damage in Alzheimer's disease. *Neuroscience Bulletin, 37*, 281–283. https://doi.org/10.1007/s12264-020-00596-2.
146. Moon, Y., Han, S. H., & Moon, W. J. (2016). Patterns of brain iron accumulation in vascular dementia and Alzheimer's dementia using quantitative susceptibility mapping imaging. *American Journal of Alzheimer's Disease, 5*(3), 737–745. https://doi.org/10.3233/JAD-151037.
147. Gong, N. J., Dibb, R., Bulk, M., van der Weerd, L., & Liu, C. (2019). Imaging beta amyloid aggregation and iron accumulation in Alzheimer's disease using quantitative susceptibility mapping MRI. *Neuroimage, 191*, 176–185. https://doi.org/10.1016/j.neuroimage.2019.02.019.
148. Sharma, S., & Mandal, P. K. (2022). A comprehensive report on machine learning-based early detection of Alzheimer's disease using multi-modal neuroimaging data. *ACM Computing Surveys, 55*(2), 1–44. https://doi.org/10.1145/3492865.

149. Brüggen, K., Dyrba, M., Barkhof, F., Hausner, L., Filippi, M., Nestor, P. J., Hauenstein, K., Klöppel, S., Grothe, M. J., Kasper, E., & Teipel, S. J. (2015). Basal forebrain and hippocampus as predictors of conversion to Alzheimer's disease in patients with mild cognitive impairment–a multicenter DTI and volumetry study. *Journal of Alzheimer's Disease, 48*(1), 197–204. https://doi.org/10.3233/JAD-150063.
150. Teipel, S. J., Grothe, M., Lista, S., Toschi, N., Garaci, F. G., & Hampel, H. (2013). Relevance of magnetic resonance imaging for early detection and diagnosis of Alzheimer disease. *Medical Clinics of North America, 97*(3), 399–424. https://doi.org/10.1016/j.mcna.2012.12.013.
151. Hoy, A. R., Ly, M., Carlsson, C. M., Okonkwo, O. C., Zetterberg, H., Blennow, K., Sager, M. A., Asthana, S., Johnson, S. C., Alexander, A. L., & Bendlin, B. B. (2017). Microstructural white matter alterations in preclinical Alzheimer's disease detected using free water elimination diffusion tensor imaging. *PLOS ONE, 12*(3), e0173982. https://doi.org/10.1371/journal.pone.0173982.
152. Doustar, J., Torbati, T., Black, K. L., Koronyo, Y., & Koronyo-Hamaoui, M. (2017). Optical coherence tomography in Alzheimer's disease and other neurodegenerative diseases. *Frontiers in Neurology, 8*, 701. https://doi.org/10.3389/fneur.2017.00701.
153. Song, A., Johnson, N., Ayala, A., & Thompson, A. C. (2021). Optical coherence tomography in patients with Alzheimer's disease: What can it tell us? *Eye and Brain, 13*, 1–20. https://doi.org/10.2147/EB.S235238.
154. Ossenkoppele, R., Smith, R., Mattsson-Carlgren, N., Groot, C., Leuzy, A., Strandberg, O., Palmqvist, S., Olsson, T., Jögi, J., Stormrud, E., & Cho, H. (2021). Accuracy of tau positron emission tomography as a prognostic marker in preclinical and prodromal Alzheimer disease: A head-to-head comparison against amyloid positron emission tomography and magnetic resonance imaging. *JAMA Neurology, 78*(8), 961–971. https://doi.org/10.1001/jamaneurol.2021.1858.
155. Benussi, A., Di Lorenzo, F., Dell'Era, V., Cosseddu, M., Alberici, A., Caratozzolo, S., Cotelli, M. S., Micheli, A., Rozzini, L., Depari, A., & Flammini, A. (2017). Transcranial magnetic stimulation distinguishes Alzheimer disease from frontotemporal dementia. *Neurology, 89*(7), 665–672. https://doi.org/10.1212/WNL.0000000000004232.
156. Benussi, A., Dell'Era, V., Cantoni, V., Ferrari, C., Caratozzolo, S., Rozzini, L., Alberici, A., Padovani, A., & Borroni, B. (2018). Discrimination of atypical parkinsonism's with transcranial magnetic stimulation. *Brain Stimulation, 11*(2), 366–373. https://doi.org/10.1016/j.brs.2017.11.013.
157. Cassani, R., Falk, T. H., Fraga, F. J., Cecchi, M., Moore, D. K., & Anghinah, R. (2017). Towards automated electroencephalography-based Alzheimer's disease diagnosis using portable low-density devices. *Biomedical Signal Processing and Control, 33*, 261–271. https://doi.org/10.1016/j.bspc.2016.12.009.

CHAPTER 2

Tangled Connection of Gut Microbiome and Alzheimer's Disease

ROHINI PUJARI,[1] SATISH SHILPI,[2] KAMAL DUA,[3,4] SHREYA SHARMA,[1] and SHVETANK BHATT[1*]

[1]*School of Health Sciences and Technology, Dr. Vishwanath Karad MIT World Peace University, Pune, Maharashtra India*

[2]*Faculty of Pharmacy, DIT University, Dehradun, Uttarakhand, India*

[3]*Discipline of Pharmacy, Graduate School of Health, University of Technology Sydney, NSW, Australia*

[4]*Faculty of Health, Australian Research Center in Complementary and Integrative Medicine, University of Technology Sydney, Ultimo, NSW, Australia*

*Corresponding author.

ABSTRACT

Several preclinical and clinical investigations have proved that the human gut microbiome plays a crucial role in the pathobiology of central nervous system (CNS) disorders. Recent studies suggest correlations between the altered gut microbiota and major Alzheimer's Disease (AD). AD is characterized by the formation of Aβ plaques and neurofibrillary tangles. It is proposed that normalization of the gut microbiota alleviates AD. The imbalance in levels of normal gut microbiota has a crucial role in the pathogenesis of AD. Treatment strategies with certain antibiotics lead to the depletion of useful microbes and thereby induce AD-like effects in subjects. The microbiota is also involved in the synthesis of various neurotransmitters (NTs) like acetylcholine (ACh), 5-hydroxytryptamine (5-HT; serotonin), norepinephrine (NE), and dopamine (DA). Probiotics, prebiotics, synbiotics, and a healthy

Neuro-Nutraceuticals and Drug Discovery and Delivery in Alzheimer's Disease, Volume 1: Targeting Key Pathological Pathways. Varinder Singh, Amit Kumar, Parul Sood (Eds.)

diet have been found to have positive benefits in controlling the etiology of AD. The control of brain-gut microbiota is developing as a potential AD therapy approach in light of the history of the limited therapeutic advantages of cholinesterase inhibitors. The importance of the brain-gut-microbiota axis in the development of AD is discussed in detail in this review, with an emphasis on the regulation of the gut microbiota as an important intervention for the treatment of AD.

2.1 INTRODUCTION

Alzheimer's disease (AD) is an untreatable, progressive neurological ailment that causes memory loss, odd behavior, personality changes, and a deterioration in mental capacity. With almost 70% of all dementia in people over 60, AD is the most prevalent kind of dementia among the elderly [1, 2]. Around 40 million people worldwide are already affected by AD, and by 2050 that number will have risen to over 100 million. Age increases the prevalence of AD, according to estimates from studies [3]. The World Alzheimer Report (2015) and other investigations have predicted that the direct cost of dementia care worldwide (including ADRDs and other dementias) will reach $2 trillion by 2030 and reach $9.12 trillion (including lost earnings of carers) by 2050 [4, 5]. N-methyl D-aspartate receptor antagonists (memantine) and acetylcholinesterase inhibitors (donepezil, galantamine, rivastigmine) are two major categories of drugs used in the treatment of AD. These medications can help with symptoms, but they don't change the course of the disease [6, 7].

Numerous elements of human health, including the immune system, metabolism, and neurobehavioral characteristics, depend on gut bacteria [8]. The human microbiome is made up of these microbes and their genomes, and it has been suggested that it is an "essential organ" of the human body and that it is a crucial modulator of human health [9]. The gut microbiota-brain axis is real, according to scientific investigations that have revealed a direct correlation between the brain and the intestinal microbiota. Normal brain and emotional functioning depend on a healthy gut with a variety of microorganisms. Additionally, the majority of GI physiology is managed by the CNS [10, 11].

In order to maintain gut homeostasis and appropriate digestion, there is a complicated, two-way molecular connection between the gut microbiome and CNS. The quantities of related neurotransmitters, their precursors, or both in the brain can be influenced by the neuroactive metabolites that the gut bacteria also produce [12]. It has lately become clear that these bacteria, notably those in the gut, have a significant impact on numerous physiological factors, including cognitive processes like memory, learning, and decision-making [11, 12].

2.2 PATHOPHYSIOLOGY OF ALZHEIMER'S DISEASE

According to scientific theory, the neurodegeneration brought on by Alzheimer's disease is an age-dependent condition that inevitably results in dendritic and neuronal damage, as well as deterioration of the synaptic afferent system and the development of aberrant protein aggregates throughout the brain [13]. The regions of the brain crucially involved in learning memory and other mental functions are frequently affected. Diffuse neuronal loss, deposits of extracellular amyloid (Aβ) (senile plaques) encircled by dystrophic neurites, and intracellular neurofibrillary tangles (NFT) made up of hyperphosphorylated tau protein are the three main structural changes in the brain associated with AD [14, 15].

There may be neuronal loss or illness in the hippocampal formation, entorhinal cortex, amygdala, frontal, parietal, and temporal cortices, subcortical nuclei like the cholinergic basal nucleus, noradrenergic locus coeruleus, and serotonergic dorsal raphe. Tangles first start to build up in the trans-entorhinal cortex, followed by the entorhinal cortex, the CA1 hippocampal region, and eventually, the cortical association areas, which are most severely affected in the frontal, parietal, and temporal lobes [15, 16].

The degree and location of tangle growth correlate to a greater extent with the severity of dementia than the number of amyloid plaques. The shrinkage of the hippocampal neuronal network, cognitive decline, and brain atrophy are all negatively linked with tau protein accumulation. The temporofrontal cortex exhibits shrinkage and neuronal loss in the neuropathology of Alzheimer's disease, resulting in inflammation and the development of amyloid plaques, an abnormal accumulation of tangled bundles of fibers and protein fragments. Monocytes and macrophages are more prevalent in the cortical region as a result of activated parenchymal microglial cells [17, 18].

2.2.1 AMYLOID B AND HYPERPHOSPHORYLATED TAU PROTEIN HYPOTHESIS

One of the major pathogenic characteristics of AD is the emergence of senile plaques (SP), which are brought on by the accumulation of amyloid beta (Aβ). The enzymes α-secretase, β-secretase, and γ-secretase convert the precursor protein of amyloid (APP) into soluble little peptides termed A. Protofibrils, fibrils, and plaques are three distinct types of dangerous oligomers that develop from an imbalance between β-amyloid (Aβ) formation and clearance, depending on the degree of oligomerization [19, 20]. Although the precise reason for Aβ's production is still a mystery, its sequence, concentration, and stabilizing conditions all have a big impact. There are a variety of factors hypothesized to be involved in the etiology of Alzheimer's disease including Aβ amyloid/tau toxicity, oxidative stress, cholinergic dysfunction, and mitochondrial dysfunctions [21].

2.2.2 OXIDATIVE STRESS HYPOTHESIS

Humans produce reactive nitrogen species (RNS) and reactive oxygen species (ROS) in both normal and disordered conditions. These two species play complementary roles in cellular signaling pathways and engage in hazardous actions that can harm cellular structures [22]. The brain is highly susceptible to oxidative stress because of its high oxygen consumption. The neuron, which is the basic structural and functional unit of the brain, is mostly composed of polyunsaturated fatty acids. One of the causes of oxidative stress is lower levels of glutathione in neurons which facilitates ROS to cause molecular apoptosis and lipid peroxidation [23, 24].

2.2.3 METAL ION HYPOTHESIS

Dyshomeostasis of metal ions has a role in the development and pathophysiology of several ailments including neurodegenerative disorders. A number of these compounds are employed in clinical studies. Several agents involved in the modulation of transition metal homeostasis include the metal and ionosphere chelators [25]. Other medications besides metal-binding ones can also target the homeostasis of transition metals. According to current findings, the homeostasis of redox transition metals, such as iron (Fe), copper (Cu), and other trace metals, has been altered frequently due to several etiological factors. In AD, their brain levels are observed to be elevated. Other neurological diseases also involve Cu, manganese, aluminum, and zinc [26, 27].

2.2.4 CHOLINERGIC THEORY

The mainstay of AD treatment is AchEI medicine, and the major risk factor for the development of AD is the APOE genotype. Given that cholinergic neurons are not the primary target of AD, the lack of a significant effect of APOE is examined in relation to the cholinergic hypothesis of AD. Reduced cholinergic receptor binding in certain brain regions is related to neuropsychiatric symptoms in mild to severe AD [28]. In elderly, healthy individuals, slower processing speed may be caused by lower receptor binding. A significant reduction in cholinergic neurons made in the medial forebrain nuclei, together with a concomitant decline in neurotransmission mediated by acetylcholine, is linked to clinical decline [29].

2.3 ENDOCRINE DYSFUNCTION

As one of the main physiological regulators of brain growth, hormones play a crucial role. Any disturbance of the endocrine system may contribute to the onset or progression of AD. The Hypothalamic-pituitary-adrenal (HPA) axis is involved in the regulation of the release of glucocorticoids from the adrenal cortex, adrenocorticotrophic hormone (ACTH) from the anterior pituitary, and corticotropin-releasing factor (CRF) from the hypothalamus. It is considered to be gradually dysregulated in AD [30].

Additionally, the HPA system is a prominent endocrinal target in several neurological conditions, most notably AD. The adrenal cortex releases glucocorticoids when the HPA axis triggers the stress response. These hormones attach to the glucocorticoid (GR) and mineralocorticoid receptors after passing through the blood-brain barrier. Through modest hypercortisolemia and dysregulated GR in AD, the involved HPA axis leads to cognitive impairment and hence plays a crucial role in the etiology and pathophysiology of the disease.

The sensitivity of cerebral neurons is increased by the ongoing high levels of glucocorticoids, which further supports the pathology of AD. The hypothalamic-pituitary-gonadal (HPG) axis, releasing activins, gonadotropin-releasing hormone (GnRH), and luteinizing hormone (LH), is another regulator of neuronal function. The expression of these receptors, which are present in a variety of cell types throughout the limbic system, is controlled by negative feedback loops [31, 32].

The structure and wide variety of functions of the brain are regulated by these hormones and their receptors. Through a variety of signaling pathways, the HPG axis dysregulation associated with andropause, and menopause induces changes to the structure and activities of neuronal cells [33]. Other characteristics of the endocrine abnormalities seen in AD pathology include insulin dysregulation and insulin resistance, which may hasten the disease development. Aβ metabolism is mechanistically relevant to insulin resistance because elevated Aβ levels induce the removal of cell surface insulin receptors which further exaggerates AD progression. High Aβ levels promote the loss of cell surface insulin receptors, which further accelerates the course of AD and thus, Aβ metabolism is mechanistically linked to insulin resistance. With age, insulin-like growth factor-1 (IGF-1)/growth hormone levels significantly decline which further contributes to the pathogenesis of AD [34, 35].

2.4 GUT MICROBIOTA IN THE DEVELOPMENT OF THE BRAIN

According to several studies, the mother implants the fetal microbiome before delivery, and it is subsequently strengthened by the maternal microbiome when the baby is born and breastfed. It is generally acknowledged that the early-life programming of brain circuits and host physiology that regulate motor activity, stress response, cognitive functions, and anxiety-like behavior are affected by gut bacteria [36]. In the first few years of life, the brain's structure and function undergo significant and quick changes. Huge dendritic and axon growth, the development of synapses (synaptogenesis), an expansion of glial cells, and myelination are examples of how this presents itself. Additionally, during this time, there is a rapid synthesis of synaptic connections, which, depending on the cortical region, culminate between 3 and 24 months later [37]. The end of the second year is often when myelination is formed. Even so, this furthers its colonization. The developing fetus receives vital nutrients from the mother's circulation throughout the prenatal stage, while at the same time, metabolic waste products from the gut microbiota penetrate the placental barrier and affect fetal brain development. Numerous studies on animals treated with broad-spectrum antibiotics showed the ill effects of certain microbiota on CNS neurochemistry and physiology [38].

2.4.1 THE MICROBIOTA GUT BRAIN AXIS

A channel for communication between the central and enteric neural systems is the gut-brain axis (GBA), which connects the emotional and cognitive regions of the brain to the peripheral activities of the intestine. Recent scientific developments have emphasized how crucial it is for the gut flora to affect these interactions [39].

Different channels of communication between the brain and the gut bacteria have been proposed such as:

- Via the vagus nerve's incoming and outgoing branches, which constitute the main modulatory pathway.

- As a result of the microbiota's modification of transmitters (serotonin and acetylcholine) and the production of bioactive peptides (such as short-chain fatty acids) and metabolites.
- The HPA's release of cortisol in stress response, can impair intestinal motility, integrity, and mucus production and alter the makeup of the gut microbiota. The modulation of stress hormones by this modification could thus have an impact on the CNS.
- Using chemokines and cytokines that promote inflammation.
- Immunity also plays a crucial role. Toll-like receptors (TLRs) and peptidoglycans (PGNs) specifically serve as sensors of microbial components to mediate the immune response to microorganisms [40, 41].

This association between GBA and microbiota is documented to be bidirectional because of signals from the gut microbiota to the brain and vice versa through endocrine, neurological, humoral, and immunological links. Therefore, a local immune activation may result in an immunological activation in other organs, including the brain, via several pathways. The biology of various forms of depression and neurodegenerative diseases such as Parkinson's and Alzheimer's disease has been linked to this low-grade immunological activation (PD). It is not unexpected, given this complex interplay, that the gut-brain axis and consequently, the gut microbiota, which acts as the major constituent of this crosstalk, have an indirect or direct effect on neuropsychiatric disorders [42, 43].

2.5 FACTORS CAUSING DYSBIOSIS OF GUT MICROBIOTA

2.5.1 BACTERIAL AMYLOIDS

An important source of amyloids is the gut microbiome. Bacterial amyloids have a tertiary structure that is comparable to that of CNS amyloids. The exposure of the gut to bacterial amyloid proteins may prime the immune system, improving the immune reaction to the endogenous neuronal amyloid generation by the brain [44].

Friedland and Chapman have even come up with a brand-new name, "mapranosis," to characterize the neuroinflammation and proteopathy caused by the microbiota. Bacterial amyloids may mimic prion proteins through molecular mimicry, triggering a process known as cross-seeding, wherein one amyloidogenic protein such as tau, curli, prion, and A causes other structurally different host proteins to take on a pathogenic beta-sheet form. Several *in vivo* and *in vitro* studies regarding the cross-seeding of amyloidogenic proteins by bacterial amyloids have been documented [45].

2.5.2 LIPOPOLYSACCHARIDES

Several *in vivo* and *in vitro* studies have proven that bacterial LPS encourages the formation of amyloid fibrils. Bacterial LPS has recently been found in brain lysates from AD patients' hippocampus and neocortex. Additionally, LPS colocalizes with Aβ1–40/42 in blood arteries and amyloid plaques (Figure 2.1) [46]. Furthermore, compared to healthy individuals, AD patients have plasma concentrations of LPS that are substantially greater. Moreover, more *E. coli* nucleic acids or pili proteins were discovered in human brains commonly in AD patients. The innate immune system's microglial cells, which express TLRs, especially TLR4 and TLR2, and recognize common damage or pathogen-related molecular patterns, are activated by LPS which initiates the inflammatory response leading to neurodegeneration [47, 48].

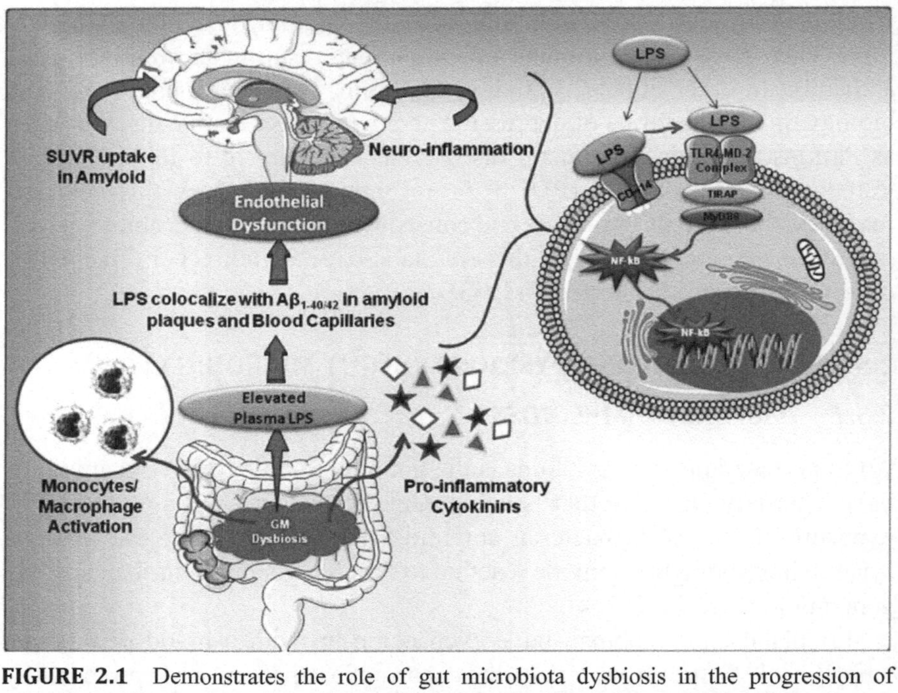

FIGURE 2.1 Demonstrates the role of gut microbiota dysbiosis in the progression of Alzheimer's disease through the involvement of LPS and proinflammatory cytokines.

2.5.3 ANTIBIOTICS

Without specifically targeting any particular bacteria, antibiotics are often used to get rid of or stop bacterial colonization in the human body. Therefore, broad-spectrum antibiotics can significantly alter the gut microbiota's makeup, diminish its variety, and postpone colonization for a considerable amount of time following administration. Numerous research studies have revealed that different antibiotic therapies alter the gut microbiota in both humans and animals in the short- and/or long term. Additionally, it has been shown in both animal and human research that the consumption of antibiotics and the ensuing dysbiosis is linked to alterations in behavior and neurochemistry [49]. Antibiotic use in humans has been shown to be linked to neurological problems such as anxiety and panic attacks, significant depression, psychosis, and delirium when given as a cocktail therapy. A number of antibiotics cause high glucocorticoid levels, which are then linked to memory issues and a decrease in hippocampus BDNF, two typical signs of AD pathology. Antibiotic-induced gut dysbiosis reduces the production of transmembrane proteins including occludin and claudin-5 and microbial metabolites (SCFAs), which makes the blood-brain barrier more permeable to neuroinflammatory mediators [50].

2.6 ROLE OF DYSBIOSIS OF GUT MICROBIOTA IN THE DEVELOPMENT OF AD

2.6.1 EFFECT DYSBIOSIS OF GUT MICROBIOTA ON BRAIN NEUROTRANSMITTERS

Microbiota stimulates neurotransmitters and their precursors. The metabolites that bacteria create have the ability to send out signals that influence the production and transmission of neurotransmitters. Local transmission of these signals can take place in the gut through vagus nerve transmission to the brain. Neurotransmitters including glutamate, gamma-aminobutyric acid (GABA), dopamine, and serotonin do not pass through the blood-brain barrier; instead, they are produced locally in the central nervous system by precursors that frequently come from the gastrointestinal tract [51]. Several studies have reported that altered gut microbiota affect the neurotransmitter release and alter the CNS neurotransmission leading to several neurological disorders. Gut dysbiosis has been documented to be strongly involved in the neuropathogenesis of AD [52].

2.6.2 EFFECT DYSBIOSIS OF GUT MICROBIOTA ON GUT BARRIER FUNCTION

Polymorphonuclear leukocytes migrate from the blood to the gut mucosa during intestinal inflammation, especially if mucosal architecture is disturbed, to the gut lumen. This little calcium-binding protein, which is an S100A8/A9 heterodimer, makes about 60% of the proteins in neutrophils' cytoplasm and possesses anti-bacterial capabilities. The S100A8 and S100A9 proteins can produce amyloid fibrils and oligomers that mimic amyloid polypeptides like α-syn and Aβ and, *in vitro*, monomeric and dimeric S100A9 may promote Aβ fibrillization due to their intrinsically amyloidogenic amino acid sequences [53].

In addition to inducing its expression in neuronal cells, S100A9 is released by macrophages and microglia after the production of amyloid plaques. These cells may then activate microglia through the receptor for advanced glycation end products (RAGE) and TLR4 mechanistic pathways. Calprotectin levels are markedly elevated in the brain and CSF of AD patients, which encourages calprotectin's amyloid aggregation and co-aggregation with Aβ. The production of amyloid fibrils in the gut or directly in the brain may be influenced by this intestinal supply of calcium-binding proteins. The mucus layer, lamina propria, and intestinal epithelium make up the intestinal barrier which when broken leads to an increase in permeability that allows dangerous substances and germs to enter the bloodstream (a process called atopobiosis) [54, 55]. Increased intestinal permeability (also known as "leaky gut") and gut dysbiosis and inflammation are both closely related to gut barrier dysfunction and may have an impact on the neurodegenerative process. In addition to changes in the makeup of the gut microbiota, the increased quantity of bacteria in the small intestine also affects permeability, as seen in small intestinal bacterial overgrowth (SIBO). Preliminary findings indicate that AD patients have a higher prevalence of SIBO [56].

2.6.3 EFFECT DYSBIOSIS OF GUT MICROBIOTA ON BLOOD-BRAIN-BARRIER PERMEABILITY

Microvascular endothelial cells and tight junction proteins form the static and selective BBB, which controls the integrity, stability, and homeostasis of the barrier. While permitting the nutritive vital fibers to carry out fundamental physiological activities of the brain, this barrier prevents the paracellular passage of hazardous constituents from the blood to the central nervous system [57]. Any significant alterations to the complex gut microflora's environment have a negative impact on the BBB's permeability. Altering the expression of tight junction proteins compromises the BBB's integrity and makes it possible for dangerous chemicals from the periphery to enter, which can cause neurological disturbances like AD [58].

2.6.4 DYSBIOSIS OF GUT MICROBIOTA AND NEUROINFLAMMATION

One typical early pathogenic change in AD is the emergence of neuroinflammation, a chronic inflammatory response in the brain. Recently, it has been proven that the gut microbiota plays a significant part in the homeostasis and dysfunction of the CNS. Aging, long-term antibiotic use, an unrestricted calorie diet, and lifestyle modifications that lead to gut contamination all have an impact on the community of gut bacteria. Additionally, an increase in amyloid plaques in the brain may also lead to systemic and gastrointestinal inflammation [59]. An increasing body of research indicates that alterations in the gut milieu and gut microbiota predominantly mediate immune functions and low-grade inflammation (inflammaging). Along with the known link between altered gut microbiota and gastrointestinal illnesses, intestinal and blood-brain-barrier (BBB) permeabilities may also rise [60]. A framework for the pathogenesis of AD is set by these altered permeabilities that may promote the accumulation of metabolites and molecules from the gut microbiota in the brain, like lipopolysaccharides and SCFA. Additional pathological changes brought on by the microbiota might depend on the elevation of concentrations of metabolites in the blood as well as cellular or humoral peripheral immune effectors. The pathogenesis of AD and the detrimental effects associated with it are thought to be strongly impacted by such inflammatory modulation. In keeping with this, microbiota influences the induction of regulatory T-cells (Treg) and the functionality of microglia, which physiologically correlate to macrophages residing in the brain. This overall interaction between the central neuroinflammatory response and the peripheral immune system may contribute to the neuropathogenesis of AD (Figure 2.2) [61].

2.6.5 DYSBIOSIS OF GUT MICROBIOTA AND NEURODEGENERATION

Increasing evidence points to the importance of gut microorganisms in the process of neurogenesis. A healthy gut is essential for the growth of behavioral and brain processes because the microbiota symbionts living in the gut support the host in a way that benefits both parties [62]. Using several models of gut microbiota modulation, scientists have recently increased their efforts in understanding the characteristics and complexity of these symbionts in the neurodegeneration associated with AD. The production of neurodegenerative markers such as inflammatory cytokines, Aβ, NFT, and other molecules involved in neurodegeneration and AD pathogenesis is sensitive to changes in gut microbial diversity in a healthy gut [63].

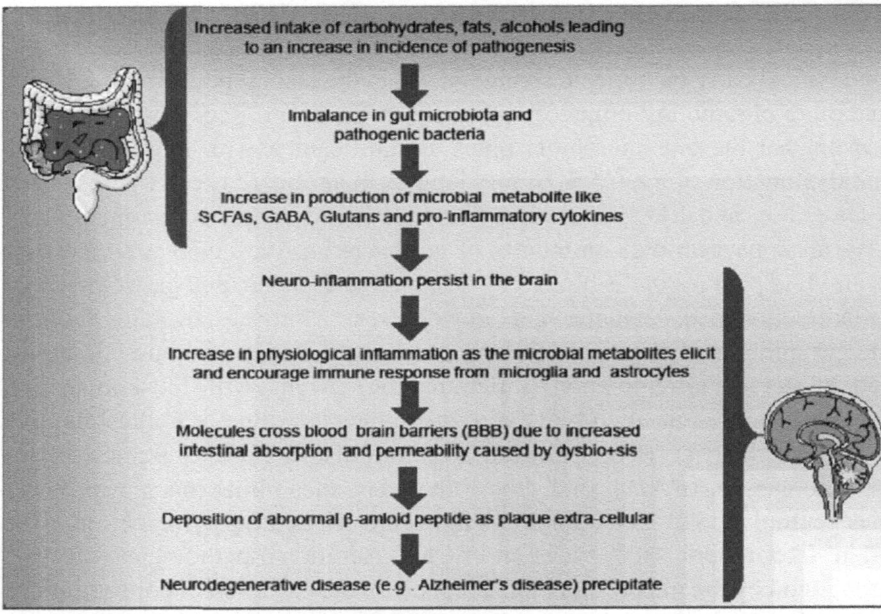

FIGURE 2.2 Role of gut microbiota in Alzheimer's disease.

2.7 TARGETING MICROBIOTA RESTORATION FOR TREATMENT OF ALZHEIMER'S DISEASE

2.7.1 PREBIOTICS

Prebiotics are organic, non-digestible compounds (short-chain carbohydrates) that can specifically promote the development and/or effect of good bacteria in the gut. They serve as food products for the gut flora, which in turn stimulates the creation of short-chain fatty acids (SCFAs), affecting both gastrointestinal and extraintestinal functionality. They can also enhance serotonin levels, which can help with behavior and neurological function. They may be effective as adjuvant therapy for a variety of neurological and psychiatric diseases, including AD, according to mounting data [64]. An obvious treatment target for enhancing gut barrier function, reducing inflammation, and enhancing cognitive and behavioral results is encouraging the proliferation and activity of advantageous, SCFA-producing microorganisms like bifidobacteria. Numerous prebiotic kinds, particularly fructans, have been discovered to be efficient in adjusting the composition of the gut microbiota and the generation of metabolites of gut bacteria, as well as altering health outcomes that are pertinent for people with AD. The ability of these molecules to maintain the diversity and stability of the gut microbiota may be the reason for these advantages, even if the exact mechanistic approach of these molecules is not completely clear [65].

2.7.2 PROBIOTICS

When ingested in sufficient amounts, probiotics are living bacteria that offer health benefits. The two genera of probiotic bacteria that are most frequently utilized are *Lactobacillus* and *Bifidobacterium*. According to studies using human and animal models, by assisting in the maintenance of the epithelial barrier, generating SCFAs, inhibiting the release of pro-inflammatory cytokines, promoting survival of cells, and increasing the protective immune response, probiotics can modify the homeostasis of the intestinal environment and regulate the physiology of intestinal epithelia [66]. Since they are not composed of any lipopolysaccharides, their consumption does not result in any inflammatory reactions. They serve as antibiotics, maintain the integrity of the intestinal lining, control the body's pH level, and boost the brain-derived neurotrophic factor (BDNF). Neurotrophic factors aid in the survival and development of neurons in the brain. As a result, they are essential for neurological development. If these components of the brain are absent, problems such as learning deficits and memory impairments frequently result. By altering the makeup of helpful bacteria in the gut microbiota and enhancing CNS processes, probiotics have favorable impacts on the central nervous system (CNS) [67]. Probiotics, in addition to brain neurotrophic factors, have an excellent prognosis for treating memory loss and mental problems by directly altering brain biochemical substances like serotonin, dopamine, and γ-aminobutyric acid (GABA). Probiotics have been shown to slow the progression of AD, notably the inflammatory response and oxidative stress, and to improve cognitive decline. Probiotics work by restoring the balance of the gut flora. Numerous studies have also demonstrated that certain probiotics possess the capability to decrease mucosal inflammation and modify local immune reactions by altering the cytokine network and macrophage tissue architecture [68].

Many of these reactions are brought on by probiotics controlling particular intracellular signaling pathways in intestinal epithelial cells, like nuclear factor (NF)-κB and mitogen-activated protein kinases (MAPK). Probiotic bacteria have demonstrated their ability to control the immune response by stimulating NK and B cells, Th1, Th2, and Th17 cells, as well as altering the intestinal microbial ecosystem [69].

2.7.3 SYNBIOTICS

Probiotic and prebiotic ingredients are combined to form synbiotics. In a randomized, double-blind, placebo-controlled crossover research, consumption of a synbiotic including *B. longum* as a probiotic and an insulin-based prebiotic in older adults showed considerable benefits. Synbiotic supplementation successfully controlled the pro-inflammatory response [70]. The metabolic activities and composition of colonic bacterial populations and immunological factors in aged adults can be promoted by synbiotic treatments [71]. The synbiotics boost AChE activity, motility, and viability, and prevent Aβ deposition. The synbiotics combined activity on the gut-brain axis signaling pathways, like metabolic stability, immunological signaling, oxidative and mitochondrial stress, and perhaps over networks linking PPARγ, was responsible for these effects [72]. A recent study identified a novel synbiotic with beneficial effects in a transgenic APP/PS1 mice model of AD. This synbiotic contained *L. plantarum, L. fermentum,* and *Bifidobacterium longum* subspecies *infantis* along with a polyphenol plant extract from the GI tonic *Triphala* (TFLA; *Terminalia chebula, Terminalia bellirica*, and *Emblica officinalis*) [73]. Through the use of an *in vitro* GI tract model, probiotics including *L. plantarum, B. infantis*, and *L. salivarius* were combined with the 3-(3′-hydroxyphenyl) propionic acid from grape seed polyphenolic extract (GSPE) and polyphenolic metabolites 3-hydroxybenzoic acid. The synbiotic may cross the blood-brain barrier and stop the accumulation of Aβ, tauopathy, and neuroinflammation [73]. Patients with AD chosen using appropriate sampling were investigated in a recent uncontrolled clinical study. The proposed synbiotic contained *Candida famata, C. krusei, Acetobacter sp., Acetobacter aceti, Enterococcus faecium, L. fermentum, L. delbrueckii, L. fructivorans, Leuconostoc* sp., and *L. kefiranofaciens* in the form of fermented milk grains. Kefir reduced systemic inflammation, oxidative stress, mitochondrial dysfunction, DNA damage, and apoptosis, which in turn reduced cognitive impairments. As a result, kefir could be an acceptable adjuvant treatment for the development of AD [75].

2.7.4 DIETARY REGULATORS OF MICROBIOTA

The gut microbiota has various roles to play in the host body. They are able to do so by interacting with substrates, such as food, that they encounter in the gastrointestinal tract. They derive their nutrition directly from the water and the nutrients. To fulfill their energy requirements, they metabolize the remnants of carbs and proteins after the host's digestion. Thus, the food we eat is largely responsible for the maintenance and diversity of the gut microbiota [76]. Further, the host's peristalsis, digestive enzymes, and excretion all affect the microbiome diversity and density in the gut. The eating rhythms and specific dietary patterns can control the availability of by-products of microbiota metabolism, which are used in the normal physiological functioning of the body. The gut microbiome, due to its symbiotic relationship with the host, directs the host's circadian rhythm (or diurnal rhythm) by acting as both the trigger and the responding element. The food we consume can be divided into a few major components: carbohydrates, proteins, fats, and polyphenols (Figure 2.3 and Table 2.1) [77].

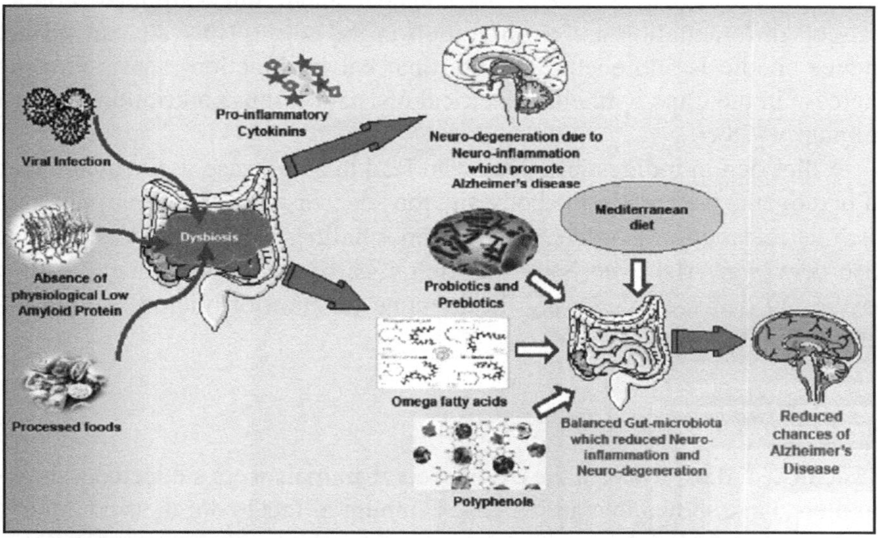

FIGURE 2.3 Dietary interventions for restoration of gut microbiota in treatment of AD.

TABLE 2.1 Dietary Factors Responsible for Gut Dysbiosis and Balanced Gut Microbiota

Dietary Factors Promoting Gut Dysbiosis in Alzheimer's Disease	Dietary Factors Promoting a Balanced Gut Microbiota in Alzheimer's Disease
Protein imbalance (hyperproteinemia)	Optimum intake of polyphenols
Increased blood glucose levels	Prebiotics
Increased intake of indigestible carbohydrates	Antibiotics
Bacterial dysbiosis in the gut	Antimicrobial peptides (physiological amyloid protein)
Consumption of processed/ultra-processed food	Increased intake of dietary fibers
High saturated fatty acid intake	High intake of omega-3 fatty acids
High alcohol intake	Synbiotics (onion, garlic, radish, etc.)

2.7.5 DIETARY COMPONENT: CARBOHYDRATES

The carbohydrates that are present in our food can be further divided into digestible and indigestible carbohydrates. The digestible carbs get broken down into simple sugars which get directly absorbed into the bloodstream. It's the indigestible carbs, better known as dietary fibers (or microbiota-accessible fibers), that are acted upon by the non-pathogenic bacteria in the gut. These MAFs include pectin, cellulose, resistant starches, oligosaccharides that evade digestion, and undigested alcohols and sugars. The gut bacteria ferment these dietary fibers to short-chain fatty acids (SCFAs). The three major fatty acids – acetate, propionate, and butyrate – stimulate epithelial cell differentiation and proliferation in the colon. Butyrate can further induce apoptosis and encourage intestinal barrier function measured as an increase in the trans-epithelial electrical resistance, thus contributing to host immunity [78].

A diet rich in indigestible fibers can lead to a decrease in the abundance of pathogenic bacteria in the body and thus decrease the chances of diseases such as metabolic disorders, enteric abnormalities, and neurodegenerative disorders (e.g., Alzheimer's). A diet rich in carbs, on the other hand, causes severe gut damage by altering the immune function of microbiota and the antioxidant capacity [79].

2.7.5.1 DIETARY COMPONENT: FATS

Basically, studies, wherein the experimental animals were subjected to high-fat diets, have shown that an increased amount of fats in our diets could lead to an increased abundance of pathogenic bacteria, contrary to the desirable gut microbiota. This could then lead to opportunistic obesity disorders and pathogenic low-grade chronic inflammation by virtue of the release of lipopolysaccharides by the pathogens, which elicit an immune response. A diet consisting of high saturated fatty acids leads to an increased abundance of bacterial species (e.g., *Campylobacter*) which are associated with the development of obesity and pro-inflammatory diseases [80]. Healthy fats like omega-3 polyunsaturated fatty acids can encourage the growth of butyrate-producing bacteria (*Bifidobacterium* and *Lactobacillus* species) and produce anti-inflammatory effects, followed by subsequent SCFA productions. Thus, the maintenance of good gut bacteria depends on the diet of the host individual, but gut homeostasis is its regulator, ensuring that despite a diet based on high-fat consumption, the gut microbiota thrives well [81].

2.7.5.2 DIETARY COMPONENT: POLYPHENOLS

Polyphenol sources in the diet comprise fruits, vegetables, wine, cereals, tea, and coffee. These can be of two types – flavonoids and non-flavonoids. The low molecular weight polyphenols are easily absorbed in the small intestine. It is the oligomeric and polymeric polyphenols (e.g., tannins) that are acted upon by the gut microbiota present in the colon. The effects of polyphenols are subjective; the effects produced depend on the polyphenol [82]. Mostly, polyphenols alter the composition of gut microbiota by favoring the growth of one species over another. Some polyphenols, like those present in red wine and tea, strongly inhibit the VacA toxin, which is the major virulence factor of *Helicobacter pylori*. They are anti-inflammatory in nature and promote a reduction in carcinogenic potential by increasing apoptosis and reducing cell proliferation. Regular intake of red wine polyphenols helps keep hypertension and cholesterol levels in check [82, 83].

2.7.5.3 DIETARY COMPONENT: ALCOHOLS

The current lifestyle of most human beings has them consuming alcohol occasionally at least, if not regularly. Like all other dietary components, alcohols too, have an effect on the gut microbiota. A high alcohol level can lead to the demise or decrease of non-pathogenic gut bacteria while promoting the growth of their pathogenic rivals, producing a condition known as dysbiosis (imbalance of gut microbial species). They increase intestinal permeability and exacerbate inflammation. Moderate amounts of alcohol can act as a substrate for energy production, which aids in microbial proliferation and the production of microbial metabolites like SCFAs [86].

2.7.5.4 DIETARY COMPONENT: SPECIAL DIETS

The host diet influences the gut bacteria and hence it's important to study which diet works in favor of the microbiota. A diet similar to the Western diet with high-fat content and low fiber content leads to a decrease in the bloom of bacteria associated with gut well-being. The Western diet basically includes ultra-processed food and drinks available on-the-go in most countries. These food items are lacking in essential dietary fibers. This has led to a high incidence of diet-induced obesity (DIO). It led to an increase in the diversity and abundance of bacteria (e.g., *Firmicutes, Proteobacteria, Actinobacteria*) which precipitated patterns that can be taken as an early forecast of inflammatory diseases. As the dietary fibers are absent and the molecules required for energy generation by the bacteria are readily available, this leads to a bloom in the growth of gut bacteria. This can be interpreted as an increased production of virulence factors. This can further harm the host by eliciting neuroinflammation [87].

Many studies have linked antibiotic treatment with increased episodes of epilepsy. A ketogenic diet comprising a very low carb content and a high-fat content has proven to enhance the neurovascular state. The ketogenic diet alters the gut diversity, and it is this altered gut bacteria that provides an anti-epileptic effect by increasing GABA levels relative to glutamate levels in the central nervous system. Increased ketosis and metabolism are also observed [88].

The Mediterranean diet (MD) consists of cereals, legumes, vegetables, and extra-virgin olive oil followed by animal resources – fish, eggs, poultry, and dairy products. It is light on refined sugar and red meat. Herbs and spices flow freely with the inclusion of red wine too. Individuals following this diet are subject to a reduction in cardiovascular and total mortality and risk of neurodegenerative disorders including Alzheimer's disease. The dietary components, like extra-virgin olive oil, promote anti-inflammatory activity. Potatoes, included in MD, are a good source of dietary fiber [89].

2.7.5.5 FECAL MICROBIOTA TRANSPLANTATION (FMT)

FMT is a treatment strategy wherein a solution of fecal matter from a donor is transported into the recipient's intestinal tract (through colonoscopy, nasogastric tube, or oral tablets), with the goal of directly altering the composition of the gut microbiota. Researchers have verified that treatments aiming at modifying gut bacteria have an impact on mental diseases. In fact, fecal microbiota transplants from healthy wild-type mice to animal models of AD showed a reduction in amyloid buildup, blood levels of pro-inflammatory biomarkers, and cognitive impairment [74]. Another study supported these findings, finding improvements in cognition, decreased amyloid buildup and tau expression, increased gut endobacteria, and greater synaptic plasticity that produces SCFAs. In another study, FMT was shown to be beneficial in improving the microglia and Aβ deposition profiles and restoring the composition of the gut microbiome in the APP/PS1 transgenic mice model of AD. Only two case studies involving people have so far produced encouraging findings; in these studies, FMT therapy was found to increase cognitive function, microbial diversity, and SCFA production [84].

2.8 CONCLUSION

The gut microbiota has been recognized as a major disease state regulator, and its dysregulation is linked to the etiology of several gastrointestinal and extraintestinal illnesses. GMBA impairment has been documented as the basic etiological factor of AD, a neurodegenerative condition that frequently affects the aged. More recently, changes in the gut microbiome have been connected to neurodegeneration in Alzheimer's disease via the gut microbiota-brain axis. This relationship generally results from neuroinflammation brought on by bacterial brain migration or bacterium products, paving the door for novel microbiota-based therapy approaches. Given the strong relationship between gut bacteria and the brain, we highlighted the role of gut microbiota dysregulations in Alzheimer's disease and how this dysbiosis may be exploited as a novel therapeutic strategy with the possibility of prebiotics, probiotics, synbiotics, fecal microbiota transplantation, and diets as supplementary therapeutic interventions on disease development and progression, thereby bringing new insights into the treatment of this tragic and degenerative illness. Despite encouraging results, further research is needed to reduce interstudy discrepancies and improve repeatability before contemplating therapeutic use.

KEYWORDS

- **acetylcholine**
- **Alzheimer's disease**
- **degenerative illness**
- **microbiome**
- **neurofibrillary tangles**
- **oxidative stress**
- **synbiotics**
- **therapeutic use**

REFERENCES

1. Knopman, D. S., Amieva, H., Petersen, R. C., Chételat, G., Holtzman, D. M., Hyman, B. T., Nixon, R. A., & Jones, D. T. (2021). Alzheimer disease. Nature Reviews Disease Primers, 7(1), 33.
2. Breijyeh, Z., & Karaman, R. (2020). A comprehensive review on Alzheimer's disease: Causes and treatment. Molecules, 25(24), 5926. https://doi.org/10.3390/molecules25245926.
3. Mayeux, R., & Stern, Y. (2012). Epidemiology of Alzheimer's disease. Cold Spring Harbor Perspectives in Medicine, 2(8), a006239. https://doi.org/10.1101/cshperspect.a006239.
4. Nandi, A., Counts, N., Chen, S., Seligman, B., Tortorice, D., Vigo, D., & Bloom, D. E. (2022). Global and regional projections of the economic burden of Alzheimer's disease and related dementias from 2019 to 2050: A value of statistical life approach. eClinicalMedicine, 51, 101580. https://doi.org/10.1016/j.eclinm.2022.101580.
5. Wimo, A., Guerchet, M., Ali, G. C., Wu, Y. T., Prina, A. M., Winblad, B., Jönsson, L., Liu, Z., & Prince, M. (2017). The worldwide costs of dementia 2015 and comparisons with 2010. Alzheimer's & Dementia, 13(1), 1–7. https://doi.org/10.1016/j.jalz.2016.10.006.
6. Kerwin, D., Abdelnour, C., Caramelli, P., Ogunniyi, A., Shi, J., Zetterberg, H., & Traber, M. (2022). Alzheimer's disease diagnosis and management: Perspectives from around the world. Alzheimer's & Dementia: Translational Research & Clinical Interventions, 14(1), e12334. https://doi.org/10.1002/trc2.12334.
7. Hampel, H., Au, R., Mattke, S., van der Flier, W. M., Aisen, P., Apostolova, L., Chen, C., Cho, M., De Santi, S., Gao, P., Iwata, A., Kurzman, R., Saykin, A. J., Teipel, S., Vellas, B., Vergallo, A., Wang, H., & Cummings, J. (2022). Designing the next-generation clinical care pathway for Alzheimer's disease. Nature Aging, 2(8), 692–703. https://doi.org/10.1038/s43587-022-00264-6.
8. Fan, Y., & Pedersen, O. (2021). Gut microbiota in human metabolic health and disease. Nature Reviews Microbiology, 19(1), 55–71. https://doi.org/10.1038/s41579-020-0433-9.
9. de Vos, W. M., Tilg, H., Van Hul, M., & Cani, P. D. (2022). Gut microbiome and health: Mechanistic insights. Gut, 71(5), 1020–1032. https://doi.org/10.1136/gutjnl-2021-324283.
10. Galland, L. (2014). The gut microbiome and the brain. Journal of Medicinal Food, 17(12), 1261–1272. https://doi.org/10.1089/jmf.2014.7000.
11. Liu, L., Huh, J. R., & Shah, K. (2022). Microbiota and the gut-brain-axis: Implications for new therapeutic design in the CNS. eBioMedicine, 77, 103908. https://doi.org/10.1016/j.ebiom.2022.103908.
12. Zhu, S., Jiang, Y., Xu, K., Cui, M., Ye, W., Zhao, G., Jin, L., & Chen, X. (2020). The progress of gut microbiome research related to brain disorders. Journal of Neuroinflammation, 17(1), 25. https://doi.org/10.1186/s12974-020-1705-z.
13. Tiwari, S., Atluri, V., Kaushik, A., Yndart, A., & Nair, M. (2019). Alzheimer's disease: Pathogenesis, diagnostics, and therapeutics. International Journal of Nanomedicine, 14, 5541–5554. https://doi.org/10.2147/IJN.S200490.
14. Fan, L., Mao, C., Hu, X., Zhang, S., Yang, Z., Hu, Z., Sun, H., Fan, Y., Dong, Y., Yang, J., Shi, C., & Xu, Y. (2020). New insights into the pathogenesis of Alzheimer's disease. Frontiers in Neurology, 10. https://doi.org/10.3389/fneur.2019.01312.

15. dos Santos Picanco, C. L., Ozela, F. P., de Fatima de Brito Brito, M., Pinheiro, A. A., Padilha, C. E., Braga, S. F., de Paula da Silva, H. T. C., dos Santos, B. R. C., Rosa, M. C. J., & da Silva Hage-Melim, I. L. (2018). Alzheimer's disease: A review from the pathophysiology to diagnosis, new perspectives for pharmacological treatment. Current Medicinal Chemistry, 25(26), 3141–3159. https://doi.org/10.2174/0929867325666180228124703.
16. Long, J. M., & Holtzman, D. M. (2019). Alzheimer disease: An update on pathobiology and treatment strategies. Cell, 179(2), 312–339. https://doi.org/10.1016/j.cell.2019.09.001.
17. Alves, L., Correia, A., Miguel, R., Alegria, P., & Bugalho, P. (2012). Alzheimer's disease: A clinical practice-oriented review. Frontiers in Neurology, 3. https://doi.org/10.3389/fneur.2012.00063
18. Kaur, D., Behl, T., Sehgal, A., Singh, S., Sharma, N., & Bungau, S. (2021). Multifaceted Alzheimer's disease: Building a roadmap for advancement of novel therapies. Neurochemical Research, 46(11), 2832–2851. https://doi.org/10.1007/s11064-021-03435-4.
19. Thal, D. R., & Fändrich, M. (2015). Protein aggregation in Alzheimer's disease: Aβ and τ and their potential roles in the pathogenesis of AD. Acta Neuropathologica, 129(2), 163–165. https://doi.org/10.1007/s00401-015-1379-9.
20. Gallardo, G., & Holtzman, D. M. (2019). Amyloid-β and Tau at the crossroads of Alzheimer's disease. Advances in Experimental Medicine and Biology, 1184, 187–203. https://doi.org/10.1007/978-981-32-9358-8_15.
21. Ashrafian, H., Zadeh, E. H., & Khan, R. H. (2021). Review on Alzheimer's disease: Inhibition of amyloid beta and tau tangle formation. International Journal of Biological Macromolecules, 167, 382–394. https://doi.org/10.1016/j.ijbiomac.2020.12.083.
22. Huang, W. J., Zhang, X., & Chen, W. W. (2016). Role of oxidative stress in Alzheimer's disease. Biomedical Reports, 4(5), 519–522. https://doi.org/10.3892/br.2016.630.
23. Cassidy, L., Fernandez, F., Johnson, J. B., Naiker, M., Owoola, A. G., & Broszczak, D. A. (2020). Oxidative stress in Alzheimer's disease: A review on emergent natural polyphenolic therapeutics. Complementary Therapies in Medicine, 49, 102294. https://doi.org/10.1016/j.ctim.2020.102294.
24. Misrani, A., Tabassum, S., & Yang, L. (2021). Mitochondrial dysfunction and oxidative stress in Alzheimer's disease. Frontiers in Aging Neuroscience, 13. https://doi.org/10.3389/fnagi.2021.617588.
25. Greenough, M. A., Camakaris, J., & Bush, A. I. (2013). Metal dyshomeostasis and oxidative stress in Alzheimer's disease. Neurochemistry International, 62(5), 540–555. https://doi.org/10.1016/j.neuint.2012.08.014.
26. Yang, G. J., Liu, H., Ma, D. L., & Leung, C. H. (2019). Rebalancing metal dyshomeostasis for Alzheimer's disease therapy. JBIC Journal of Biological Inorganic Chemistry, 24(8), 1159–1170. https://doi.org/10.1007/s00775-019-01715-5.
27. Wang, L., Yin, Y. L., Liu, X. Z., Shen, P., Zheng, Y. G., Lan, X. R., Lu, C. B., & Wang, J. Z. (2020). Current understanding of metal ions in the pathogenesis of Alzheimer's disease. Translational Neurodegeneration, 9(1), 10. https://doi.org/10.1186/s40035-020-0183-x.
28. Terry, A. V., Jr., & Buccafusco, J. J. (2003). The cholinergic hypothesis of age and Alzheimer's disease-related cognitive deficits: Recent challenges and their implications for novel drug development. Journal of Pharmacology and Experimental Therapeutics, 306(3), 821–827. https://doi.org/10.1124/jpet.102.041920.

29. Hampel, H., Mesulam, M. M., Cuello, A. C., Khachaturian, A. S., Vergallo, A., Farlow, M. R., Snyder, P. J., Giacobini, E., Khachaturian, Z. S., & Cholinergic System Working, G.; for the Alzheimer Precision Medicine, I. (2019). Revisiting the cholinergic hypothesis in Alzheimer's disease: Emerging evidence from translational and clinical research. The Journal of Prevention of Alzheimer's Disease, 6(1), 2–15. https://doi.org/10.14283/jpad.2018.43.
30. Matsunaga, A., & Yoneda, M. (2016). Dementia due to endocrine diseases. Brain and Nerve, 68(4), 399–405. https://doi.org/10.11477/mf.1416200534.
31. Calsolaro, V., Bottari, M., Coppini, G., Lemmi, B., & Monzani, F. (2021). Endocrine dysfunction and cognitive impairment. Minerva Endocrinologica (Torino), 46(3), 335–349. https://doi.org/10.23736/S2724-6507.20.03427-6.
32. Vercruysse, P., Vieau, D., Blum, D., Petersén, Å., & Dupuis, L. (2018). Hypothalamic alterations in neurodegenerative diseases and their relation to abnormal energy metabolism. Frontiers in Molecular Neuroscience, 11, 2. https://doi.org/10.3389/fnmol.2018.00002.
33. Wafik Said, B., Yasser, A. E. H., & Ehab, A. E. S. (2017). Sex hormones and Alzheimer's disease. In Gorazd, D. (Ed.), Sex Hormones in Neurodegenerative Processes and Diseases (Ch. 7). IntechOpen. https://doi.org/10.5772/intechopen.69210.
34. Davidson, M., Bastiaens, L., Davis, B. M., Shah, M. B., & Davis, K. L. (1988). Endocrine changes in Alzheimer's disease. Neurologic Clinics, 6(1), 149–157. https://doi.org/10.1016/S0733-8619(18)30657-5.
35. Pasqualetti, G., Calsolaro, V., & Monzani, F. (2016). Editorial (Thematic issue: Endocrine disorders and cognitive function in the elderly). Recent Patents on Endocrine, Metabolic & Immune Drug Discovery, 10(1), 2–3. https://doi.org/10.2174/1872214810 01160429103143.
36. Dash, S., Syed, Y. A., & Khan, M. R. (2022). Understanding the role of the gut microbiome in brain development and its association with neurodevelopmental psychiatric disorders. Frontiers in Cell and Developmental Biology, 10, 880544. https://doi.org/10.3389/fcell.2022.880544.
37. Maiuolo, J., Gliozzi, M., Musolino, V., Carresi, C., Scarano, F., Nucera, S., Scicchitano, M., Oppedisano, F., Bosco, F., Ruga, S., Zito, M. C., Macri, R., Palma, E., Muscoli, C., & Mollace, V. (2021). The contribution of gut microbiota–Brain axis in the development of brain disorders. Frontiers in Neuroscience, 15, 616883. https://doi.org/10.3389/fnins.2021.657179.
38. Varier, K. M., Karandikar, A., Liu, W., Chen, J., Ben-David, Y., Shen, X., Chinnasamy, A., & Gajendran, B. (2020). Chapter 18 – Gut microbiota and brain development: A review. In S. De Mandal & P. Bhatt (Eds.), Recent Advancements in Microbial Diversity (pp. 423–444). Academic Press. https://doi.org/10.1016/B978-0-12-821265-3.00018-1.
39. Cryan, J. F., O'Riordan, K. J., Cowan, C. S. M., Sandhu, K. V., Bastiaanssen, T. F. S., Boehme, M., Codagnone, M. G., Cussotto, S., Fulling, C., Golubeva, A. V., Guzzetta, K. E., Jaggar, M., Long-Smith, C. M., Lyte, J. M., Martin, J. A., Molinero-Perez, A., Moloney, G., Morelli, E., Morillas, E., & Dinan, T. G. (2019). The microbiota-gut-brain axis. Physiological Reviews, 99(4), 1877–2013. https://doi.org/10.1152/physrev.00018.2018.
40. Rutsch, A., Kantsjö, J. B., & Ronchi, F. (2020). The gut-brain axis: How microbiota and host inflammasome influence brain physiology and pathology. Frontiers in Immunology, 11, 604179. https://doi.org/10.3389/fimmu.2020.604179.

41. Dinan, T. G., & Cryan, J. F. (2017). Gut instincts: Microbiota as a key regulator of brain development, aging, and neurodegeneration. *The Journal of Physiology, 595*(2), 489–503. https://doi.org/10.1113/JP273106.
42. Cenit, M. C., Sanz, Y., & Codoñer-Franch, P. (2017). Influence of gut microbiota on neuropsychiatric disorders. *World Journal of Gastroenterology, 23*(30), 5486–5498. https://doi.org/10.3748/wjg.v23.i30.5486.
43. Blanco, L. P., Evans, M. L., Smith, D. R., Badtke, M. P., & Chapman, M. R. (2012). Diversity, biogenesis and function of microbial amyloids. *Trends in Microbiology, 20*(2), 66–73. https://doi.org/10.1016/j.tim.2011.11.005.
44. Hill, J. M., & Lukiw, W. J. (2015). Microbial-generated amyloids and Alzheimer's disease (AD). *Frontiers in Aging Neuroscience, 7*, 9. https://doi.org/10.3389/fnagi.2015.00009.
45. Bu, X. L., Yao, X. Q., Jiao, S. S., Zeng, F., Liu, Y. H., Xiang, Y., Liang, C. R., Wang, Q. H., Wang, X., Cao, H. Y., Yi, X., Deng, B., Liu, C. H., Xu, J., Zhang, L. L., Gao, C. Y., Xu, Z. Q., Zhang, M., Wang, L., & Wang, Y. J. (2015). A study on the association between infectious burden and Alzheimer's disease. *European Journal of Neurology, 22*(12), 1519–1525. https://doi.org/10.1111/ene.12754.
46. Zhan, X., Stamova, B., & Sharp, F. R. (2018). Lipopolysaccharide associates with amyloid plaques, neurons, and oligodendrocytes in Alzheimer's disease brain: A review. *Frontiers in Aging Neuroscience, 10*, 42. https://doi.org/10.3389/fnagi.2018.00042.
47. Kim, H. S., Kim, S., Shin, S. J., Park, Y. H., Nam, Y., Kim, C. W., Lee, K. W., Kim, S. M., Jung, I. D., Yang, H. D., Park, Y. M., & Moon, M. (2021). Gram-negative bacteria and their lipopolysaccharides in Alzheimer's disease: Pathologic roles and therapeutic implications. *Translational Neurodegeneration, 10*(1), 49. https://doi.org/10.1186/s40035-021-00272-6.
48. Zhao, Y., Jaber, V. R., Pogue, A. I., Sharfman, N. M., Taylor, C., & Lukiw, W. J. (2022). Lipopolysaccharides (LPSs) as potent neurotoxic glycolipids in Alzheimer's disease (AD). *International Journal of Molecular Sciences, 23*(20), 12671. https://doi.org/10.3390/ijms232012671.
49. Angelucci, F., Cechova, K., Amlerova, J., & Hort, J. (2019). Antibiotics, gut microbiota, and Alzheimer's disease. *Journal of Neuroinflammation, 16*(1), 108. https://doi.org/10.1186/s12974-019-1494-4.
50. Kim, M., Park, S. J., Choi, S., Chang, J., Kim, S. M., Jeong, S., Park, Y. J., Lee, G., Son, J. S., Ahn, J. C., & Park, S. M. (2022). Association between antibiotics and dementia risk: A retrospective cohort study. *Frontiers in Pharmacology, 13, 888333*. https://doi.org/10.3389/fphar.2022.888333.
51. Chen, Y., Xu, J., & Chen, Y. (2021). Regulation of neurotransmitters by the gut microbiota and effects on cognition in neurological disorders. *Nutrients, 13*(6), 2099. https://doi.org/10.3390/nu13062099.
52. Huang, F., & Wu, X. (2021). Brain neurotransmitter modulation by gut microbiota in anxiety and depression. *Frontiers in Cell and Developmental Biology, 9, 649103*. https://doi.org/10.3389/fcell.2021.649103
53. Takiishi, T., Fenero, C. I. M., & Câmara, N. O. S. (2017). Intestinal barrier and gut microbiota: Shaping our immune responses throughout life. *Tissue Barriers, 5*(4), e1373208. https://doi.org/10.1080/21688370.2017.1373208.
54. Stolfi, C., Maresca, C., Monteleone, G., & Laudisi, F. (2022). Implication of intestinal barrier dysfunction in gut dysbiosis and diseases. *Biomedicines, 10*(2), 289. https://doi.org/10.3390/biomedicines10020289.

55. Qiao, J., Chen, R., Wang, M., Bai, R., Cui, X., Liu, Y., Wu, C., & Chen, C. (2021). Perturbation of gut microbiota plays an important role in micro/nanoplastics-induced gut barrier dysfunction. *Nanoscale, 13*(19), 8806–8816. https://doi.org/10.1039/D1NR01103K.
56. Régnier, M., Van Hul, M., Knauf, C., & Cani, P. D. (2021). Gut microbiome, endocrine control of gut barrier function and metabolic diseases. *Journal of Endocrinology, 248*(2), R67–R82. https://doi.org/10.1530/JOE-20-0615.
57. Braniste, V., Al-Asmakh, M., Kowal, C., Anuar, F., Abbaspour, A., Tóth, M., Korecka, A., Bakocevic, N., Ng, L. G., Kundu, P., Gulyás, B., Halldin, C., Hultenby, K., Nilsson, H., Hebert, H., Volpe, B. T., Diamond, B., & Pettersson, S. (2014). The gut microbiota influences blood-brain barrier permeability in mice. *Science Translational Medicine, 6*(263), 263ra158. https://doi.org/10.1126/scitranslmed.3009759.
58. Tang, W., Zhu, H., Feng, Y., Guo, R., & Wan, D. (2020). The impact of gut microbiota disorders on the blood-brain barrier. *Infection and Drug Resistance, 13*, 3351–3363. https://doi.org/10.2147/IDR.S274883.
59. Bairamian, D., Sha, S., Rolhion, N., Sokol, H., Dorothée, G., Lemere, C. A., & Krantic, S. (2022). Microbiota in neuroinflammation and synaptic dysfunction: A focus on Alzheimer's disease. *Molecular Neurodegeneration, 17*(1), 19. https://doi.org/10.1186/s13024-022-00508-1.
60. Cerovic, M., Forloni, G., & Balducci, C. (2019). Neuroinflammation and the gut microbiota: Possible alternative therapeutic targets to counteract Alzheimer's disease? *Frontiers in Aging Neuroscience, 11*, 284. https://doi.org/10.3389/fnagi.2019.00284.
61. Yu, X., Zhou, G., Shao, B., Zhou, H., Xu, C., Yan, F., Wang, L., Chen, G., Li, J., & Fu, X. (2021). Gut microbiota dysbiosis induced by intracerebral hemorrhage aggravates neuroinflammation in mice. Frontiers in Microbiology, 12, 647304. https://doi.org/10.3389/fmicb.2021.647304.
62. Zhang, H., Chen, Y., Wang, Z., Xie, G., Liu, M., Yuan, B., Chai, H., Wang, W., & Cheng, P. (2022). Implications of gut microbiota in neurodegenerative diseases. Frontiers in Immunology, 13, 785644. https://doi.org/10.3389/fimmu.2022.785644.
63. Padhi, P., Worth, C., Zenitsky, G., Jin, H., Sambamurti, K., Anantharam, V., Kanthasamy, A., & Kanthasamy, A. G. (2022). Mechanistic insights into gut microbiome dysbiosis-mediated neuroimmune dysregulation and protein misfolding and clearance in the pathogenesis of chronic neurodegenerative disorders. Frontiers in Neuroscience, 16, 836605. https://doi.org/10.3389/fnins.2022.836605.
64. D'Argenio, V., & Sarnataro, D. (2021). Probiotics, prebiotics and their role in Alzheimer's disease. Neural Regeneration Research, 16(9), 1768–1769. https://doi.org/10.4103/1673-5374.306095.
65. Pluta, R., Ułamek-Kozioł, M., Januszewski, S., & Czuczwar, S. J. (2020). Gut microbiota and pro/prebiotics in Alzheimer's disease. Aging (Albany NY), 12(6), 5539–5550. https://doi.org/10.18632/aging.102935.
66. Naomi, R., Embong, H., Othman, F., Ghazi, H. F., Maruthey, N., & Bahari, H. (2021). Probiotics for Alzheimer's disease: A systematic review. Nutrients, 14(1), 20. https://doi.org/10.3390/nu14010020.
67. Xiang, S., Ji, J. L., Li, S., Cao, X. P., Xu, W., Tan, L., & Tan, C. C. (2022). Efficacy and safety of probiotics for the treatment of Alzheimer's disease, mild cognitive impairment, and Parkinson's disease: A systematic review and meta-analysis. Frontiers in Aging Neuroscience, 14, 730036. https://doi.org/10.3389/fnagi.2022.730036.

68. Chyn Boon, W., Yodai, K., & Jin-zhong, X. (2018). Probiotics for preventing cognitive impairment in Alzheimer's disease. In E. Alper & Ü. Barış Önen (Eds.), Gut Microbiota (Ch. 6). IntechOpen. https://doi.org/10.5772/intechopen.77073.
69. Guo, L., Xu, J., Du, Y., Wu, W., Nie, W., Zhang, D., Luo, Y., Lu, H., Lei, M., Xiao, S., & Liu, J. (2021). Effects of gut microbiota and probiotics on Alzheimer's disease. Translational Neuroscience, 12(1), 573–580. https://doi.org/10.1515/tnsci-2021-0007.
70. Macfarlane, S., Cleary, S., Bahrami, B., Reynolds, N., & Macfarlane, G. T. (2013). Synbiotic consumption changes the metabolism and composition of the gut microbiota in older people and modifies inflammatory processes: A randomized, double-blind, placebo-controlled crossover study. Alimentary Pharmacology & Therapeutics, 38(7), 804–816. https://doi.org/10.1111/apt.12436.
71. Talebi, M., Ebrahimi, V., Rasouli, A., Farjami, A., Razi, S., Soleimanian, A., Forouhandeh, H., & Tarhriz, V. (2022). A new insight on feasibility of pre-, pro-, and synbiotics based therapies in Alzheimer's disease. Journal of Reports in Pharmaceutical Sciences, 11(2), 141–155. https://doi.org/10.4103/jrptps.JRPTPS_170_21.
72. Westfall, S., Lomis, N., & Prakash, S. (2019). A novel synbiotic delays Alzheimer's disease onset via combinatorial gut-brain-axis signaling in Drosophila melanogaster. PLoS One, 14(4), e0214985. https://doi.org/10.1371/journal.pone.0214985.
73. Pasinetti, G. (2022). Symbiotic-derived metabolites reduce neuroinflammatory symptoms of Alzheimer's disease. Current Developments in Nutrition, 6(Supplement_1), 804–804. https://doi.org/10.1093/cdn/nzac061.004.
74. Gupta, S., Allen-Vercoe, E., & Petrof, E. O. (2016). Fecal microbiota transplantation: In perspective. Therapeutic Advances in Gastroenterology, 9(2), 229–239. https://doi.org/10.1177/1756283X15607414.
75. Ton, A. M. M., Campagnaro, B. P., Alves, G. A., Aires, R., Côco, L. Z., Arpini, C. M., Guerra, E. O. T., Campos-Toimil, M., Meyrelles, S. S., Pereira, T. M. C., & Vasquez, E. C. (2020). Oxidative stress and dementia in Alzheimer's patients: Effects of symbiotic supplementation. Oxidative Medicine and Cellular Longevity, 2020, 2638703. https://doi.org/10.1155/2020/2638703.
76. Frausto, D. M., Forsyth, C. B., Keshavarzian, A., & Voigt, R. M. (2021). Dietary regulation of gut-brain axis in Alzheimer's disease: Importance of microbiota metabolites. Frontiers in Neuroscience, 15, 736814. https://doi.org/10.3389/fnins.2021.736814.
77. Romanenko, M., Kholin, V., Koliada, A., & Vaiserman, A. (2021). Nutrition, gut microbiota, and Alzheimer's disease. Frontiers in Psychiatry, 12, 712673. https://doi.org/10.3389/fpsyt.2021.712673.
78. Shi, H., Wang, Q., Zheng, M., Hao, S., Lum, J. S., Chen, X., Huang, X. F., Yu, Y., & Zheng, K. (2020). Supplement of microbiota-accessible carbohydrates prevents neuroinflammation and cognitive decline by improving the gut microbiota-brain axis in diet-induced obese mice. Journal of Neuroinflammation, 17(1), 77. https://doi.org/10.1186/s12974-020-01779-8.
79. Kincaid, H. J., Nagpal, R., & Yadav, H. (2021). Diet-microbiota-brain axis in Alzheimer's disease. Annals of Nutrition and Metabolism, 77(suppl 2), 21–27. https://doi.org/10.1159/000510073.
80. Zhang, M., Zhao, D., Zhou, G., & Li, C. (2020). Dietary pattern, gut microbiota, and Alzheimer's disease. Journal of Agricultural and Food Chemistry, 68(46), 12800–12809. https://doi.org/10.1021/acs.jafc.0c06234.

81. Bonfili, L., Cuccioloni, M., Gong, C., Cecarini, V., Spina, M., Zheng, Y., Angeletti, M., & Eleuteri, A. M. (2022). Gut microbiota modulation in Alzheimer's disease: Focus on lipid metabolism. Clinical Nutrition, 41(3), 698–708. https://doi.org/10.1016/j.clnu.2021.09.038.
82. Reddy, V. P., Aryal, P., Robinson, S., Rafiu, R., Obrenovich, M., & Perry, G. (2020). Polyphenols in Alzheimer's disease and in the gut-brain axis. Microorganisms, 8(2), 199. https://doi.org/10.3390/microorganisms8020199.
83. Shabbir, U., Tyagi, A., Elahi, F., Aloo, S. O., & Oh, D. H. (2021). The potential role of polyphenols in oxidative stress and inflammation induced by gut microbiota in Alzheimer's disease. Antioxidants, 10(9), 1370. https://doi.org/10.3390/antiox10091370.
84. Wang, J. W., Kuo, C. H., Kuo, F. C., Wang, Y. K., Hsu, W. H., Yu, F. J., Hu, H. M., Hsu, P. I., Wang, J. Y., & Wu, D. C. (2019). Fecal microbiota transplantation: Review and update. Journal of the Formosan Medical Association, 118, S23–S31. https://doi.org/10.1016/j.jfma.2018.08.011.
85. Frausto, D. M., Engen, P. A., Naqib, A., Jackson, A., Tran, L., Green, S. J., Shaikh, M., Forsyth, C. B., Keshavarzian, A., & Voigt, R. M. (2022). Impact of alcohol-induced intestinal microbiota dysbiosis in a rodent model of Alzheimer's disease. Frontiers in Aging, 3, 916336. https://doi.org/10.3389/fragi.2022.916336.
86. Yussof, A., Yoon, P., Krkljes, C., Schweinberg, S., Cottrell, J., Chu, T., & Chang, S. L. (2020). A meta-analysis of the effect of binge drinking on the oral microbiome and its relation to Alzheimer's disease. Scientific Reports, 10(1), 19872. https://doi.org/10.1038/s41598-020-76762-1.
87. Solch, R. J., Engler-Chiurazzi, E., Harper, C., Wasson, S., Ogbonna, S., Ouvrier, B., McDonald, K., Wang, H., Biose, I. J., Bix, G. J., & Maraganore, D. M. (2022). Effect of diet on cognitive function and gut microbiota. Alzheimer's & Dementia, 18(S11), e061639. https://doi.org/10.1002/alz.061639.
88. Nagpal, R., Neth, B. J., Wang, S., Craft, S., & Yadav, H. (2019). Modified Mediterranean-ketogenic diet modulates gut microbiome and short-chain fatty acids in association with Alzheimer's disease markers in subjects with mild cognitive impairment. EBioMedicine, 47, 529–542. https://doi.org/10.1016/j.ebiom.2019.08.032.
89. Solch, R. J., Aigbogun, J. O., Voyiadjis, A. G., Talkington, G. M., Darensbourg, R. M., O'Connell, S., Pickett, K. M., Perez, S. R., & Maraganore, D. M. (2022). Mediterranean diet adherence, gut microbiota, and Alzheimer's or Parkinson's disease risk: A systematic review. Journal of the Neurological Sciences, 434, 120166. https://doi.org/10.1016/j.jns.2022.120166.

CHAPTER 3

Epigenetic Modifications in Alzheimer's Disease

RAHUL KUMAR,[1] PRACHI PARVATIKAR,[2] INDRANI MAJI,[3]
SHASHI BALA SINGH,[1] and PANKAJ KUMAR SINGH[3*]

[1]*Department of Biological Science, National Institute of Pharmaceutical Education and Research (NIPER), Hyderabad, Telangana, India*

[2]*Department of Biotechnology, Allied Health Sciences BLDE (DU), Vijayapura, Karnataka, India*

[3]*Department of Pharmaceutics, National Institute of Pharmaceutical Education and Research (NIPER), Hyderabad, Telangana, India*

*Corresponding author.

ABSTRACT

Alzheimer's disease (AD) is the most common neurodegenerative disorder, characterized by the progressive loss of neurons with aging, synaptic alterations, and memory loss. Genomic, epigenomic changes, and environmental factors in the brain interact with external and internal toxins, directing the pathophysiology of AD. Epigenetic modification refers to changes in phenotype due to alterations in DNA sequence and includes histone modification, DNA methylation, and modification of noncoding RNA (ncRNA). The epigenetic changes observed in AD involve DNA hypermethylation, histone deacetylation, and dysregulation of ncRNA, leading to chromatin repression. These markers regulate the expression of genes such as APP, SERT1, and GSK3β at the transcriptional level, either up-regulating or down-regulating them and silencing the target gene. Up-regulation of these genes, APP, SERT1, and GSK3β, is implicated in the pathogenesis of AD. Furthermore, these epigenetic markers influence the expression of genes that play a role

Neuro-Nutraceuticals and Drug Discovery and Delivery in Alzheimer's Disease, Volume 1: Targeting Key Pathological Pathways. Varinder Singh, Amit Kumar, Parul Sood (Eds.)

in the pathophysiology of Alzheimer's disease. Evidence from various studies using human, rodent, and *in-vitro* models suggests that epigenetic modifications significantly impact cognitive impairment by down-regulating the expression of CREB, BDNF, and synaptic genes. However, the direct contribution of the epigenetic mechanism to cognitive dysfunction and neuronal loss remains unclear. Studies over the past decades have highlighted the potential role of epigenetic markers in the pathophysiology of AD, suggesting that these markers could be used as therapeutic targets for managing AD. In this chapter, we have discussed the role of epigenetic markers and their mechanisms altered in AD, which could potentially serve as therapeutic targets.

3.1 INTRODUCTION

Alzheimer's disease (AD) is the most common progressive neurodegenerative disorder with the progression of age and is characterized by the loss of neurons. The critical hallmark for AD includes extracellular accumulation of senile plaques made by amyloid beta (Aβ) peptides and intracellular deposition of neurofibrillary tangles made by hyper-phosphorylated twisted filaments of the microtubule-associated protein tau in neurons of different brain regions [1]. As the disease progresses, these pathogenic changes directly or indirectly trigger other pathways, including inflammation mediated by microglia, oxidative stress, mitochondrial dysfunction, excitotoxicity caused by calcium, and vascular damage [2]. These processes cause neuronal damage, synaptic malfunction, and dysfunctions in neurotransmission, which in turn cause affected individuals to develop clinical dementia [3]. However, AD is a multifarious disease resulting from many prominent risk factors such as aging, genetic, epigenetic, environmental, and vascular factors [4]. AD is clinically characterized by memory impairment and cognitive dysfunction that eventually affect several other functions, including sleep, behavior, and speech alteration, resulting in neuropsychological manifestations [5]. The pathogenesis of AD is the result of the mutation of three genes: PSEN1 (presenilin-1), PSEN2 (presenilin-2), and APP (amyloid precursor protein). These genes encode proteins that are involved in the maturation and aggregation of Aβ, which further cause familial early-onset forms of AD that affect people under the age of 65 years [6]. Additionally, the enzymatic components of the γ-secretase complex are presenilin-1, two proteins made of a catalytic presenilin, and three components, whereas β-secretase is an aspartic acid protease that is encoded by the BACE1 gene [7]. Furthermore, the expression of APP, PSEN1, PSEN2, and BACE1 genes is regulated by epigenetic modifications [8]. Epigenetic modification is a post-transcriptional mechanism that positively or negatively regulates gene expression at the mRNA level through chromatin remodeling. Chromatin remodeling results from histone modification, DNA methylation, and non-coding RNA [9, 10]. The results from several studies based on epigenetic modification and neurodegenerative disease revealed that DNA methylation and histone deacetylase (HDAC) globally increase in different regions of the human brain suffering from AD compared to the normal brain [11, 12]. Additionally, non-coding RNA also regulates the expression of genes concerned with memory, synaptic plasticity, neuroinflammation, and neurodegeneration [10, 13]. An increasing number of studies have confirmed these epigenetic changes in AD. Although it is unclear whether these epigenetic changes are the cause or effect of AD, they offer medical researchers around the world a new path for a cure [14, 15].

This chapter describes the different epigenetic alterations associated with AD, such as DNA methylation, histone modification, and miRNA. We conclude that Epigenetics has enormous potential as a novel therapeutic avenue. Additionally, we aim to discuss the epigenetic mechanisms in AD and their role in the pathogenesis of AD. Furthermore, we discuss the potential epigenetic markers that may be further used as therapeutic targets for managing AD. Moreover, these epigenetic markers will lead to a better understanding of the disease etiopathogenesis.

3.2 ALZHEIMER'S DISEASE (AD)

Globally, 47 million individuals already have dementia; by 2050, that number is expected to more than triple (to 131 million). One of the leading causes of increasing dementia is Alzheimer's disease (AD) [14]. The Alzheimer's Association attributes 60–80% of dementia cases to Alzheimer's disease (AD), a degenerative brain illness. Depending on the disease's stage, symptoms include apathy, depression, decreased communication, confusion, poor judgment, difficulties swallowing and walking, and behavioral changes that might make it challenging to complete daily tasks (Alzheimer's Disease Facts and Figures, 2022). Alzheimer's disease (AD) is a chronic neurological disorder affecting different brain regions. People suffering from AD impair one's ability to function independently and cognitively. The progressive loss of neurons characterizes AD, especially in the brain's hippocampus, temporal lobe, frontal lobes, and frontal cortex regions [16]. These brain regions gradually affected by the disease experience neuronal loss. Neurodegeneration in different brain regions imposes AD clinical indices, including memory impairment and cognitive alteration [17, 18]. Several factors concern the pathophysiology of AD, including genetic factors, environmental factors, head injury, age, gender, and others like diabetes and obesity [16]. The pathology of AD is characterized by the deposition of extracellular amyloid beta (Aβ) plaques and neurofibrillary tangles (NFT) of tau that result from the hyperphosphorylation of tau protein within neurons [19]. Prior to the onset of clinical symptoms and cognitive impairment by several years, the hippocampus and entorhinal cortex show the earliest pathological changes. Currently, several studies based on the drug targets for mimicking the pathophysiology of AD have ended in failure. In comparison, the FDA approves some drugs that indirectly act on AD with very low efficacy and higher side effects. Thus, the creation of a new AD treatment strategy is urgently needed.

3.3 EPIGENETIC MODIFICATION

Epigenetic modification alters heritable and non-heritable changes in phenotype without changes in primary DNA sequences. Thus, employing a common genetic code for all cells, epigenetic modification enables the different cellular phenotypes and functions the organism requires [20, 21]. Usually, to achieve these effects, transcriptional access to different genes is inhibited, which results in their suppression or silencing. Epigenetic modification is a study of how environment and behaviors cause changes in the pattern of gene expression. 'Epi' means on or above in Greek and Epigenetics is defined as modification beyond the genetic code.

In contrast to genetic changes, epigenetic changes are reversible without changes in the primary DNA sequence. Additionally, genetic changes are typically independent of environmental stimuli, while epigenetic changes involve the response produced by environmental influences [22, 23]. Furthermore, genetic modification alters which protein is synthesized, while epigenetic modifications regulate the expression of genes to turn off or on [24]. Therefore, epigenetic modification also regulates the production of proteins in cells by controlling the turning on or off of genes [25]. These modifications ensure tissue-specific gene/protein expression. For example, muscle cells do not synthesize the proteins that promote bone growth. Three main epigenetic mechanisms control the interaction between genes and environmental variables, including DNA methylation, histone modification, and non-coding RNA molecules-mediated regulation of gene expression [26]. The patterns of epigenetic markers vary among individuals, in different tissues of the same individual, and different cells of a tissue. Epigenetic markers are stable from cell to cell and can be inherited through generations. These epigenetic markers are critical in the regulation of gene expression and in maintaining genomic homeostasis [17].

3.4 EPIGENETIC MECHANISM INVOLVES IN AD PATHOGENESIS

Epigenetic modification regulates the expression of genes in different ways, such as DNA methylation, histone modification (histone methylation, acetylation, and phosphorylation), and miRNA modifications [17]. Abnormal epigenetic alteration is associated with various complex diseases, including AD. The epigenetic mechanism that becomes altered in AD is characterized by DNA hypermethylation, histone deacetylation, and transcriptional repression of chromatin, resulting in altered gene expression at the mRNA level through transcriptional activation or repression [22]. Therefore, these differentially expressed epigenetic markers reveal vast potential as a therapeutic target for AD treatment. Here, we first describe how these two epigenetic alterations generally work before discussing how they relate to neurology in general and Alzheimer's disease.

3.4.1 DNA METHYLATION

DNA methylation is a common and most studied epigenetic modification and is becoming a very interesting subject for researchers because it can make more accessible the unknown aspects of the pathophysiology of a complex disease like AD [27]. DNA methylation is reported at the cytosine nucleotide that precedes a guanine nucleotide (CpG) of the genome. It plays an imperative role in maintaining cell functions, genetic imprinting, and gene expression [28]. The site of the genome composed of the CpG cluster is determined as a CpG island. If the CpG island present at the gene's promoter undergoes methylation, that results in the transcriptional inactivation of the gene [29]. DNA methylation is catalyzed by DNA methyltransferases (DNMTs), further classified as DNMT1, DNMT3b, and DNMT3b. DNMTs have a similar structure with a large N-terminal as a regulatory site, while the C-terminal works as a catalytic site [30]. DNMT1 is associated with the maintenance of DNA methylation, while DNMT3a and 3b are associated with de novo methylation [31]. DNMT catalyzes the transfer of a methyl group (–CH_3) on the C5 position from 5-methylcytosine. DNA methylation regulates gene expression by providing the binding site for proteins involved in the transcriptional repression of a gene or by restricting the binding of transcription factors to DNA [32]. Although brain tissue is comprised of a higher level of DNA methylation than other body tissues.

Interestingly, there is evidence of DNA methylation at the non-CpG nucleotide in mouse and human embryonic stem cells, but this methylation is temporary and lost in mature tissues [33]. Methylation of CpG islands results in the transcriptional inactivation of gene expression. Another epigenetic modification of cytosine facilitated by oxidation, defined as hydroxy methylcytosine (5-hmC), is generally distributed in the CNS and associated with several neurodegenerative disorders and neuronal development abnormalities [34].

3.4.2 ROLE OF DNA METHYLATION IN AD

AD disease is an age-dependent and most common neurodegenerative disorder. AD's complex pathophysiology symptoms result from the interaction between genetic and epigenetic factors, modified by epigenetic pathways [35]. DNA methylation is a significant epigenetic marker change in several complex diseases, including AD. Specific changes in brain DNA methylation patterns are hallmarks of Alzheimer's disease (AD). Although it is well established that age and sex, two key risk factors for AD, have a significant impact on the epigenetic profiles in the brain, little is known about how these factors contribute to DNA changes associated with AD [27]. Studies based on epigenetic modification have reported the relationship between DNA methylation and AD, which engages with the progression of AD pathophysiology. A recent study reported that the accumulation of Aβ reduces the expression of 5-hydroxymethylcytosine, which results in hypomethylation and concerns with the progression of AD pathophysiology [36].

Differential changes in DNA methylation may play a key role in the cognitive function of AD. A study on aged mice exhibited a lower level of DNA methyltransferase DNMT3a2 mRNA expression, which may cause a lower degree of DNA methylation in these animals [4]. In aged mice, cognitive performance like fear conditioning and object-place identification tasks was improved by DNMT3a2 ectopic expression in their brains via viral delivery. In contrast, younger mice's performance in the same tasks was additionally lowered when their DNMT3a2 levels were lowered with shRNA [37]. According to studies that targeted the genome, SNPs in DNMT3A are linked to moderate memory impairment [38], and immunohistochemical analysis of aged mice reveals a decrease in the density of DNMT3-positive cells in the hippocampus [39]. Another study reported that DNMT1 does not display any association with Alzheimer's disease, while DNMT3B expression is associated with AD. Additionally, reduction in the level of DNMT1 and 5mC in the temporal cortex and decreases in 5mC and 5hmC have been reported in the hippocampus of AD patients [41]. In contrast, some studies reported an elevated level of 5mC and 5mC in the temporal cortex, frontal cortex, and hippocampus of AD [42, 43]. Moreover, the level of 5mC decreases at the promoter region of APP, PSEN1, and SIRT1 genes, resulting in the upregulation of these genes in brain and blood samples of AD patients [44, 45]. Increases in the expression of these genes, especially APP, are a risk factor associated with AD pathophysiology. Along with these genes, differential methylation is also found at the promoter region of the following genes: microtubule-associated protein tau, GSK3B, and beta-secretase 1 precursor, or apolipoprotein E (Figure 3.1) [46].

In conclusion, it is becoming clear that patterns of global DNA methylation alter consistently with age and that those with Alzheimer's experience

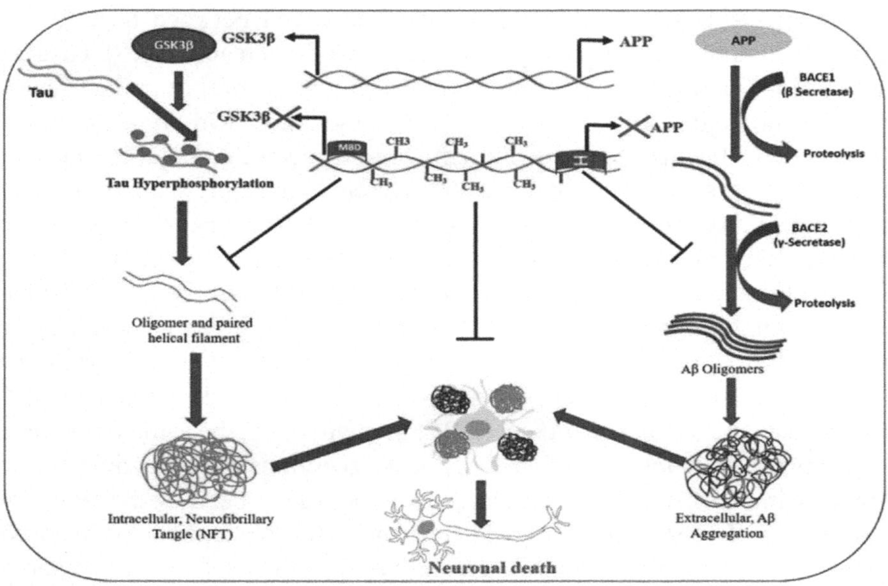

FIGURE 3.1 Depicts the involvement of GSK3β and APP gene expression in the aggregation of extracellular Aβ and intracellular neurofibrillary tangles deposition in the brain. The expression of GSK3β and APP genes is regulated by epigenetic modification, i.e., DNA methylation. This aggregation of proteins activates the microglial cells that further release cytokines and neuronal death.

these changes earlier. Although there is significantly less proof currently available that DNA methylation alterations cause the neuronal loss found in AD, it is logical to assume some effect on neuronal cell survival given that change in DNA methylation leads to significant changes in gene expression. However, there is strong evidence that DNA methylation and demethylation have a significant role in memory. There is experimental proof that changing the methylation-modifying enzymes can affect learning and memory.

3.4.3 HISTONE ACETYLATION/DEACETYLATION

Epigenetic modifications are a key regulator of gene expression and determine the cellular properties of the cells. Histone acetylation is a principal epigenetic marker that influences gene expression by providing the binding site for transcription factors in chromatin. Histone acetylation homeostasis in cells is maintained by two distinct enzymes, histone acetyltransferases (HATs) and histone deacetylases (HDACs) [47]. Histone acetylation catalyzes the addition of an acetyl group on the ε-amino group of lysine using acetyl CoA as a cofactor at the core histone tail, which neutralizes the charge of histone and decreases the interaction between histone and DNA. In contrast, HDAC catalyzes the reverse of this reaction [48]. Histone acetylation is associated with transcriptional activation of the targeted genes, while histone deacetylases (HDAC) are associated with transcriptional repression of the targeted gene by removing the acetyl group at the histone tail that favors heterochromatin [49]. Deregulations of histone acetylation and HDAC are frequently associated with several neurodegenerative diseases, such as AD and PD [50]. Histone acetylation involved in learning is proven by incorporating 4C-acetate which becomes an insert in histone after learning to histones of different brain regions [51]. The mechanism for memory formation proves that the knockdown of HAT in mice demonstrates memory impairment [52, 53]. An earlier study first reported the role of cAMP response element-binding protein (CBP) in memory. At the same time, mice that express a mutant form of CBP that lacks acetyltransferase activity show memory impairment. However, that phenotype was rescued by the administration of an HDAC inhibitor [54]. More than 30 HATs have been reported in humans and classified into two groups based on their subcellular location. Type-A HATs are localized in the nucleus and associated with the transcription regulation of genes in the nucleus [55]. Type-A HATs are further classified into five families based on their sequence homology and mechanism of acetylation: 1. GNAT family composed of P300/CBP-associated factor

(PCAF), Gnc5, and ELP3 [56], 2. MYST family included Tip60, MOZ, MORF, HBO1, and HMOF [57], 3. CBP/p300 family comprised CBP and p300 [58], 4. HAT family comprised of TAF1 and TIFIIIC90 [59, 60], 5. Steroid receptor co-activator steroid receptor co-activators (SRC)/nuclear receptor co-activators (NCoA) family included p600, SRC1, CLOCK, and AIB1/ACTR/SCR3 [59, 61]. While Type-B HATs are localized in the cytoplasm, associated with the acetylation of newly synthesized histone in the cytoplasm. Type-B, composed of HAT1, involves repairing damaged DNA and accumulating histones [62]. A list of various Histone acetyltransferases Enzymes and their role in Alzheimer's is summarized in Table 3.1.

TABLE 3.1 List of Histone Acetyl Transferases Enzymes

Type of HATs	Location in Cells	Families	HATs	References
Type A HATs	Nucleus	1. GNAT Family (involved in cellular growth).	p300/CBP-associated factor (PCAF), Gnc5 and Elp3.	[56]
		2. MYST Family (involved in transcriptional regulation, cell growth, and survival.	Tip60, MOZ, MORF, HBO1, and HMOF.	[57]
		3. CBP/p300 family.	CBP and p300 form.	[58]
		4. HAT family.	TAf1 and TIFIIIC90	[60]
		5. Steroid receptor co-activator (SRC)/ nucleus receptor co-activator (NCoA).	P600, SRC1, CLOCK, and AIB1/ACTR/SCR3.	[59]
Type B HATs	Cytoplasm	HAT1	Involvement in damaged DNA repairing and accumulation of histone proteins.	[64]

Histone acetylation in cells results from HAT/HDAC homeostasis and increases in the level of HDAC result in the interruption of HAT/HDAC homeostasis that leads to disruption of cellular integrity and progression of several diseases, including AD. Mammalian HDACs are classified into four groups: Class I HDACs composed of HDACs 1, 2, 3, and 8 exclusively located in the nucleus [65]. Class II HDAC is further classified into two sub-classes: Class IIa, composed of HDACs 4, 5, 7, and 9, and Class IIb, composed of HDACs 6, 10 [66], located in both the nucleus and cytoplasm. Class III HDACs are classified as the sirtuins (Sirt) family and consist of

Sirt 1–7 located in the nucleus, cytoplasm, as well as mitochondria, and Class IV composed of HDAC 11, located predominantly in the cytoplasm. HDACs Class I, II, and IV are zinc (Zn) dependent enzymes, while HDAC Class III are nicotinamide adenine dinucleotide (NAD+) dependent enzymes [32]. A list of various Histone deacetyl transferase enzymes and their role in Alzheimer's is summarized in Table 3.2.

TABLE 3.2 List of Histone Deacetyl Transferases Enzymes

Type of HDACs	Families	Location in Cells	Respective Functions	References
Class I HDACs	HDAC1	Nucleus	Regulate neuronal survival/death and is also a negative regulator of fear memory and mood disorder.	[67]
	HDAC2		Upregulated in AD and negative regulator of neuronal survival and memory.	[68, 69]
	HDAC3		Cause neuronal death by interacting with HDAC1 and cause neurotoxicity by mutant huntingtin (htt) in Huntington's disease.	[70]
	HDAC8		Negative regulator of declarative and non-declarative memory.	[66]
Class Ia HDACs	HDAC4	Both in nucleus and cytoplasm	It is a risk factor for autism spectrum disorders, and neuronal survival and is involved in synaptic alterations, memory impairment, and depression.	[71]
	HDAC5		Increases in a mouse model of AD and courses fear memory impairment.	[72]
	HDAC7		Neuroprotective against apoptosis.	[73]
	HDAC9		Expressed exclusively in post-mitotic and mature neurons.	[74]
Class Ib HDACs	HDAC6	Predominately in nucleus	Down-regulate BDNF expression and increase Tau expression.	[75]
	HDAC10	Both in nucleus and cytoplasm	Not much is reported for the brain functions.	[76]
Class III HDACs	Sirt1	–	Sirt1 increases in the brain of AD patients and increases Aβ accumulation by increasing the activity of α-secretase.	[77]
			Upregulation of BDNF, CREB, and downregulation of mi134.	
			Involvement in memory formation and acts as neuroprotective.	

TABLE 3.2 *(Continued)*

Type of HDACs	Families	Location in Cells	Respective Functions	References
	Sirt2	Both in nucleus and cytoplasm	Inhibition of microglial activation as well as neuroinflammation. Negative regulator of neuronal cholesterol.	[78]
	Sirt3	Mitochondria	Increases in response to ROS synthesis in AD and neuroprotective.	[79]
	Sirt4		Involvement in glial cell development.	[80]
	Sirt5		Increases in brain and spinal cord of ALS patient.	[80]
	Sirt6		Decreases in cerebral ischemia, involve in HMGB1 mediated neuroinflammation after cerebral ischemia.	[81, 82]
	Sirt7	Predominately in nucleus	Still not reported	–
Class IV HDAC	HDAC11	Predominately in cytoplasm	Regulates the expression of brain-specific N-acetylglucosaminyltransferases-IX.	[83, 84]

3.4.3.1 ROLE OF HISTONE ACETYLATION IN AD

Progressive loss of neurons and memory impairment are the key symptoms of AD. Epigenetic modification, particularly histone acetylation, is the most studied histone modification that regulates synaptic plasticity, learning, and memory. It also regulates the process of neuroprotection and neurodegeneration [85]. The expression of CREB-Binding Protein (CBP), P300/CBP-associated protein (PCAF), Histone Deacetylase 1 (HDAC1), and HDAC2 significantly decreases in the F2 region while CBP and HDAC1 decrease in the hippocampus of AD patients [86]. Additionally, total histone (H3 and H2B) acetylation increases in the frontal cortex, whereas H3 decreases in cell nuclei of the frontal cortex of AD patients. These findings suggest abnormalities in the acetylation of histones and associated enzymes in AD brains, which may cause transcriptional dysregulation and AD-related cognitive deficits [87]. Another study reported that HDAC2 is commonly expressed in the brain and negatively regulates memory and synaptic transmission. The overexpression of HDAC2 in mice hippocampus accompanied by hypo-acetylation of histone H4 on lysine 12 and 5 (H4K12, H4K5) but not H3K14, along with a reduction in the synaptic density and synaptic plasticity, which are involved in memory impairment. HDAC2 negatively regulates synaptic plasticity by binding HDAC2 at the promoter region of genes related to synaptic plasticity and negatively regulates their transcription. HDAC2 expression increases in the postmortem brain samples of AD patients while the knockdown of HDAC2 restores memory and synaptic plasticity [88, 89].

Additionally, HDAC6 protein increases in the hippocampus and cortices of AD postmortem brain samples, and reduction in HDAC6 expression restores memory deficit and α-tubulin acetylation in a mouse model of AD [90, 91]. One crucial step contributing to neurofibrillary tangles in AD, tau metabolism, is the cytoplasmic deacetylase HDAC6 [92]. In contrast, HDAC6 expression positively correlates with tau phosphorylation, and a reduction in HDAC6 activity or expression significantly inhibits tau aggregation and speeds up tau clearance by acetylating tau on KXGS motifs [88].

3.4.3.2 HISTONE METHYLATION

Histone methylation involves the addition of methyl groups ($-CH_3$) at the N-terminal of lysine or arginine by the action of histone methyltransferases (HMTs) [93]. Lysine can undergo mono-methylation, di-methylation, and tri-methylation, while arginine can undergo either mono- or di-methylation, resulting in the regulation of gene expression, especially those involved in the maintenance of brain function and memory formation [94]. Arginine methyltransferases (PRMT1) associated with monomethylate and asymmetrically dimethylate arginine residues catalyze methylation at the arginine position, resulting in transcriptional activation of gene expression [95]. At the same time, PRMT2 suppresses gene expression through mono-methylation and symmetric dimethylation of arginine residues [96]. Lysine methyltransferases (KMTs) catalyze lysine amino acids' methylation in other proteins and histone proteins. They are distinguished from histone methyltransferases (HMT) by their broad enzymatic activity and finely tuned substrate selectivity [94]. The KMTs that catalyze the addition of methyl groups on H3K9, H3K27, and H4K20 are associated with transcriptional repression. In contrast, KMTs that catalyze the addition of methyl groups on H3K4, H3K14, and H3K36 are associated with the transcriptional activation of targeted genes [97]. The most researched form of histone methylation is H3K4 methylation, which is associated with the activation of gene transcription (or up-regulation of gene expression). Furthermore, H3K4Me3 is linked to the up-regulation of genes such as BDNF and ZIF268 involving memory and other brain functions. ZIF268 is crucial for maintaining long-term potentiation (LTP) in the hippocampus, while knockout of this gene during object recognition memory (ORM) reintegration causes active recognition memory traces to be deleted. The levels of H3K4me2 and H3K4me3, which control the differential expression of several genes, including Egr1, c-Fos, and GluR1, in the hippocampus, can be considerably reduced by the deletion of H3K4 methyltransferases KMT2B [98, 99].

3.4.3.3 ROLE OF HISTONE METHYLATION IN AD

Histone methylation is another epigenetic marker that controls the expression of genes involved in pathogenesis and AD pathophysiology. Numerous experimental findings have demonstrated that histone methylation primarily affects the transcription and translation of genes and proteins associated with learning and memory, which in turn interferes with AD [100]. While a decrease in histone methylation or hypermethylation, consequently associated with alteration in several gene expressions, has been reported in aging and dementia brains [101]. However, the role of different histone methylation, even in AD, needs to be better reported. In light of several experimental studies, it has been reported that histone methylation interferes with AD pathophysiology by modulating the transcription and translation of genes and proteins, which involve the regulation of cognitive functions like learning and memory, synaptic plasticity, and neuronal growth [101]. Methylation plays a significant function in neurodegenerative disorders not only as a PTM of Tau but also in terms of its role in metabolic and epigenetic control. Various epigenetic alterations in neural cells, such as neurons, microglia, and astrocytes, are linked to Alzheimer's disease. Enhancer of zest homolog 2 (EZH2) collaborates with polycomb repressive complex, i.e., catalytic subunit, to silence transcription in microglia. The tri-methylation of H3K27 (H3K27me3) is a function of this complex [102]. The epigenetic makeup of microglia frequently changes, and they exhibit phenotypic alterations in response to stimulation. In their primed and unprimed stages, microglia previously exposed to lipopolysaccharides (LPS) and a toll-like receptor 4 (TLR4) ligand undergo significant alterations in their epigenetic makeup [102, 103].

On the other hand, it is reported that histone (H3) tri-methylation at arginine 9 (H3K9Me3) is downregulated in an immunosuppressed state. Another study based on postmortem brain tissue from an AD patient and AD mouse model reported that the H3K4me3 marker and its catalyzing enzyme significantly increase in the prefrontal cortex (PFA) [104]. Inhibition of H3K4Me3 with the WDR5-0103 compound improves synaptic transmission and memory behavior in AD [99].

Furthermore, a clinical study reported histone methylation of H2BK108 and H4K54 in the frontal cortex of the human AD brain, signifying that histone methylation is a potential therapeutic target for treating AD-induced memory impairment [105]. A study based on AD patient postmortem brain showed increases in the level of H3K9Me2 protein in the occipital cortex. At the same time, prevention of G9a/GLP activity through BIX 01294 prevents Aβ-induced synaptic tagging and capture (STC) and long-term potentiation (LTP) in hippocampal deficit by transcriptional repression of BDNF gene [106, 107]. In the same way, an additional study reported increases in H3K9Me2, Emt1 (G9a), and Emt2 (GLP) in the prefrontal cortex and hippocampus in human AD patients and late-stage FAD mice. Global increases in H3K9Me2 in FAD mice negatively regulate the expression of glutamate receptor (Gria2/GluA2 and Grin2b/NR2B) genes in AD that indicate downregulation of glutamate receptors by the binding of H3K9Me2 at the promoter of these genes. In comparison, inhibition of H3K9Me2 synthesis by GLP/G9a improves Gria2/GluA2, Grin2b/NR2B genes, and SHANK2 gene expression is impaired in AD. Another more specific GLP/G9a inhibitor UNC0642 significantly improved the expression of NRF2 (nuclear factor erythroid-2-related factor 2), Hmox1 (Heme oxygenase decycling 1), NGF (Nerve growth factor), BDNF, and Synaptophysin (SYN) [106–108].

Additionally, a current study has shown that the expression of H3K9Me3, a marker of transcriptional activation, increases in the PFC of human and mouse AD brains. PFC is a critical region involved in working memory and decision-making. At the same time, inhibition of H3K4-specific methyltransferases leads to significant memory improvement in mutant Tau transgenic mice. These findings suggest methylation may be a potential intervention for treating neurodegenerative diseases, including AD. These epigenetic markers offer strong experimental support using a variety of AD models. They suggest that re-establishing the homeostasis of histone methylation, which G9a/GLP and KMT2A-D significantly mediate, maybe a potential therapeutic approach to treat neurodegenerative disorders associated with AD [106, 107]. Due to the complex nature of AD, pathophysiological and behavioral problems are unlikely to be prevented by targeting only one or a few faulty genes. Histone methylation-targeted pharmacotherapy may benefit from extensive, multifunctional actions and the capacity to target a network of genes crucial for neuronal survival and function [99, 100].

3.4.4 HISTONE PHOSPHORYLATION

Histone phosphorylation refers to the addition of phosphate groups to the proteins and intermediate metabolites in a reaction catalyzed by phosphotransferase. Phosphorylation is usually reported at serine (Ser) and threonine (Thr) amino acids, which is associated with either activation or transcription inactivation of genes that depend on the specific amino acid undergoing phosphorylation and the cellular environment state [98]. Histone phosphorylation has been reported at the N-terminal sequence of all core histones. H2A is phosphorylated at Ser1, H2B at Ser14 and 32, H3 at Ser10 and 28, and H4 at Ser1 [109].

3.4.5 HISTONE PHOSPHORYLATION IN AD

Histone (H3) phosphorylation at site Serine 10 (H3S10P) has been frequently studied as epigenetic markers associated with chromatin condensation during mitosis and minor in neurodegenerative diseases such as AD. The immunoreactivity of H3S10P increases in the cytoplasm of hippocampal neurons of AD compared to control animals, suggesting neurons in AD are mitotically activated [110]. An increased level of H3S10P was found in the perikaryal cytoplasm of pyramid neurons that limited neurofibrillary tangles in CA1 of the hippocampus and subiculum. Conclusively, H3 phosphorylation is associated with chromatin condensation and its level increases in neuronal populations susceptible to neurodegeneration in AD. In addition to other cell cycle abnormalities, the abnormal expression and location of phosphorylated H3 suggest that a mitotic catastrophe contributes to the pathophysiology of AD. Thus, alterations in histone distribution, probably due to mitotic processes, maybe a frequent modification in neurodegenerative illnesses [110]. Phosphorylation of H2A and H2B on Ser 139 and 32, respectively, seems to increase in response to the diversity of apoptotic agents. Other different histone phosphorylation's have been reported depending on the variety of apoptotic agents used [111]. For instance, H3S10p, H1, and H4 phosphorylation increases in response to the apoptotic agent. Several studies reported that the role of H3 phosphorylation at Ser10 increases in other stimuli such as UV irradiation [112]. The phosphorylation level of H3S57p decreased by 40%, and H3S58p decreased by 45%, while double phosphorylated H3S57 decreased by 30% in the brain hemisphere of rapid amyloid deposition (5XFAD) mouse model compared to the control. Additionally, the production of Amyloid-β (Aβ) and amyloid precursor protein increases in the 5XFAD model of AD. Decreases in phosphorylation of the H3S57 and H3S58 site may lead to stabilizing the interaction between DNA and histone, which is further associated with chromatin condensation state and consistent with the epigenetic blockade coupled with the pathogenesis of neurodegeneration [105].

3.4.6 NON-CODING RNA

Non-coding RNAs are an immense and diverse family of non-protein coding RNA that regulate the various functions of cells by regulating the expression of genes via the mechanism of microRNAs (miRNAs), long non-coding RNAs (lncRNAs), and circular RNAs (circRNAs) [113]. The majority of the non-coding sequences are transcribed into various ncRNAs, including miRNAs, lncRNAs, and circRNAs. MicroRNAs are a class of non-coding RNAs that control the repression of messenger RNAs translated in a particular order. Most microRNAs found in the brain are crucial for forming neurons, glial cells, differentiation, proliferation, and metabolism [114]. Furthermore, lncRNAs are RNAs with transcript lengths longer than 200 nucleotides but do not translate into proteins [115]. A wide variety of lncRNAs have been proven to control cellular functions like regulation of gene expression, transcription activation and interference, and nuclear transport, which has prompted more researchers to investigate how lncRNAs affect human biology [116]. The mechanism by which they regulate the expression of a gene is complicated. It is found that they directly bind to DNA or transcription factors, target mRNAs, or proteins and modify their activity and stability, resulting in either transcriptional activation or repression of genes [117–119]. A growing body of research has started highlighting the modulation of lncRNAs in different physiological and pathological processes. Neurological research is one of those that is of considerable importance, especially in AD. The low-throughput tests revealed that several lncRNAs, including BACE1-AS, 51A, BC200, and NDM29, were abnormally expressed in AD compared to healthy controls and were concerned with AD pathophysiology [120].

Additionally, non-coding RNAs (ncRNAs) are concerned with the pathogenesis of several neurodegenerative illnesses and have the ability to alter gene expression and the creation of proteins. Circular RNAs (circRNAs) and mRNAs were recently studied using microarray analysis to differentiate the expression patterns in hippocampus tissue from an AD rat model. The results revealed that 555 circRNAs, 183 miRNAs, and 319 mRNAs were notably dysregulated in the hippocampus [121].

3.4.7 ROLE OF NON-CODING RNA IN AD

Post-transcriptional gene silencing elements known as microRNAs (miRNAs) are a type of 22-nucleotide-long non-coding regulatory RNA molecules. MiRNAs have the ability to silence genes by inducing mRNA degradation or inhibiting translation by attaching to the 3′-untranslated region (UTR) of particular gene mRNAs. Up to 90% of human genes may be regulated by miRNAs, which also have the potential to govern all cellular activity in all body cells and tissues [122]. About 70% of all known miRNAs are expressed in the brain [123]. The evidence from several studies suggests that altered miRNA expression is linked to the regulation of critical AD-related genes, such as APP, BACE1, and microtubule-associated protein tau. Growing evidence suggests that changes in the miRNA network may increase the risk of developing AD. Mis regulated miRNA may indirectly contribute to AD development [33]. A recent study has shown that the brain's parietal and frontal lobes, which are most likely to experience AD, are discovered to have differently expressed miRNAs and target genes. The downregulation of miR-26b-5p, miR-26a-5p, miR-107, and miR-103a-3p in the parietal lobe and the upregulation of HA-miR-7, HA-miR-128, HA-miR-29c, and HA-miR-136 in the frontal lobe were later discovered to be strongly associated with AD through additional functional analysis and data mining [124]. Moreover, it has been reported that the superior temporal lobe, i.e., the neocortex of AD patients, had considerably higher levels of the microRNAs miRNA-7, miRNA-9-1, miRNA-23a/miRNA-34a, miRNA-125b-1, miRNA-146a, and miRNA-155 [125].

Additionally, miRNA-188-downregulation 5p causes synaptic and cognitive impairment, which overexpression reverses [126]. It has been reported that HSA-miR-219 stimulates neurodegeneration via post-transcriptionally controlling the tau protein. Inhibiting extracellular signal-regulated kinase (ERK) 1/2 and tau protein phosphorylation can reduce degenerative damage to the hippocampus in AD animals, improve cognitive impairment in mice, and prevent hippocampal neuronal apoptosis [127].

3.5 EPIGENETIC MODIFICATION AND AB DEPOSITION

Amyloid beta (Aβ) is the primary element of senile plaques, pathology hallmarks of Alzheimer's disease. Aβ aggregation-induced neurotoxicity is revealed by apoptosis, mitochondrial dysfunction, neuroinflammation, and oxidative stress, which subsequently aggravate the pathogenesis of AD. Earlier studies reveal that epigenetic modification, especially DNA methylation and demethylation, play a vital role in regulating gene expression associated with the production, clearance, and aggregation of Aβ and may contribute to the appearance of senescence [128, 129]. Aβ-induced oxidative stress, which further leads to DNA hypermethylation; however, contrasting to this, DNA hypomethylation has been reported in aging brains. Therefore, whether Aβ causes DNA methylation or demethylation is still completely uncertain. Additionally, histone modification, especially histone acetylase PCAF (CBP/p300 associated factor), another crucial epigenetic marker, increases after Aβ treatment and further up-regulates NFkB expression by increasing the level of histone acetylation at its promoter region. Contrarily, the PCAF inhibitor C-30–27 decreases NFkB expression by decreasing histone acetylation at its promoter, further suppressing NFkB-mediated inflammatory response induced by Aβ in BV2 and Neuroblastoma cells [50, 130]. However, valproic acid (VPA), an HDAC inhibitor, downregulates NFkB mRNA in the blood and hippocampus of AD transgenic (Tg6799) mice [131]. These contradictory findings imply that further investigation and explanation are needed to determine how acetylation-induced regulation of NFkB expression contributes to AD pathogenesis. Another deacetylase, SIRT1, similarly closely regulates NFkB expression in an AD *in-vitro* model [132]. The transcription factor p53 is up-regulated in AD brain tissue by increasing histone acetylation (CBP/p300) levels. Thus, it has been concluded that CBP/p300 hyperacetylates p53 at the neuronal outgrowth and maturation [133]. The details of histone DNA methylation and histone acetylation, methylation, and phosphorylation in the regulation of Alzheimer's disease-related gene expression are depicted in Figure 3.2.

3.6 APPLICATION OF EPIGENETIC MARKERS AS THERAPEUTICS TARGETS IN AD

Epigenetic alterations can occur before disease pathology manifests, serving as diagnostic risk markers as well as prognostic markers for disease development. Clinically effective inhibitors of DNA methylation and histone deacetylase have been FDA-approved for a number of years [99]. Histone methylation and microRNAs have also drawn interest as possible therapeutic targets in neurodegenerative diseases. Combination therapy may be most helpful, as evidenced by the existence of several epigenetic abnormalities within a sick tissue and the capacity of cells to build resistance. The most recent clinical advancements in epigenetic therapies focus on treatments that combine epigenetic therapeutics and cytotoxicity agents to increase the effectiveness of the treatment [134].

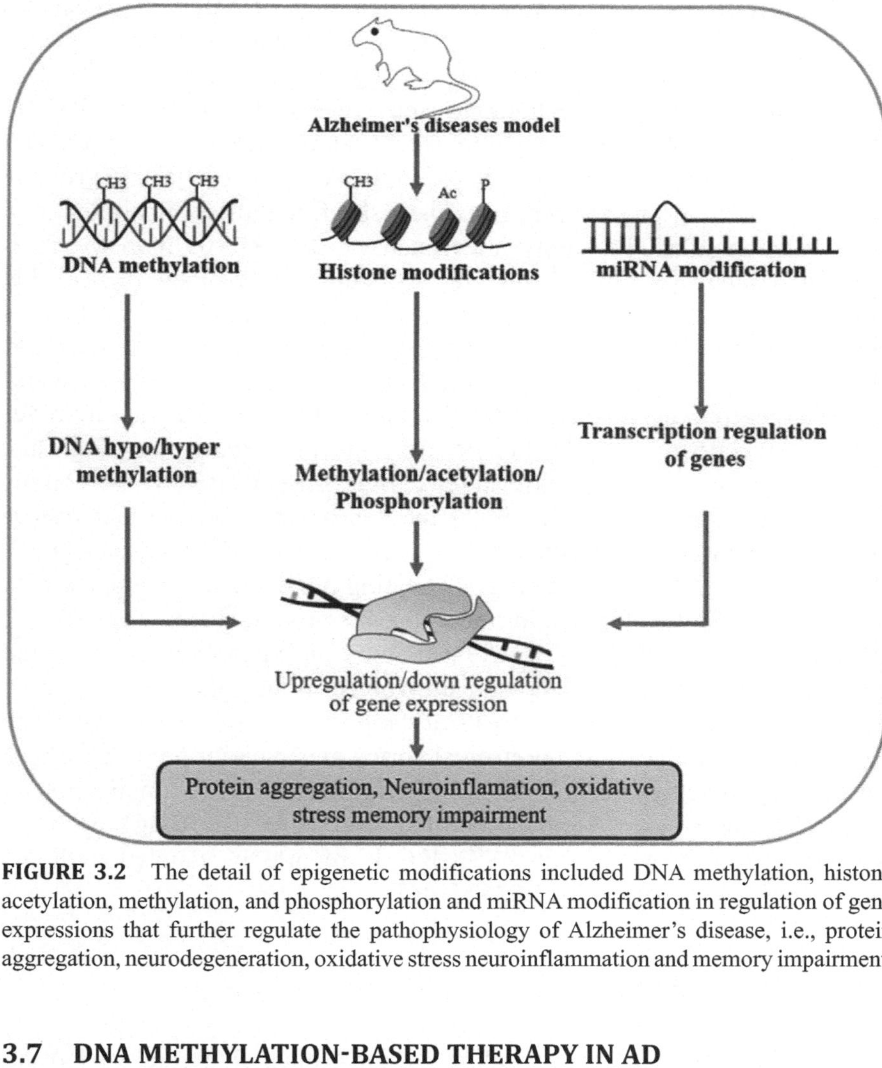

FIGURE 3.2 The detail of epigenetic modifications included DNA methylation, histone acetylation, methylation, and phosphorylation and miRNA modification in regulation of gene expressions that further regulate the pathophysiology of Alzheimer's disease, i.e., protein aggregation, neurodegeneration, oxidative stress neuroinflammation and memory impairment.

3.7 DNA METHYLATION-BASED THERAPY IN AD

DNA methylation plays a vital role in cognitive functions like learning and memory in AD. A study has revealed that hypomethylation at the APP, PSEN1, and PSEN2 genes leads to the upregulation of these genes, which are further involved in the pathogenesis of AD and have consequences on neurodegeneration, learning, and memory [8, 135]. Increases in S-adenosyl-L-methionine (SAM) lead to down-regulating APP and PSEN1 expression by hypermethylation of these genes' promoter region [120]. Furthermore, in applications of DNA methylation for the treatment of AD, some successes have been accomplished by adding DNA methylation donors in AD patients [27, 136]. The addition of supplementary ingredients in the diet, like B12, Folate, and a source of methionine, may reverse the APP and PSEN1 gene expression. Another study found that supplementation of folate for three years improves cognitive function in AD. Similarly, the growing Vita B12 in blood plasma decreases the risk of cognitive impairment and homocysteine-induced memory impairment [137, 138]. Additionally, additions of S-adenosyl-L-methionine and L-methyl-folate supplement in diet improve idiopathic dementia, while S-adenosyl-L-methionine also improves depression-like behavior [139]. Tet1, which reserves the methylation status [140], in the brain by regulating the production of 5hmC, is a potential therapeutic target for managing AD pathophysiology. Inhibition of Tet1 improves cognitive functions, while deletion of Tet1 improves cognitive functions like memory consolidation and retrieval [141, 142]. Several studies based on the DNMT inhibitor (DNMTi) highlight the neuroprotective role and restore memory impairment by modulating the expression of AD risk genes [143]. DNMTi is an FDA-approved drug for treating tumors and leukemia, which may be used further for treating neurodegenerative diseases like AD and Friedreich's ataxia [144, 145]. A recent study on human patients reported differential methylation of HOX gene involved in the pathogenesis of AD. Based on independent cohorts, this study reported hypermethylation of the HOXA cluster in the human prefrontal cortex and superior temporal gyrus. Besides, hypomethylation of the APP gene links with the implication in AD pathogenesis [146]. Methylation of several genes like ANK1, MCF2L, S100B, LRRC8B, MAP2, and STK32C is reportedly coupled with the pathogenesis and progression of AD [146].

3.8 HISTONE MODIFICATION-BASED THERAPY IN AD

HDAC inhibitors (HDACi), including sodium 4-phenylbutyrate, Vorinostat, and Valproic acid, are most extensively studied and have shown a promising effect in AD. The HDACi reduce hyperphosphorylation of tau protein and Aβ deposition [137]. Valproic acid increases GSK3β-mediated α-secretase expression that further cleaves amyloid precursor protein (APP) and improves cognitive functions like memory [147]. Another HDACi, Sodium 4-phenylbutyrate, increases histone acetylation status in the brain and dendrite density in the hippocampus, alleviates endoplasmic reticulum (ER) stress, and improves synaptic transmission in AD transgenic mice [148]. Similarly, another study showed that Sodium 4-phenyl-butyrate decreases Aβ deposition and tau hyperphosphorylation in AD transgenic mice [149]. Whereas FDA-approved HDACi, Vorinostat, restores the expression of genes related to memory and synaptic plasticity by increasing H4K12 acetylation in AD [150]. Vorinostat further regulates the expression of the PU.1 transcription factor, which has been significantly possible for treating AD pathogenesis. The PU.1 transcription factor is crucial for expressing microglia genes and myeloid cell development. Reduction in the expression of PU.1 in microglia leads to delaying AD onset. Vorinostat, along with other HDACi, reduces the level of PU.1, which further reduces microglia-mediated response that primarily includes excessive neuroinflammation. Therefore, Vorinostat may be a promising therapeutic agent for the management of AD [151]. HDAC Class II inhibitors Vorinostat, Sodium valproic acid, and Sodium butyrate restore contextual memory by increasing histone (H4) acetylation in AD [149]. Despite several concluding pieces of evidence that revealed the contribution of histone acetylation in AD pathogenesis, clinical studies of this gained limited success due to several issues like toxicity, which is a key concern.

Although several cancer studies have shown HDACi-induced cell death, apoptosis, and cell cycle arrest, similar expected results were reported in the Brain study. Other limiting factors for HDACi application are annoying consequences on the immune system and reduced permeability of HDACi for the blood-brain barrier [152].

3.9 NON-CODING RNA-BASED THERAPY IN AD

Non-coding RNA (ncRNA) is extensively reported in the brain and is the principal regulator of various brain functions, such as neuronal development and memory, by regulating the expression of genes [119]. Several studies have reported the therapeutic potential of ncRNA. The expression of ncRNA becomes altered in the brain and other regions, such as blood and CSF in AD. MiRNA is most extensively studied in several diseases, including AD, and these miRNA mRNAs may be used as promising biomarkers for early diagnosis or as a therapeutic target for treating AD [153]. A study has reported that over-expression of miR-124 and miR-195 prevents the deposition of Aβ by regulating the BACE1 expression in AD. An *in-vitro* study found the potential role of miR-16 that down-regulated the expression of APP and BACE1, which further prevented the production of Aβ peptide and tau hyper-phosphorylation [154, 155]. Neutralizing inhibitors of miR-206 called AM206 improve memory, hippocampus neurogenesis, and synaptic density in an AD mouse model. Another study reported that miR3c robustly increases in the hippocampus of AD patients, and it may be used as a biomarker for diagnosing AD. Additionally, a study based on a Genome-wide association study (GWAS) reported Hsa-miR-199a-5p, has-miR-199b-5p, has-miR-423-5p, and has-miR-3184-5p are the most significant miRNAs, while NEAT1, XIST, and KCNQ1OT1 are three important lncRNAs that have been identified as new candidate biomarkers in AD and diabetes mellitus [156].

3.10 DISCUSSION AND FUTURE PROSPECTIVE

AD is a neurological condition that worsens with time and is marked by cognitive decline. Although amyloid plaques and neurofibrillary tangles, the pathological indicators of AD, have received extensive research, viable treatments for AD are still unavailable. The pathogenesis of AD may be significantly influenced by transcriptional gene alterations brought on by aging-related epigenetic abnormalities. Epigenetic modifications play an essential role in the pathogenesis of AD by regulating genes that concern AD [157]. Histone modification, including histone methylation and acetylation, is a key element of the epigenetic mechanisms that control gene expression [158]. A recent study discovered that the prefrontal cortex (PFC) of the P301S Tau AD mouse model has elevated histone H3 dimethylation at lysine 9 (H3K9me2, a restrictive histone mark), and its catalytic enzyme euchromatic histone-lysine N-methyltransferase 2. Consistently, the PFC of a family AD mouse with APP/PS1 mutations similarly exhibits increased H3K9me2 and EHMT1/2, as well as excessive repression of glutamate receptor genes [157, 159]. It reveals a potential mechanism driving the decreased expression of synaptic genes crucial for cognitive stability in AD patients, which was discovered by bioinformatics analysis. During a brief course of therapy, the EHMT inhibitor UNC0642 improves synaptic and memory and reduces hyperphosphorylation in the AD model. A study based on transcriptomics reported down-regulation of several genes that are concerned with synaptic alteration has recovered after treatment with UNC0642. These studies suggested potential therapeutic targets for AD management by targeting epigenetic enzymes [159].

Even though decades of research in the genetics of AD, there is still widespread agreement in the field of AD risk, which progresses with age and is characterized by the overexpression of three essential genes PSEN1, PSEN2, and APP. As a result, AD research has expanded to include the evaluation of other molecular biomarkers, including epigenetic markers implicated in the condition that may be influenced by aging or gene-environment interactions [63]. Epigenetic variation, specifically differential methylation, has emerged as an area of particular interest in AD, as epigenetic markers from specific chromatin loci collectively can reflect influences of multiple genetic and environmental factors and result in differential gene expression patterns. Additionally, identifying novel epigenetic markers based on histone acetylation, methylation, and DNA methylation that directly or indirectly contribute to the pathogenesis of AD may be further used for diagnosis and therapeutic targets for managing AD.

KEYWORDS

- **Alzheimer disease**
- **cognitive impairment**
- **dementia**
- **epigenetic modification**
- **neurodegeneration**
- **pathogenesis**
- **therapeutic targets**

REFERENCES

1. Tarawneh, R. (2020). Biomarkers: Our path towards a cure for Alzheimer disease. Biomarker Insights, 15, 1177271920976367. https://doi.org/10.1177/1177271920976367.
2. Hardy, J., & Selkoe, D. J. (2002). The amyloid hypothesis of Alzheimer's disease: Progress and problems on the road to therapeutics. Science, 297(5580), 353–356. https://doi.org/10.1126/science.1072994.
3. Reddy, P. H. (2017). A critical assessment of research on neurotransmitters in Alzheimer's disease. Journal of Alzheimer's Disease, 57(4), 969–974. https://doi.org/10.3233/JAD-160960.

4. Gharipour, M., et al. (2021). How are epigenetic modifications related to cardiovascular disease in older adults? International Journal of Molecular Sciences, 22(18), 9949. https://doi.org/10.3390/ijms22189949.
5. Villa, C., Ferini-Strambi, L., & Combi, R. (2015). The synergistic relationship between alzheimer's disease and sleep disorders: An update. Journal of Alzheimer's Disease, 46(3), 571–580. https://doi.org/10.3233/JAD-150075.
6. Hampel, H., et al. (2021). The amyloid-β pathway in Alzheimer's disease. Molecular Psychiatry, 26(10), 5481–5503. https://doi.org/10.1038/s41380-021-01148-0.
7. De Strooper, B., Iwatsubo, T., & Wolfe, M. S. (2012). Presenilin's and γ-secretase: Structure, function, and role in Alzheimer disease. Cold Spring Harbor Perspectives in Medicine, 2(1), a006304. https://doi.org/10.1101/cshperspect.a006304.
8. Xiao, X., Liu, X., & Jiao, B. (2020). Epigenetics: Recent advances and its role in the treatment of Alzheimer's disease. Frontiers in Neurology, 11, 538301. https://doi.org/10.3389/fneur.2020.538301.
9. Breton, C. V., et al. (2021). Exploring the evidence for epigenetic regulation of environmental influences on child health across generations. Communications Biology, 4(1), 769. https://doi.org/10.1038/s42003-021-02186-w.
10. Stoccoro, A., & Coppedè, F. (2018). Role of epigenetics in Alzheimer's disease pathogenesis. Neurodegenerative Disease Management, 8(3), 181–193. https://doi.org/10.2217/nmt-2018-0001.
11. Rasmi, Y., et al. (2022). The role of DNA methylation in progression of neurological disorders and neurodegenerative diseases as well as the prospect of using DNA methylation inhibitors as therapeutic agents for such disorders. IBRO Neuroscience Reports, 12, 217–227. https://doi.org/10.1016/j.ibneur.2022.03.001.
12. Fernandez, A., et al. (2021). Epigenetic mechanisms in DNA double strand break repair: A clinical review. Frontiers in Molecular Biosciences, 8, 685440. https://doi.org/10.3389/fmolb.2021.685440.
13. Liu, Y., et al. (2022). Non-coding RNAS as novel regulators of neuroinflammation in Alzheimer's disease. Frontiers in Immunology, 13, 908076. https://doi.org/10.3389/fimmu.2022.908076.
14. Abubakar, M. B., et al. (2022). Alzheimer's disease: An update and insights into pathophysiology. Frontiers in Aging Neuroscience, 14, 742408. https://doi.org/10.3389/fnagi.2022.742408.
15. Yang, Y., et al. (2023). Epigenetic and integrative cross-omics analyses of cerebral white matter hyperintensities on MRI. Brain, 146(2), 492–506. https://doi.org/10.1093/brain/awac374.
16. Breijyeh, Z., & Karaman, R. (2020). Comprehensive review on Alzheimer's disease: Causes and treatment. Molecules, 25(24), 5789. https://doi.org/10.3390/molecules25245789.
17. Wang, E., et al. (2022). Non-coding RNAs in Alzheimer's disease: Perspectives from omics studies. Human Molecular Genetics, 31(R1), R54–R61. https://doi.org/10.1093/hmg/ddac083.
18. Lane, C. A., Hardy, J., & Schott, J. M. (2018). Alzheimer's disease. European Journal of Neurology, 25(1), 59–70. https://doi.org/10.1111/ene.13439.
19. Vlassenko, A. G., Benzinger, T. L., & Morris, J. C. (2012). PET amyloid-beta imaging in preclinical Alzheimer's disease. Biochimica et Biophysica Acta (BBA)–Molecular Basis of Disease, 1822(3), 370–379. https://doi.org/10.1016/j.bbadis.2011.08.007.

20. Lacal, I., & Ventura, R. (2018). Epigenetic inheritance: Concepts, mechanisms and perspectives. Frontiers in Molecular Neuroscience, 11, 292. https://doi.org/10.3389/fnmol.2018.00292.
21. Trerotola, M., et al. (2015). Epigenetic inheritance and the missing heritability. *Human Genomics, 9*, 1–12. https://doi.org/10.1186/s40246-015-0107-x.
22. Sharma, V. K., Mehta, V., & Singh, T. G. (2020). Alzheimer's disorder: Epigenetic connection and associated risk factors. *Current Neuropharmacology, 18*(8), 740–753. https://doi.org/10.2174/1570159X18666200608l6588.
23. Mirbahai, L., & Chipman, J. K. (2014). Epigenetic memory of environmental organisms: A reflection of lifetime stressor exposures. *Mutation Research/Genetic Toxicology and Environmental Mutagenesis, 764*, 10–17. https://doi.org/10.1016/j.mrgentox.2014.07.007.
24. Dhar, G. A., et al. (2021). DNA methylation and regulation of gene expression: Guardian of our health. *The Nucleus, 64*(3), 259–270. https://doi.org/10.1007/s13237-021-00539-2.
25. Retis-Resendiz, A. M., et al. (2021). The role of epigenetic mechanisms in the regulation of gene expression in the cyclical endometrium. *Clinical Epigenetics, 13*(1), 116. https://doi.org/10.1186/s13148-021-01097-x.
26. Al Aboud, N. M., Tupper, C., & Jialal, I. (2018). Genetics, epigenetic mechanism. *2018*.
27. Shireby, G., et al. (2022). DNA methylation signatures of Alzheimer's disease neuropathology in the cortex are primarily driven by variation in non-neuronal cell-types. *Nature Communications, 13*(1), 5620. https://doi.org/10.1038/s41467-022-33453-8.
28. Zeng, Y., et al. (2022). DNA methylation: An important biomarker and therapeutic target for gastric cancer. *Frontiers in Genetics, 13*. https://doi.org/10.3389/fgene.2022.971217.
29. Christopher, M. A., Kyle, S. M., & Katz, D. J. (2017). Neuroepigenetic mechanisms in disease. *Epigenetics & Chromatin, 10*, 1–18. https://doi.org/10.1186/s13072-017-0422-7.
30. Mattei, A. L., Bailly, N., & Meissner, A. (2022). DNA methylation: A historical perspective. *Trends in Genetics, 38(7), 676–707*. https://doi.org/10.1016/j.tig.2022.03.010.
31. LD, M., LeT, & Fan, G. (2013). DNA methylation and its basic function. *Neuropsychopharmacology, 38*(1), 23–38. https://doi.org/10.1038/npp.2012.130.
32. Kumar, V., et al. (2022). Understanding the role of histone deacetylase and their inhibitors in neurodegenerative disorders: Current targets and future perspective. *Current Neuropharmacology, 20*(1), 158. https://doi.org/10.2174/1570159X19666220929l6195.
33. Xie, T., et al. (2022). Identification of miRNA-mRNA pairs in the Alzheimer's disease expression profile and explore the effect of miR-26a-5p/PTGS2 on amyloid-β induced neurotoxicity in Alzheimer's disease cell model. *Frontiers in Aging Neuroscience, 14, 909222*. https://doi.org/10.3389/fnagi.2022.909222.
34. Cheng, Y., et al. (2015). 5-Hydroxymethylcytosine: A new player in brain disorders? *Experimental Neurology, 268*, 3–9. https://doi.org/10.1016/j.expneurol.2015.03.006.
35. Nunes, G. H. P., de Lima, M. F. L., & Orsolin, P. C. (2023). A cooperação entre fatores genéticos e epigenéticos na patogênese da Doença de Alzheimer. *Research, Society and Development, 12*(2), e5312238806–e5312238806. https://doi.org/10.33448/rsd-v12i2.38806.
36. Pellegrini, C., et al. (2021). A meta-analysis of brain DNA methylation across sex, age, and Alzheimer's disease points for accelerated epigenetic aging in neurodegeneration. *Frontiers in Aging Neuroscience, 13*, 639428. https://doi.org/10.3389/fnagi.2021.639428.

37. Oliveira, A. M. (2016). DNA methylation: A permissive mark in memory formation and maintenance. *Learning & Memory, 23*(10), 587–593. https://doi.org/10.1101/lm.041830.116.
38. Chouliaras, L., et al. (2015). DNMT3A moderates cognitive decline in subjects with mild cognitive impairment: Replicated evidence from two mild cognitive impairment cohorts. *Epigenomics, 7*(4), 533–537. https://doi.org/10.2217/epi.15.5.
39. Chouliaras, L., et al. (2012). Age-related increase in levels of 5-hydroxymethylcytosine in mouse hippocampus is prevented by caloric restriction. *Current Alzheimer Research, 9*(5), 536–544. https://doi.org/10.2174/156720512801661860.
40. Pezzi, J. C., et al. (2014). DNA methyltransferase haplotype is associated with Alzheimer's disease. *Neuroscience Letters, 579*, 70–74. https://doi.org/10.1016/j.neulet.2014.06.023.
41. Wang, J., et al. (2013). Epigenetic mechanisms in Alzheimer's disease: Implications for pathogenesis and therapy. *Ageing Research Reviews, 12*(4), 1024–1041. https://doi.org/10.1016/j.arr.2013.03.005.
42. Lyubartseva, G., et al. (2010). Alterations of zinc transporter proteins ZnT-1, ZnT-4 and ZnT-6 in preclinical Alzheimer's disease brain. *Brain Pathology, 20*(2), 343–350. https://doi.org/10.1111/j.1750-3639.2009.00333.x.
43. Lashley, T., et al. (2015). Alterations in global DNA methylation and hydromethylation are not detected in Alzheimer's disease. *Neuropathology and Applied Neurobiology, 41*(4), 497–506. https://doi.org/10.1111/nan.12177.
44. Hou, Y., et al. (2013). Changes in methylation patterns of multiple genes from peripheral blood leucocytes of Alzheimer's disease patients. *Acta Neuropsychiatrica, 25*(2), 66–76. https://doi.org/10.1111/np.12012.
45. Wang, S. C., Oelze, B., & Schumacher, A. (2008). Age-specific epigenetic drift in late-onset Alzheimer's disease. *PLOS ONE, 3*(7), e2698. https://doi.org/10.1371/journal.pone.0002698.
46. Toral-Rios, D., et al. (2020). GSK3β and tau protein in Alzheimer's Disease and epilepsy. *Frontiers in Cellular Neuroscience, 14*, 19. https://doi.org/10.3389/fcell.2020.00019.
47. Milazzo, G., et al. (2020). Histone deacetylases (HDACs): Evolution, specificity, role in transcriptional complexes, and pharmacological actionability. *Genes, 11*(5), 556. https://doi.org/10.3390/genes11050556.
48. Kim, J. Y., et al. (2022). Pathological role of HDAC8: Cancer and beyond. *Cells, 11*(19), 3161. https://doi.org/10.3390/cells11193161.
49. Cavalieri, V. (2021). The expanding constellation of histone post-translational modifications in the epigenetic landscape. *Genes, 12*(10), 1596. https://doi.org/10.3390/genes12101596.
50. Park, S. Y., et al. (2015). Selective PCAF inhibitor ameliorates cognitive and behavioral deficits by suppressing NF-κB-mediated neuroinflammation induced by Aβ in a model of Alzheimer's disease. *International Journal of Molecular Medicine, 35*(4), 1109–1118. https://doi.org/10.3892/ijmm.2015.2100.
51. Schmitt, M., & Matthies, H. (1979). [Biochemical studies on histones of the central nervous system. III. Incorporation of [14C]-acetate into the histones of different rat brain regions during a learning experiment]. *Acta Biologica et Medica Germanica, 38*(4), 683–689.

52. McNulty, S. E., et al. (2012). Differential roles for Nr4a1 and Nr4a2 in object location vs. object recognition long-term memory. *Learning & Memory, 19*(12), 588–592. https://doi.org/10.1101/lm.028539.112.
53. Barrett, R. M., et al. (2011). Hippocampal focal knockout of CBP affects specific histone modifications, long-term potentiation, and long-term memory. *Neuropsychopharmacology, 36*(8), 1545–1556. https://doi.org/10.1038/npp.2011.73.
54. Alarcón, J. M., et al. (2004). Chromatin acetylation, memory, and LTP are impaired in CBP+/− mice: A model for the cognitive deficit in Rubinstein-Taybi syndrome and its amelioration. *Neuron, 42*(6), 947–959. https://doi.org/10.1016/j.neuron.2004.06.007.
55. Roth, S. Y., Denu, J. M., & Allis, C. D. (2001). Histone acetyltransferases. *Annual Review of Biochemistry, 70*(1), 81–120. https://doi.org/10.1146/annurev.biochem.70.1.81.
56. Zhang, Y., et al. (1998). The dermatomyositis-specific autoantigen Mi2 is a component of a complex containing histone deacetylase and nucleosome remodeling activities. *Cell, 95*(2), 279–289. https://doi.org/10.1016/S0092-8674(00)81737-3.
57. Utley, R. T., & Cote, J. (2003). The MYST family of histone acetyltransferases. *Protein Complexes That Modify Chromatin, 274*, 203–236. https://doi.org/10.1007/978-1-4615-0096-7_10.
58. Bowers, E. M., et al. (2010). Virtual ligand screening of the p300/CBP histone acetyltransferase: Identification of a selective small molecule inhibitor. *Chemistry & Biology, 17*(5), 471–482. https://doi.org/10.1016/j.chembiol.2010.03.013.
59. Chen, H., et al. (1997). Nuclear receptor coactivator ACTR is a novel histone acetyltransferase and forms a multimeric activation complex with P/CAF and CBP/p300. *Cell, 90*(3), 569–580. https://doi.org/10.1016/S0092-8674(00)80592-6.
60. Spencer, T. E., et al. (1997). Steroid receptor coactivator-1 is a histone acetyltransferase. *Nature, 389*, 194–198. https://doi.org/10.1038/38454.
61. Torchia, J., Glass, C., & Rosenfeld, M. G. (1998). Co-activators and co-repressors in the integration of transcriptional responses. Current Opinion in Cell Biology, 10(3), 373–383. https://doi.org/10.1016/S0955-0674(98)80012-0.
62. Blanco-García, N., et al. (2009). Autoacetylation regulates P/CAF nuclear localization. Journal of Biological Chemistry, 284(3), 1343–1352. https://doi.org/10.1074/jbc.M804873200.
63. Xiao, X., et al. (2021). APP, PSEN1, and PSEN2 variants in Alzheimer's disease: Systematic re-evaluation according to ACMG guidelines. *Frontiers in Aging Neuroscience, 13*, 695808. https://doi.org/10.3389/fnagi.2021.695808.
64. Blanco Garcia, J., et al. (2009). Physiopathological effects of the NO donor 3-morpholinosydnonimine on rat cortical synaptosomes. Neurochemical Research, 34, 931–941. https://doi.org/10.1007/s11064-009-9973-3.
65. Zhang, W., et al. (1998). Essential and redundant functions of histone acetylation revealed by mutation of target lysines and loss of the Gcn5p acetyltransferase. The EMBO Journal, 17(11), 3155–3167. https://doi.org/10.1093/emboj/17.11.3155.
66. Fischle, W., et al. (2002). Enzymatic activity associated with class II HDACs is dependent on a multiprotein complex containing HDAC3 and SMRT/N-CoR. Molecular Cell, 9(1), 45–57. https://doi.org/10.1016/S1097-2765(01)00421-2.
67. Johnstone, S. E., et al. (2022). Epigenetic clocks, aging, and cancer. Science, 378(6626), 1276–1277. https://doi.org/10.1126/science.abn2094.

68. Morris, M. J., et al. (2013). Loss of histone deacetylase 2 improves working memory and accelerates extinction learning. Journal of Neuroscience, 33(15), 6401–6411. https://doi.org/10.1523/JNEUROSCI.3874-12.2013.
69. Schroeder, F. A., et al. (2013). A selective HDAC 1/2 inhibitor modulates chromatin and gene expression in brain and alters mouse behavior in two mood-related tests. PLOS ONE, 8(8), e71323. https://doi.org/10.1371/journal.pone.0071323.
70. Bardai, F. H., et al. (2013). Disassociation of histone deacetylase-3 from normal huntingtin underlies mutant huntingtin neurotoxicity. Journal of Neuroscience, 33(29), 11833–11838. https://doi.org/10.1523/JNEUROSCI.0413-13.2013.
71. Pinto, J. T., et al. (2011). Chemopreventive mechanisms of α-keto acid metabolites of naturally occurring organoselenium compounds. Amino Acids, 41, 29–41. https://doi.org/10.1007/s00726-010-0511-3.
72. Host, L., et al. (2011). Cocaine self-administration alters the expression of chromatin-remodeling proteins; modulation by histone deacetylase inhibition. Journal of Psychopharmacology, 25(2), 222–229. https://doi.org/10.1177/0269881110370696.
73. Ma, C., & D'Mello, S. R. (2011). Neuroprotection by histone deacetylase-7 (HDAC7) occurs by inhibition of c-jun expression through a deacetylase-independent mechanism. Journal of Biological Chemistry, 286(6), 4819–4828. https://doi.org/10.1074/jbc.M110.180636.
74. Pinto, D., et al. (2014). Convergence of genes and cellular pathways dysregulated in autism spectrum disorders. The American Journal of Human Genetics, 94(5), 677–694. https://doi.org/10.1016/j.ajhg.2014.03.019.
75. Fass, D. M., et al. (2013). Crebinostat: A novel cognitive enhancer that inhibits histone deacetylase activity and modulates chromatin-mediated neuroplasticity. Neuropharmacology, 64, 81–96. https://doi.org/10.1016/j.neuropharm.2012.05.058.
76. Oehme, I., et al. (2013). Histone deacetylase 10 promotes autophagy-mediated cell survival. Proceedings of the National Academy of Sciences, 110(28), E2592–E2601. https://doi.org/10.1073/pnas.1301378110.
77. Gao, J., et al. (2010). A novel pathway regulates memory and plasticity via SIRT1 and miR-134. Nature, 466(7310), 1105–1109. https://doi.org/10.1038/nature09271.
78. Pais, T. F., et al. (2013). The NAD-dependent deacetylase sirtuin 2 is a suppressor of microglial activation and brain inflammation. The EMBO Journal, 32(19), 2603–2616. https://doi.org/10.1038/emboj.2013.190.
79. Weir, H. J., et al. (2012). CNS SIRT3 expression is altered by reactive oxygen species and in Alzheimer's disease. PLOS ONE, 7(11), e48225. https://doi.org/10.1371/journal.pone.0048225.
80. Komlos, D., et al. (2013). Glutamate dehydrogenase 1 and SIRT4 regulate glial development. Glia, 61(3), 394–408. https://doi.org/10.1002/glia.22473.
81. Schwer, B., et al. (2010). Neural sirtuin 6 (Sirt6) ablation attenuates somatic growth and causes obesity. *Proceedings of the National Academy of Sciences, 107*(50), 21790–21794. https://doi.org/10.1073/pnas.1012058107.
82. Lee, J. H., et al. (2013). Development of a histone deacetylase 6 inhibitor and its biological effects. *Proceedings of the National Academy of Sciences, 110*(39), 15704–15709. https://doi.org/10.1073/pnas.1307465110.
83. Kizuka, Y., et al. (2014). Epigenetic regulation of a brain-specific glycosyltransferase N-acetylglucosaminyltransferase-IX (GnT-IX) by specific chromatin modifiers.

Journal of Biological Chemistry, 289(16), 11253–11261. https://doi.org/10.1074/jbc.M113.527879.
84. Funato, H., et al. (2011). Fasting and high-fat diet alter histone deacetylase expression in the medial hypothalamus. *PLOS ONE, 6*(4), e18950. https://doi.org/10.1371/journal.pone.0018950.
85. Stilling, R. M., & Fischer, A. (2011). The role of histone acetylation in age-associated memory impairment and Alzheimer's disease. *Neurobiology of Learning and Memory, 96*(1), 19–26. https://doi.org/10.1016/j.nlm.2011.01.007.
86. Martire, S., et al. (2020). Differential contribution of p300 and CBP to regulatory element acetylation in mESCs. *BMC Molecular and Cell Biology, 21*, 1–12. https://doi.org/10.1186/s12860-020-01452-0.
87. Schueller, E., et al. (2020). Dysregulation of histone acetylation pathways in hippocampus and frontal cortex of Alzheimer's disease patients. *European Neuropsychopharmacology, 33*, 101–116. https://doi.org/10.1016/j.euroneuro.2020.01.003.
88. Valencia, A., et al. (2021). Antisense Oligonucleotide-Mediated Reduction of HDAC6 Does Not Reduce Tau Pathology in P301S Tau Transgenic Mice. *Frontiers in Neurology, 12*, 624051. https://doi.org/10.3389/fneur.2021.624051.
89. Frankowski, H., et al. (2021). Knock-down of HDAC2 in human induced pluripotent stem cell derived neurons improves neuronal mitochondrial dynamics, neuronal maturation and reduces amyloid beta peptides. *International Journal of Molecular Sciences, 22*(5), 2526. https://doi.org/10.3390/ijms22052526.
90. Cummings, J. (2022). Disease modification is not all—We need symptomatic therapies for Alzheimer disease. *Nature Reviews Neurology, 18*(1), 3–4. https://doi.org/10.1038/s41582-021-00610-0.
91. Bai, R., et al. (2022). Oxidative stress: The core pathogenesis and mechanism of Alzheimer's disease. *Ageing Research Reviews, 73*, 101619. https://doi.org/10.1016/j.arr.2022.101619.
92. De Carvalho, L. M., et al. (2021). Increased transcription of TSPO, HDAC2, and HDAC6 in the amygdala of males with alcohol use disorder. *Brain and Behavior, 11*(2), e01961. https://doi.org/10.1002/brb3.1961.
93. Gong, F., & Miller, K. M. (2019). Histone methylation and the DNA damage response. *Mutation Research/Reviews in Mutation Research, 780*, 37–47. https://doi.org/10.1016/j.mrrev.2019.02.002.
94. Park, J., et al. (2022). The role of histone modifications: From neurodevelopment to neurodiseases. *Signal Transduction and Targeted Therapy, 7*(1), 217. https://doi.org/10.1038/s41392-022-01052-3.
95. Hwang, J. W., et al. (2021). Protein arginine methyltransferases: Promising targets for cancer therapy. *Experimental & Molecular Medicine, 53*(5), 788–808. https://doi.org/10.1038/s12276-021-00660-3.
96. Li, W. J., et al. (2021). Profiling PRMT methylome reveals roles of hnRNPA1 arginine methylation in RNA splicing and cell growth. *Nature Communications, 12*(1), 1946. https://doi.org/10.1038/s41467-021-22289-w.
97. Mozzetta, C., et al. (2015). Sound of silence: The properties and functions of repressive Lys methyltransferases. *Nature Reviews Molecular Cell Biology, 16*(8), 499–513. https://doi.org/10.1038/nrm4033.
98. Gao, X., et al. (2022). Epigenetics in Alzheimer's disease. *Frontiers in Aging Neuroscience, 14*. https://doi.org/10.3389/fnagi.2022.955338.

99. Cao, Q., Wang, W., & Yan, Z. (2022). Epigenetics-based treatment strategies for Alzheimer's disease. *Aging (Albany NY), 14*(10), 4193–4215. https://doi.org/10.18632/aging.204018.
100. Persico, G., et al. (2022). Histone H3 lysine 4 and 27 trimethylation landscape of human Alzheimer's disease. *Cells, 11*(4), 734. https://doi.org/10.3390/cells11040734.
101. Smith, A. R., et al. (2021). The histone modification H3K4me3 is altered at the ANK1 locus in Alzheimer's disease brain. *Future Science OA, 7*(4), FSO665. https://doi.org/10.2144/fsoa-2021-0011.
102. Benjaskulluecha, S., et al. (2022). Screening of compounds to identify novel epigenetic regulatory factors that affect innate immune memory in macrophages. *Scientific Reports, 12*(1), 1912. https://doi.org/10.1038/s41598-022-05971-8.
103. Buontempo, S., et al. (2022). EZH2-mediated H3K27me3 targets transcriptional circuits of neuronal differentiation. *Frontiers in Neuroscience, 16, 814144.* https://doi.org/10.3389/fnins.2022.814144.
104. Lee, M. Y., et al. (2020). Epigenome signatures landscaped by histone H3K9me3 are associated with the synaptic dysfunction in Alzheimer's disease. *Aging Cell, 19*(6), e13153. https://doi.org/10.1111/acel.13153.
105. Anderson, K. W., et al. (2015). Histone H3 Ser57 and Thr58 phosphorylation in the brain of 5XFAD mice. *FEBS Open Bio, 5*, 550–556. https://doi.org/10.1016/j.fob.2015.08.003.
106. Han, J. L. T., et al. (2021). Inhibition of lysine methyltransferase G9a/GLP reinstates long-term synaptic plasticity and synaptic tagging/capture by facilitating protein synthesis in the hippocampal CA1 area of APP/PS1 mouse model of Alzheimer's disease. *Translational Neurodegeneration, 10*(1), 1–3. https://doi.org/10.1186/s40035-021-00241-8.
107. Basavarajappa, B. S., & Subbanna, S. (2021). Histone methylation regulation in neurodegenerative disorders. *International Journal of Molecular Sciences, 22*(9), 4654. https://doi.org/10.3390/ijms22094654.
108. Sharma, M., Dierkes, T., & Sajikumar, S. (2017). Epigenetic regulation by G9a/GLP complex ameliorates amyloid-beta 1-42 induced deficits in long-term plasticity and synaptic tagging/capture in hippocampal pyramidal neurons. *Aging Cell, 16*(5), 1062–1072. https://doi.org/10.1111/acel.12616.
109. Jeffery, N. N., et al. (2021). Histone H2A.X phosphorylation and Caspase-Initiated Chromatin Condensation in late-stage erythropoiesis. *Epigenetics & Chromatin, 14*(1), 1–15. https://doi.org/10.1186/s13072-021-00411-w.
110. Ogawa, O., et al. (2003). Ectopic localization of phosphorylated histone H3 in Alzheimer's disease: A mitotic catastrophe? *Acta Neuropathologica, 105*, 524–528. https://doi.org/10.1007/s00401-003-0705-0.
111. Loury, R., & Sassone-Corsi, P. (2003). Histone phosphorylation: How to proceed. *Methods, 31*(1), 40–48. https://doi.org/10.1016/S1046-2023(03)00028-1.
112. Lo, W. S., et al. (2005). Histone H3 phosphorylation can promote TBP recruitment through distinct promoter-specific mechanisms. *The EMBO Journal, 24*(5), 997–1008. https://doi.org/10.1038/sj.emboj.7600558.
113. Wang, K., et al. (2022). Epigenetic regulation of aging: Implications for interventions of aging and diseases. *Signal Transduction and Targeted Therapy, 7*(1), 374. https://doi.org/10.1038/s41392-022-01065-y.

114. Rezai Moradali, S., et al. (2022). MicroRNA-127 and MicroRNA-132 Expression in Patients with Methamphetamine Abuse in East Azerbaijan, Iran: A Case-Control Study. *Addiction and Health, 14*(3), 214–217. https://doi.org/10.22122/ahj.v14i3.793.
115. Dahariya, S., et al. (2019). Long non-coding RNA: Classification, biogenesis and functions in blood cells. *Molecular Immunology, 112*, 82–92. https://doi.org/10.1016/j.molimm.2019.05.017.
116. Chen, Y., et al. (2021). Long non-coding RNAs: From disease code to drug role. *Acta Pharmaceutica Sinica B, 11*(2), 340–354. https://doi.org/10.1016/j.apsb.2020.07.013.
117. Zhong, Y., et al. (2022). Assessing the suitability of long non-coding RNAs as therapeutic targets and biomarkers in SARS-CoV-2 infection. *Frontiers in Molecular Biosciences, 9*, 975322. https://doi.org/10.3389/fmolb.2022.975322.
118. Fernandes, J. C., et al. (2019). Long non-coding RNAs in the regulation of gene expression: Physiology and disease. *Non-coding RNA, 5*(1), 17. https://doi.org/10.3390/ncrna5010017.
119. Statello, L., et al. (2021). Gene regulation by long non-coding RNAs and its biological functions. *Nature Reviews Molecular Cell Biology, 22*(2), 96–118. https://doi.org/10.1038/s41580-020-00315-0.
120. Gao, J., et al. (2018). S-adenosyl methionine and transmethylation pathways in neuropsychiatric diseases throughout life. *Neurotherapeutics, 15*, 156–175. https://doi.org/10.1007/s13311-017-0608-2.
121. Wang, Z., et al. (2018). Identifying circRNA-associated-ceRNA networks in the hippocampus of Aβ1-42-induced Alzheimer's disease-like rats using microarray analysis. *Aging (Albany NY), 10*(4), 775. https://doi.org/10.18632/aging.101418.
122. Miranda, K. C., et al. (2006). A pattern-based method for the identification of MicroRNA binding sites and their corresponding heteroduplexes. *Cell, 126*(6), 1203–1217. https://doi.org/10.1016/j.cell.2006.07.031.
123. Provost, P. (2010). Interpretation and applicability of microRNA data to the context of Alzheimer's and age-related diseases. *Aging (Albany NY), 2*(3), 166. https://doi.org/10.18632/aging.100077.
124. Li, J., et al. (2021). Identification of miRNA-target gene pairs in the parietal and frontal lobes of the brain in patients with Alzheimer's Disease using bioinformatic analyses. *Neurochemical Research, 46*, 964–979. https://doi.org/10.1007/s11064-021-03312-3.
125. Pogue, A. I., & Lukiw, W. J. (2018). Up-regulated pro-inflammatory microRNAs (miRNAs) in Alzheimer's disease (AD) and age-related macular degeneration (AMD). *Cellular and Molecular Neurobiology, 38*(5), 1021–1031. https://doi.org/10.1007/s10571-018-0560-1.
126. Lee, K., et al. (2016). Replenishment of microRNA-188-5p restores the synaptic and cognitive deficits in 5XFAD Mouse Model of Alzheimer's Disease. *Scientific Reports, 6*(1), 34433. https://doi.org/10.1038/srep34433.
127. Yang, S., et al. (2020). Dietary advanced glycation end products–induced cognitive impairment in aged ICR mice: Protective role of quercetin. *Molecular Nutrition & Food Research, 64*(3), 1901019. https://doi.org/10.1002/mnfr.201901019.
128. Liu, X., Jiao, B., & Shen, L. (2018). The epigenetics of Alzheimer's disease: Factors and therapeutic implications. *Frontiers in Genetics, 9*, 579. https://doi.org/10.3389/fgene.2018.00579.

129. Wood, I. C. (2018). The contribution and therapeutic potential of epigenetic modifications in Alzheimer's disease. *Frontiers in Neuroscience, 12*, 649. https://doi.org/10.3389/fnins.2018.00649.
130. Park, S. Y., et al. (2013). Selective inhibition of PCAF suppresses microglial-mediated β-amyloid neurotoxicity. *International Journal of Molecular Medicine, 32*(2), 469–475. https://doi.org/10.3892/ijmm.2013.1377.
131. Noh, H., & Seo, H. (2014). Age-dependent effects of valproic acid in Alzheimer's disease (AD) mice are associated with nerve growth factor (NGF) regulation. *Neuroscience, 266*, 255–265. https://doi.org/10.1016/j.neuroscience.2014.02.045.
132. Marwarha, G., et al. (2014). Leptin attenuates BACE1 expression and amyloid-β genesis via the activation of SIRT1 signaling pathway. *Biochimica et Biophysica Acta (BBA)–Molecular Basis of Disease, 1842*(9), 1587–1595. https://doi.org/10.1016/j.bbadis.2014.06.014.
133. Aubry, S., et al. (2015). Assembly and interrogation of Alzheimer's disease genetic networks reveal novel regulators of progression. *PLoS One, 10*(3), e0120352. https://doi.org/10.1371/journal.pone.0120352.
134. Hwang, J. Y., Aromolaran, K. A., & Zukin, R. S. (2017). The emerging field of epigenetics in neurodegeneration and neuroprotection. *Nature Reviews Neuroscience, 18*(6), 347–361. https://doi.org/10.1038/nrn.2017.46.
135. Lanoiselée, H. M., et al. (2017). APP, PSEN1, and PSEN2 mutations in early-onset Alzheimer disease: A genetic screening study of familial and sporadic cases. *PLoS Medicine, 14*(3), e1002270. https://doi.org/10.1371/journal.pmed.1002270.
136. C Silva, T., et al. (2022). Distinct sex-specific DNA methylation differences in Alzheimer's disease. *Alzheimer's Research & Therapy, 14*(1), 1–21. https://doi.org/10.1186/s13195-022-00923-0.
137. Coppedè, F. (2010). One-carbon metabolism and Alzheimer's disease: Focus on epigenetics. *Current Genomics, 11*(4), 246–260. https://doi.org/10.2174/138920110793358779.
138. Fuso, A., et al. (2005). S-adenosylmethionine/homocysteine cycle alterations modify DNA methylation status with consequent deregulation of PS1 and BACE and beta-amyloid production. *Molecular and Cellular Neuroscience, 28*(1), 195–204. https://doi.org/10.1016/j.mcn.2004.09.001.
139. Strous, R. D., et al. (2009). Improvement of aggressive behavior and quality of life impairment following S-adenosyl-methionine (SAM-e) augmentation in schizophrenia. *European Neuropsychopharmacology, 19*(1), 14–22. https://doi.org/10.1016/j.euroneuro.2008.05.009.
140. Fetrow, C., & Avila, J. R. (2001). Efficacy of the dietary supplement S-adenosyl-L-methionine. *Annals of Pharmacotherapy, 35*(11), 1414–1425. https://doi.org/10.1345/aph.1A077.
141. Jessop, P., & Toledo-Rodriguez, M. (2018). Hippocampal TET1 and TET2 expression and DNA hydroxymethylation are affected by physical exercise in aged mice. *Frontiers in Cell and Developmental Biology, 6*, 45. https://doi.org/10.3389/fcell.2018.00045.
142. Kaas, G. A., et al. (2013). TET1 controls CNS 5-methylcytosine hydroxylation, active DNA demethylation, gene transcription, and memory formation. *Neuron, 79*(6), 1086–1093. https://doi.org/10.1016/j.neuron.2013.08.014.
143. Kaur, G., et al. (2022). DNA methylation: A promising approach in management of Alzheimer's disease and other neurodegenerative disorders. *Biology, 11*(1), 90. https://doi.org/10.3390/biology11010090.

144. Rodden, L. N., et al. (2022). A non-synonymous single nucleotide polymorphism in SIRT6 predicts neurological severity in Friedreich ataxia. *Frontiers in Molecular Biosciences, 9*, 933788. https://doi.org/10.3389/fmolb.2022.933788.
145. Hu, D., Liu, Z., & Qi, X. (2021). Mitochondrial quality control strategies: Potential therapeutic targets for neurodegenerative diseases? *Frontiers in Neuroscience, 15*, 746873. https://doi.org/10.3389/fnins.2021.746873.
146. Gasparoni, G., et al. (2018). DNA methylation analysis on purified neurons and glia dissects age and Alzheimer's disease-specific changes in the human cortex. *Epigenetics & Chromatin, 11*, 1–19. https://doi.org/10.1186/s13072-018-0185-4.
147. Singh, D., et al. (2021). Hidden pharmacological activities of valproic acid: A new insight. *Biomedicine & Pharmacotherapy, 142*, 112021. https://doi.org/10.1016/j.biopha.2021.112021.
148. Rellmann, Y., et al. (2019). 4-Phenylbutyric acid reduces endoplasmic reticulum stress in chondrocytes that is caused by loss of the protein disulfide isomerase ERp57. *Oxidative Medicine and Cellular Longevity, 2019, 6404035*. https://doi.org/10.1155/2019/6404035.
149. Shukla, S., & Tekwani, B. L. (2020). Histone deacetylases inhibitors in neurodegenerative diseases, neuroprotection and neuronal differentiation. *Frontiers in Pharmacology, 11*, 537. https://doi.org/10.3389/fphar.2020.00537.
150. Xu, J., et al. (2018). Vorinostat: A histone deacetylases (HDAC) inhibitor ameliorates traumatic brain injury by inducing iNOS/Nrf2/ARE pathway. *Folia Neuropathologica, 56*(3), 179–186. https://doi.org/10.5114/fn.2018.78314.
151. Yeh, H., & Ikezu, T. (2019). Transcriptional and epigenetic regulation of microglia in health and disease. *Trends in Molecular Medicine, 25*(2), 96–111. https://doi.org/10.1016/j.molmed.2018.12.003.
152. Lu, H., et al. (2023). Histone deacetylase 3 inhibition decreases cerebral edema and protects the blood–brain barrier after stroke. *Molecular Neurobiology, 60*(1), 235–246. https://doi.org/10.1007/s12035-022-02890-8.
153. Zhang, Y., et al. (2021). Bridging the gap between morphometric similarity mapping and gene transcription in Alzheimer's disease. *Frontiers in Neuroscience, 15*, 731292. https://doi.org/10.3389/fnins.2021.731292.
154. Kou, X., Chen, D., & Chen, N. (2020). The regulation of microRNAs in Alzheimer's disease. *Frontiers in Neurology, 11*, 288. https://doi.org/10.3389/fneur.2020.00288.
155. Fang, M., et al. (2012). The miR-124 regulates the expression of BACE1/β-secretase correlated with cell death in Alzheimer's disease. *Toxicology Letters, 209*(1), 94–105. https://doi.org/10.1016/j.toxlet.2011.12.019.
156. Ghiam, S., et al. (2022). Exploring the role of non-coding RNAs as potential candidate biomarkers in the cross-talk between diabetes mellitus and Alzheimer's disease. *Frontiers in Aging Neuroscience, 14, 955461*. https://doi.org/10.3389/fnagi.2022.955461.
157. Rabaneda-Bueno, R., et al. (2021). Advances in genetics and epigenetic alterations in Alzheimer's disease: A notion for therapeutic treatment. *Genes, 12*(12), 1959. https://doi.org/10.3390/genes12121959.
158. Santana, D. A., Smith, M. d. A. C., & Chen, E. S. (2023). Histone modifications in Alzheimer's disease. *Genes, 14*(2), 347. https://doi.org/10.3390/genes14020347.
159. Wang, W., et al. (2021). Epigenetic treatment of behavioral and physiological deficits in a tauopathy mouse model. *Aging Cell, 20*(10), e13456. https://doi.org/10.1111/acel.13456.

CHAPTER 4

Drug-Induced Alzheimer's Disease

MONIKA KAUSHIK,[1*] K. ANITHA,[1] and S. VIJAYARAJ[2]

[1]*Department of Pharmacology, Amity Institute of Pharmacy, Amity University Madhya Pradesh, Gwalior, Madhya Pradesh, India*

[2]*Department of Pharmaceutical Analysis and Chemistry, Dr. Kalam College of Pharmacy, Avanam, Thanjavur, Tamil Nadu, India*

*Corresponding author.

ABSTRACT

Dementia, psychological and cognitive abnormalities, and diminished memory are symptoms of Alzheimer's disease (AD). The number of diseases being treated nowadays has expanded due to scientific advancements. New methods of illness treatment are being developed with the aid of laboratory animals. To better understand the disease's processes and possible treatments for AD, animal models of AD can be produced using chemical medicines. Several scientists have published transgenic rat models of AD in the last few years; however, these models have significant flaws and do not include all forms of AD. Although there are two forms of AD: sporadic (which accounts for 95% of cases) and familial (which accounts for 5% of cases), the transgenic model does not depict the full model of AD. Using chemical compounds like scopolamine, colchicine, streptozotocin, okadaic acid, and trimethyltin, researchers choose to present other models of Alzheimer's disease. Scopolamine administration impairs verbal recall, visuospatial praxis, visuospatial recall psychomotor speed, visual recognition memory, and visuoperceptual processes. One of the most effective and widely used medications to prevent motion sickness is this one. Colchicine can be used as a candidate for modeling AD since it causes hippocampal lesions that impair cognition and reduce ChAT. Colchicine may impair cholinergic pathways,

Neuro-Nutraceuticals and Drug Discovery and Delivery in Alzheimer's Disease, Volume 1: Targeting Key Pathological Pathways. Varinder Singh, Amit Kumar, Parul Sood (Eds.)

which reduces the number of cholinergic neurons and subsequently lowers cholinergic renewal, mainly in the hippocampal region of the brain. This may result in neurotoxicity and memory loss. Intracerebroventricular administration of streptozotocin to rodents is known to have a severe and enduring impact on the cytoarchitecture, biochemistry, metabolism, and functions of the brain.

Each chemical may work through distinct, specialized mechanisms to aggravate AD development. In order to cause severe disease in human subjects, the dosage and the duration at which the drug is administered in rodent AD models may be greater or occasionally lower. Importantly, the method of administration, nature, duration (particularly), and age and gender of the studied animals are other factors connected to the chemicals that cause Alzheimer's disease. The chapter describes various drugs and chemicals that tend to induce AD.

4.1 INTRODUCTION

Alzheimer's is a neurodegenerative disease that worsens over time and affects memory, judgment, and eventually the ability to perform even the simplest basic activities. Often, these disease victims develop late-onset symptoms, which typically begin to appear in their mid-sixties [1]. Early-onset Alzheimer's disease is quite rare and is seen between the ages of thirty and sixty. Alzheimer's disease is the most common cause of disability in older people [1]. Dr. Alzheimer first observed abnormalities in the brain tissue of a woman who died unexpectedly in 1906 from a rare mental illness, leading to the condition being named Alzheimer's disease. Oxidative stress, an imbalance in energy metabolism, trace element neurotoxicity, a lack of neurotropic agents, mitochondrial flaws, altered amyloid precursor processing, the formation of neurofibrillary tangles, and genetic abnormalities are just a few of the potential causes of AD [2]. Research has linked microtubule disruption to cognitive dysfunction and AD [3]. The hippocampus is a crucial area in neurological disorders, particularly in dementia and Alzheimer's disease. Studies suggest that cognitive impairment resulting from hippocampal damage can lead to Alzheimer's disease [4]. Cognitive deterioration was brought on by the use of cholinesterase inhibitors in both AD animal models and dementia patients [5]. Drug effectiveness has been demonstrated in behavioral tests such as the Morris Water Maze, Radial Arm Maze, Spatial Cone Field, Five Choice Serial Reaction Time, and Object Recognition Task. The use of animal models is crucial for understanding the etiology of diseases like neurodegenerative illnesses. Chemical medicines (such as colchicine, okadaic acid, streptozotocin, trimethyltin, and scopolamine) for induction of AD-like modeling that aids AD researchers are one of the AD models.

Early signs of the illness include forgetting previous interactions or events. As Alzheimer's disease progresses, a person will have extreme loss of memory and become unable to perform everyday chores.

Alzheimer's disease, the type of dementia that is most common (AD), affects 25–50% of adults aged 85 or older and accounts for 60–80% of all cases [6]. Currently, one person in America has dementia every 70 seconds, or 4,50,000 new cases every year. This number is predicted to nearly triple by 2050, primarily as a result of longer survival rates. There is a great deal of study being done to determine the actual mechanism(s) behind AD. The course of Alzheimer's disease in the brain cannot be halted by any treatment that is now available. Death occurs in the most severe stages of the illness when major loss of brain function-related issues, such as dehydration, hunger, or infection, occur [7].

4.2 PATHOPHYSIOLOGY OF AD

With an axon and several dendrites, the brain contains billions of neurons. Neurons can interact with one another, carry out metabolism, and self-repair in order to be healthy. All three of these crucial tasks are disturbed by AD [8]. Two pathological hallmarks of Alzheimer's disease are:

1. Extracellular beta-amyloid (Aβ) plaques (dense deposits of protein and cellular material that accumulate outside and around nerve cells).
2. Intraneuronal neurofibrillary tangles (NFTs) (twisted fibers that build up inside the nerve cell).

These lesions have been associated with neuronal degeneration, functional loss, brain atrophy, and disruption of neural communication pathways. However, it is still unclear what exactly causes AD [9].

4.2.1 BETA-AMYLOID (AB) PLAQUES (AMYLOIDOGENIC PATHWAY)

The outer cell membrane of neurons contains a protein termed amyloid precursor (APP). The healthy brain's α and γ secretases break down APP into smaller Aβ protein fragments that are thought to be advantageous to neurons

(Figure 4.1). In AD, β and γ secretases disassemble APP into minute pieces. Before binding together to form beta-amyloid plaques, the Aβ oligomers are considered to interfere with synaptic signaling and communication in neurons. Beta-amyloid plaques have the potential to cause an inflammatory immune response that kills neurons [10].

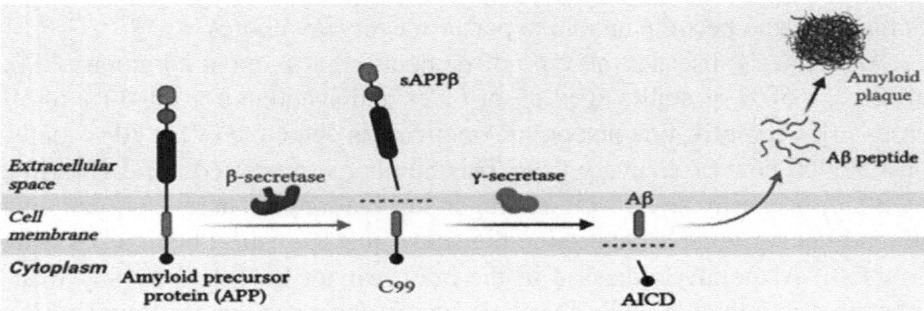

FIGURE 4.1 Amyloidogenic pathway.

The APP gene, presenilin 1 gene, and presenilin 2 gene autosomal dominant mutations are linked to the development of Aβ plaques in the early onset of AD. The Apolipoprotein E gene-allele 4 may contribute to the development of Aβ plaques in late-onset AD [11].

4.2.2 NEUROFIBRILLARY TANGLES (PROTEIN AGGREGATION PATHWAY)

Microtubules, which carry nutrients and other chemicals, are found in neurons. Tau proteins give stability and maintain the microtubules' straightness in the healthy brain. The hyperphosphorylation of tau proteins in AD causes them to separate from the microtubules (Figure 4.2). The tau proteins aggregate inside the neuron to form neurofibrillary tangles that restrict nutrient transport and hinder communication. Such knots eventually cause neuronal death because they are poisonous to the neuron [12].

The involvement of amyloid-β (Aβ) in the development of extracellular amyloid aggregates can lead to Tau clumps and neurofibrillary tangles (NFTs), both of which cause degeneration of neurons, impairment of synapses, and damaged neurons (Figure 4.3) [13].

In addition, the activation of astrocytes in plaques causes the release of numerous cytokines, as does the activation of microglia, which produces superoxide radicals. The accumulation of free radicals, which causes a

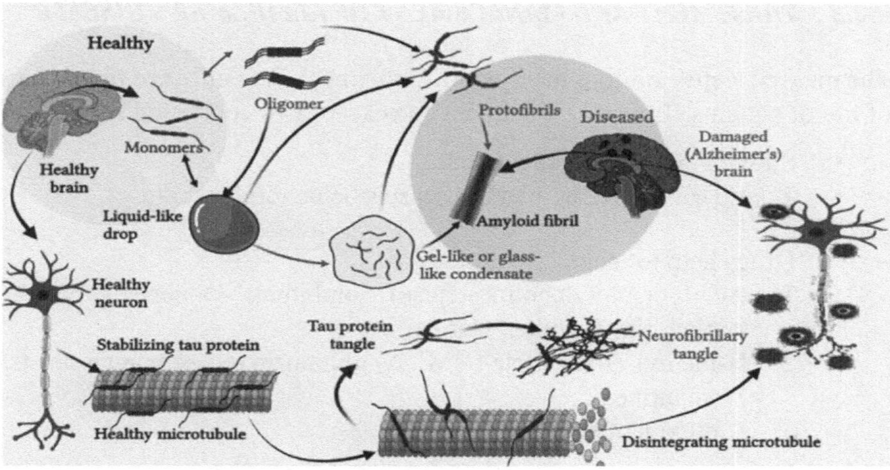

FIGURE 4.2 Protein aggregation pathways.

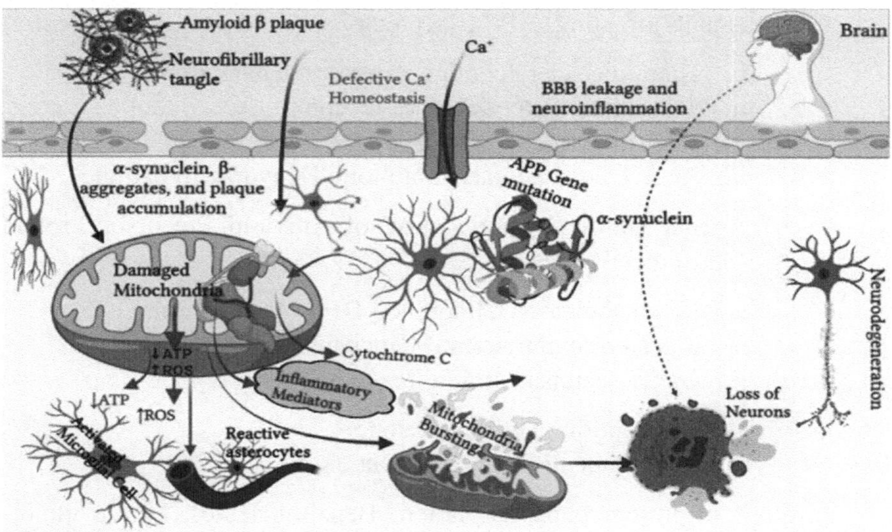

FIGURE 4.3 Pathophysiology of Alzheimer's disease.

change in the energy efficiency of neurons, is partly caused by aging-related mitochondrial damage [14]. One of the main contributing factors in the pathophysiology of AD is the loss of Ca^{2+} homeostasis, which is explained by excitotoxic activity. Alterations in the composition of the gut microbiota may also be a factor in the pathophysiology of AD [15].

4.2.3 TREATMENT AND MANAGEMENT OF ALZHEIMER'S DISEASE

The main objective of drug therapy for Alzheimer's is to enhance the quality of life of patients. Typically, treatment consists of two connected strategies:

- Slowing the development; and
- Taking care of Alzheimer's disease's behavioral symptoms.

Drugs help to manage symptoms:

1. AChE (Acetylcholinesterase) inhibitors: Donepezil, galantamine, rivastigmine, tacrine.
2. N-methyl-D-aspartate (NMDA) glutamate receptor antagonists: Memantine.
3. Antioxidants:
   i. Ginkgo-biloba, Idebenone (CoEnzQ), melatonin, Vitamin E.
   ii. MAO-B (Mono-amine Oxidase) inhibitors: Selegiline.
4. Agents affecting sAPP-a (secretary amyloid precursor protein-a)
   i. Nicotinic Acetylcholine receptors: galantamine.
   ii. Muscarinic Acetylcholine receptors: Acetylcholine, carbachol, nicotine.
   iii. Acetylcholinesterase inhibitors: Dehydroevodiamine.
5. Agents inhibiting aggregation of Amyloid Precursor Protein (APP) metabolites:
   i. Metal chelators: Clioquinol, DFO (deferoxamine).
   ii. β-secretase inhibitors: Memapsin 2.
   iii. Gama-secretase inhibitor:
      a. Peptidic: Difluoro ketone
      b. Nonpeptidic: JLK inhibitors.
6. Anti-protein phosphorylation: Benzimidazoles, kinase inhibitors, taurosporine.

4.3 MECHANISM OF ACTION OF ANTI-ALZHEIMER DRUGS

By replenishing an acetylcholine neurotransmitter that Alzheimer's disease depletes in the brain, cholinesterase inhibitors boost levels of cell-to-cell communication. Cholinesterase inhibitors increase levels of cell-to-cell communication by blocking the breakdown of acetylcholine that is depleted due to Alzheimer's disease [16]. The cholinergic pathways in the central nervous system are the target of cholinesterase inhibitors such as donepezil, galantamine, and rivastigmine. The most common side effects of anti-Alzheimer's drugs are diarrhea, nausea, appetite loss, and sleep difficulties [17]. Alkaloid galantamine functions as an allosteric modulator at nicotinic acetylcholine receptors, and all three of the medicines show anticholinesterase activity [18].

Memantine is notable for being the first AD medication to target both glutamatergic and N-methyl-D-aspartate (NMDA) receptor pathways. Glutamatergic regulation impacts dendritic spine clustering in a mouse model of AD, and excess glutamate at excitatory synapses with concomitant cytotoxicity, presumably caused by reduced glutamate absorption from microglia, has recently been proposed as a pathophysiological mechanism in AD [19] (Figure 4.4).

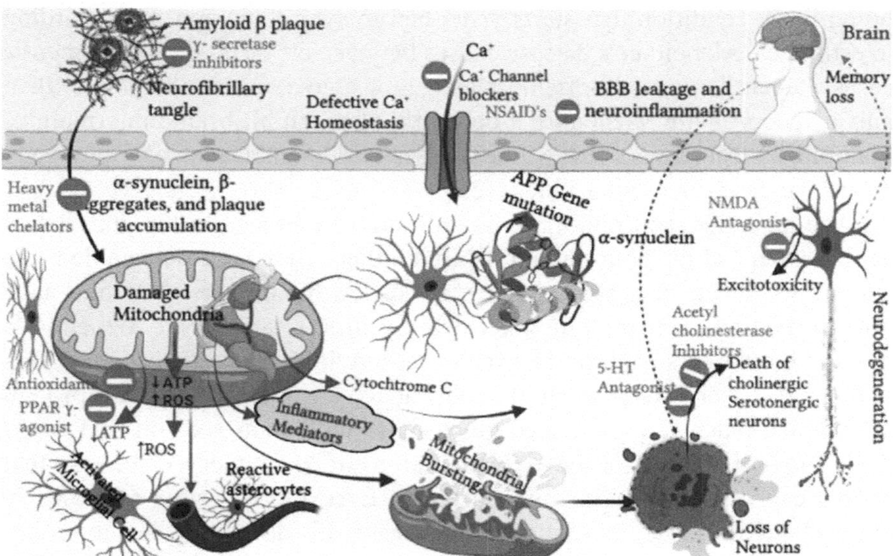

FIGURE 4.4 Main drug targets in Alzheimer's disease.

A phase II trial of the glutamate release and postsynaptic glutamate receptor signaling inhibitor riluzole is now being conducted in moderate AD patients [20]. Memantine disrupts the endocytosis pathway of APP, which is necessary for β-secretase-mediated cleavage, and lowers levels of Aβ both in AD models and in elderly animals [21].

4.4 ROLE OF CURRENT ALZHEIMER'S DRUGS

According to the Alzheimer's disease continuum, the disease develops gradually over time, starting with changes in the brain that the sick person cannot see and progressing to cognitive problems and, eventually, physical inability [22]. In general, there are three phases along this continuum: Alzheimer's also known as Alzheimer's preclinical illness, and Alzheimer's-related moderate cognitive impairment (MCI). There are three levels of stages associated with Alzheimer's disease: mild, moderate, and severe [23]. Although the length of time that people spend in each stage of the Alzheimer's disease continuum varies and leads to severe if it is untreated [24].

The hallmark conditions of Alzheimer's disease are the accumulation of the protein beta-amyloid (plaques) outside neurons and the twisted strands of the protein tau (tangles) inside neurons in the brain. Neuronal loss and brain tissue damage accompany these alterations. Alzheimer's is a slowly developing brain condition that starts years before symptoms appear. According to estimates, Alzheimer's disease causes between 60% and 80% of dementia cases. Recent large postmortem investigations have revealed that more than half of people with Alzheimer's dementia also exhibit brain abnormalities (pathology) from one or more other causes of dementia, such as Lewy body disease or cerebrovascular illness [25].

Age, genetics, and biological sex all have an impact on the duration of each segment of the continuum [26]. Individuals may have detectable brain alterations during this stage, which are called biomarkers, but they have not yet manifested symptoms like memory loss. Examples of Alzheimer's disease biomarkers include aberrant beta-amyloid levels as seen on PET scans and in cerebrospinal fluid (CSF) analyses, alterations in tau protein in CSF and plasma, and reduced glucose metabolism as seen on PET scans [27]. The brain marks for the early alterations of Alzheimer's disease so that people can continue to function normally. Even though some of the early brain changes linked to Alzheimer's disease are detectable in laboratory diagnosis, further research is necessary to increase the tools' precision before they are routinely applied in clinics, hospitals, and other clinical settings. It's important to keep in mind that not everyone who exhibits brain changes associated with Alzheimer's disease develops MCI or dementia as a result of the condition. For instance, some persons have beta-amyloid plaques when they pass away but do not have memory or cognitive problems while they are alive. Memory is disrupted: One of the most common signs of Alzheimer's is memory loss, specifically the difficulty in retaining information that has just been taught. Others include forgetting significant dates or events, repeatedly seeking the same information, and progressively requiring the assistance of family members or memory aides (such as reminder notes or technological devices) for tasks that one used to be able to complete on one's own [23].

4.5 ALZHEIMER'S DRUGS PERSPECTIVES

Present AD therapy drugs reduce symptoms and slow disease progression but do not promise a cure. There is much controversy around the drugs used to slow the course of AD, including their long-term usefulness and whether to discontinue therapy with these treatments, as well as cost and effectiveness problems. According to recent research, therapists may find the decision-making process surrounding drug discontinuation exceedingly challenging.

This reflects the current uncertainty in the literature regarding the long-term efficacy of drugs and when to discontinue treatment due to a lack of high-quality randomized controlled trials of agents' discontinuation, as well as the resulting variability in clinician decision-making [28]. It emphasizes the widely varying response to medication treatment and subsequent medication withdrawal experienced by people with AD, confirming the importance of a highly individualized and person-centered approach in clinicians' and carers' decisions about Alzheimer's drug medication withdrawal.

4.6 MECHANISMS OF DRUGS THAT INDUCE AD

The brain's atrophy is linked to Alzheimer's disease (decreased brain volume). It is believed that the presence of dangerous beta-amyloid and tau proteins activates the brain's microglia, a kind of immune cell. Microglia make an effort to remove the destructive proteins and generalized debris from dead and dying cells. When the microglia can't keep up with everything that needs to be cleaned away, chronic inflammation may develop, which then leads to atrophy. As the brain's capability to metabolize glucose reduces, Alzheimer's disease, normal brain function is further jeopardized [29].

Alzheimer's disease patients also exhibit new, subtle symptoms like memory, language, and thinking issues [30]. When the brain can no longer make up for the loss and death of neurons brought on by environmental factors, subtle issues with memory, language, and cognitive abilities arise. Dementia is known as mixed pathology if it is diagnosed later in life. Alpha-synuclein protein clumps or abnormal clusters are known as Lewy bodies in neurons. When they expand in the cortex, a part of the brain, dementia may result. Dementia with Lewy Bodies (DLB) describes this condition [31] (Table 4.1).

TABLE 4.1 Representing the Drugs/Chemical That Induce Alzheimer's Disease

Sl. No.	Drugs/Chemicals
1.	Colchicine
2.	Scopolamine
3.	OKA
4.	STZ induced model
5.	Ethanol/alcohol-induced AD
6.	Sodium azide-induced AD-like memory impairment

4.6.1 COLCHICINE

Colchicine-induced memory impairment may be due to a reduction in serotonin, dopamine, and norepinephrine levels in the caudate nucleus, hippocampus, and whole cerebral cortex. Originally used to treat gouty arthritis, colchicine is an alkaloid obtained from several plants in the lily family and used to prevent bouts of Mediterranean fever; decades later, it was also used to stop amyloidosis. The hippocampus, the part of the brain most afflicted by AD, has a threefold higher concentration of colchicine than other parts of the brain. The medication specifically inhibits acetylcholine transferase in the memory-related basal forebrain and hippocampus. Colchicine can cause symptoms like jumpy and irritable behavior, aggressiveness, and weight loss when it enters the subarachnoid space. Colchicine is a neurotoxin that disrupts microtubules and causes the loss of hippocampal granule cells [32].

Colchicine has also been shown to increase COX-1 and COX-2 expression levels, as well as ROS production. Colchicine impairs learning and memory by degenerating neurofibers via tubulin (the microtubule structural protein), which is linked to a reduction in acetylcholine transferase and the loss of cholinergic neurons. Colchicine (15 mg) was administered intracerebroventricularly (ICV), causing cognitive impairment and memory loss in the MWM and elevated plus maze (EPM) tasks. As a result, colchicine-induced dementia of the Alzheimer's type and cognitive impairment. This model's key benefit is that it reproduces various sporadic Alzheimer's-type dementia symptoms reported in real individuals, such as time-variant changes in onset, behavioral patterns, and biochemical patterns.

4.6.2 SCOPOLAMINE

Additionally, studies show that scopolamine non-selectively blocks ACh muscarinic receptors' adhesion sites in the cerebral cortex. This causes an uneven release of ACh, which kills hippocampal neurons and causes learning and memory deficits in mice in a dose-dependent way [33]. In studies on cognition in AD patients, the scopolamine model is employed as one of the models. Scopolamine alters glucose metabolism and cerebral blood flow (CBF), which have been investigated in research using PET and single photon emission computed tomography (SPECT) [34]. Left orbitofrontal and lateral occipital cortical blood flow was increased by scopolamine, but the right thalamus, precuneus, and right and left lateral premotor areas saw a decrease in rCBF. Scopolamine has been found to impair spatial learning and memory. As a result, it activates glycogen synthase kinase-3 beta (GSK-3), causes insufficient spine development, and leads to dendritic arborization linked to changes in CREC, Homer1, and amino-3-hydroxy-5-methyl-4-isoxazole propionic acid receptor (AMPA) [35].

4.6.3 OKADAIC ACID-INDUCED MODEL (OKA)

OKA is a useful model agent to examine for the screening of anti-dementia medications since it has been documented to cause memory deterioration in rats when administered intracerebroventricularly (IC). According to earlier research, OKA reduces baseline synaptic transmission and prevents the beginning of synaptic plasticity. Also, it has been discovered that OKA causes the death of neurons via increasing Ca^{2+} in cultured hippocampal neuronal cells via ionotropic excitatory amino acid receptors.

Serine/threonine phosphatases 1 and 2 are preferentially inhibited by OKA in the rat brain, according to researchers [36]. AD patients, however, exhibit decreased phosphatase activity. Additionally, OKA led to memory loss and Ca^{2+} elevations that were linked to neurotoxicity. The interference with calcium signaling changed the balance of the systems responsible for protein phosphorylation and dephosphorylation, leading to aberrant tau phosphorylation [37]. According to studies, elevated intracellular Ca^{2+} caused amyloid beta to build up, tau to become hyperphosphorylated, and neuronal death. These traits were present in AD as well [38].

OKA-induced model caused tau phosphorylation, cognitive impairment, and an increase in mRNA and protein expression of CaMKII, tau, GSK3β, and Calpain in the hippocampus [39]. Additionally, the results of rats treated with OKA showed memory impairment in the water maze test [40].

4.6.4 STZ INDUCED MODEL

Studies have demonstrated that an injection of STZ (3 mg/kg) causes cognitive deterioration, a reduction in brain mass, an increase in hippocampal A and tau levels, and a decrease in brain weight [41]. STZ induces tau hyperphosphorylation and neuronal degeneration, which releases reactive oxygen and nitrogen species (ROS and RNS) into the environment. In this model, the cytoarchitecture, biochemistry, metabolism, and functioning of the brain are known to have a significant and enduring impact (such as decreased glucose uptake and energy consumption, oxidative tissue stress, cholinergic differential, and cognitive abilities). Injection of STZ produced memory impairment and changed biochemical parameter levels (Alzheimer-like) in mouse brains, as demonstrated by Chen et al. [41]. Studies have shown that the periventricular structures, which are crucial for learning and spatial memory, as well as the axons and myelin of the fornix, are the only parts of the brain that are specifically damaged by STZ [43, 44]. Rats' memory and learning abilities were decreased after receiving ICV-STZ, which resulted in oxidative stress.

4.6.5 ETHANOL/ALCOHOL INDUCED AD

Persistent alcohol use is linked to a variety of issues, including learning disabilities, hyperactivity, language and social skill impairment, and concentration difficulties [45]. The amount of adenosine is also increased by ethanol, which may cause memory loss and shorten the route by speeding memory loss and encouraging energetic, spontaneous movements [46]. Yet, the anti-inflammatory action and the regulation of the balance of Glu and GABA can be employed to examine the memory impairment brought on by prolonged alcohol use. Although more research is still needed to fully understand the specific biochemical pathways, alcohol can seriously impair memory and learning [47, 48].

4.6.6 SODIUM AZIDE-INDUCED AD

A white crystalline substance known as sodium azide (NaN_3) has been connected to the formation of lead azide explosive as a mitochondrial poison

[49]. By inhibiting cytochrome oxidase, a vital mitochondrial enzyme, NaN_3 treatment has been shown to cause mitochondrial malfunction. In the mitochondrial respiratory chain, cytochrome oxidase is essential; its interference hinders mitochondrial complex-IV and lowers ATP levels, which contribute to metabolic impairment and ROS production and eventually result in various AD sequelae [50]. One of the crucial characteristics utilized to establish the induction of AD using minipumps to administer NaN_3 is neuronal loss in the CA3 region of the hippocampus.

4.7 PROSPECTS OF CURBING DRUG-INDUCED AD

The hippocampus may be affected by chemical medications such as colchicine, scopolamine, OKA, STZ, and TMT, which could cause AD [49]. In the past, we looked at TMT neurotoxicity in numerous research and found that TMT led to the death of neurons, anxiety, depression, memory loss, and hippocampus-induced neuronal death. Additionally, based on the research, we hypothesized that additional drugs used to induce AD, such as colchicine, scopolamine, OKA, and STZ, exhibit hippocampus-related neuronal degeneration [50].

Systematic evaluations revealed that cognitive stimulation improved various elements of well-being and cognitive performance in patients with Alzheimer's dementia [51]. Exercises for reality orientation and item classification were used to stimulate cognitive function. There was not a single form of cognitive stimulation that was found to be more efficient than another. Cognitive benefits persisted for up to three months after cognitive stimulation activities were finished [52]. Another systematic analysis found that cognitive stimulation was linked to better results on tests of depression in adults with mild-to-moderate Alzheimer's disease. Mood, challenging behaviors, or capacity to carry out everyday activities were unaffected by cognitive stimulation.

New word issues in writing or speaking: Alzheimer's patients may find it difficult to follow or participate in a discussion [53]. They can pause in the middle of a sentence and be unable to pick up where they left off, or they might speak again. They could have trouble using terminology, finding the right words, or referring to items incorrectly (such as calling a watch a "hand clock") [54].

The nerve cells in the frontal (frontal lobe) and side (temporal lobes) regions of the brain are particularly affected and considerably atrophy (shrunken). Furthermore, abnormal protein inclusions usually form in the cortex's upper layers, which also frequently become mushy and spongy (Usually, tau protein or the transactive response DNA-binding protein) [55]. Similar to Alzheimer's, FTLD symptoms may appear in adults 65 years of age and beyond, but for the most part, FTLD symptoms appear in younger patients [56]. The age range for those who have FTLD is between 45 and 60 years. Less than 10% of dementia cases are due to FTLD [57].

4.8 CONCLUSION

Among the substances that have been demonstrated to be neurotoxic and that have been utilized to make mice develop cognitive impairment resembling AD are scopolamine, STZ, etc. Each chemical may work through distinct, specialized ways to aggravate AD development. In order to cause severe illness in human patients, the dosage and the duration at which the drug is delivered in rodent AD models may be greater or occasionally lower. Notably, the method of administration, type, length (particularly), and age and gender of the studied animals are other characteristics connected to the chemicals that cause Alzheimer's disease. Designing research that incorporates cognitive impairment brought on by chemicals requires a grasp of this.

Finally, it is concluded that there are presently no effective or disease-modifying medications for AD. The course of AD is accompanied by molecular and clinical processes including amyloid accumulation, neuro-inflammation, tau accumulation, neuronal degeneration, cognitive decline, and the appearance of behavioral and psychiatric disorders. The need to create and adopt novel therapies is urgent given the increasing prevalence of dementia and the relative insufficiency of present pharmaceutical treatments. Though intriguing, recent findings from studies of AD medications with possible disease-modifying effects must also be viewed with caution. It is also stated that early administration of AD medication and patient monitoring for disease development via biomarker diagnostics are essential for its success. The development of AD pathology might be slowed in the future by treatments that specifically target tau pathology and by using combination medicines.

KEYWORDS

- **Alzheimer's disease**
- **colchicine**
- **dementia**
- **neuroinflammation**
- **pharmaceutical treatments**
- **relative insufficiency**
- **scopolamine**
- **streptozotocin**

REFERENCES

1. Barten, D. M., & Albright, C. F. (2008). Therapeutic strategies for Alzheimer's disease. Molecular Neurobiology, 37(2–3), 171–186. https://doi.org/10.1007/s12035-008-8038-8.
2. de la Torre, J. C. (2004). Is Alzheimer's disease a neurodegenerative or a vascular disorder? Data, dogma, and dialectics. The Lancet Neurology, 3(3), 184–190. https://doi.org/10.1016/S1474-4422(04)00705-5.
3. Kumar, A., Dogra, S., & Prakash, A. (2010). Protective effect of naringin, a citrus flavonoid, against colchicine-induced cognitive dysfunction and oxidative damage in rats. Journal of Medicinal Food, 13(4), 976–984. https://doi.org/10.1089/jmf.2009.0138.
4. Götz, J., & Ittner, L. M. (2008). Animal models of Alzheimer's disease and frontotemporal dementia. Nature Reviews Neuroscience, 9(7), 532–544. https://doi.org/10.1038/nrn2416.
5. Nordberg, A., & Svensson, A. L. (1998). Cholinesterase inhibitors in the treatment of Alzheimer's disease: A comparison of tolerability and pharmacology. Drug Safety, 19, 465–480. https://doi.org/10.2165/00002018-199819060-00001.
6. Jack, C. R., Jr., Albert, M. S., Knopman, D. S., McKhann, G. M., Sperling, R. A., Carrillo, M. C., Thies, B., & Phelps, C. H. (2011). Introduction to the recommendations from the National Institute on Aging-Alzheimer's Association workgroups on diagnostic guidelines for Alzheimer's disease. Alzheimer's & Dementia: The Journal of the Alzheimer's Association, 7(3), 257–262. https://doi.org/10.1016/j.jalz.2011.03.003.
7. Krell-Roesch, J., Rakusa, M., Syrjanen, J. A., van Harten, A. C., Lowe, V. J., Jack, C. R., Jr., Kremers, W. K., Knopman, D. S., Stokin, G. B., Petersen, R. C., Vassilaki, M., & Geda, Y. E. (2022). Association between CSF biomarkers of Alzheimer's disease and neuropsychiatric symptoms: Mayo Clinic Study of Aging. Alzheimer's & Dementia: The Journal of the Alzheimer's Association, 19(4), 1518–1528. https://doi.org/10.1002/alz.12795.

8. McKhann, G. M., Knopman, D. S., Chertkow, H., Hyman, B. T., Jack, C. R., Jr., Kawas, C. H., Klunk, W. E., Koroshetz, W. J., Manly, J. J., Mayeux, R., Mohs, R. C., Morris, J. C., Rossor, M. N., Scheltens, P., Carrillo, M. C., Thies, B., Weintraub, S., & Phelps, C. H. (2011). The diagnosis of dementia due to Alzheimer's disease: Recommendations from the National Institute on Aging-Alzheimer's Association workgroups on diagnostic guidelines for Alzheimer's disease. Alzheimer's & Dementia: The Journal of the Alzheimer's Association, 7(3), 263–269. https://doi.org/10.1016/j.jalz.2011.03.005.
9. Villemagne, V. L., Burnham, S., Bourgeat, P., Brown, B., Ellis, K. A., Salvado, O., Szoeke, C., Macaulay, S. L., Martins, R., Maruff, P., Ames, D., Rowe, C. C., & Masters, C. L. (2013). Amyloid β deposition, neurodegeneration, and cognitive decline in sporadic Alzheimer's disease: A prospective cohort study. The Lancet Neurology, 12(4), 357–367. https://doi.org/10.1016/S1474-4422(13)70044-9.
10. Price, J. L., Davis, P. B., Morris, J. C., & White, D. L. (1991). The distribution of tangles, plaques, and related immunohistochemical markers in healthy aging and Alzheimer's disease. Neurobiology of Aging, 12(4), 295–312. https://doi.org/10.1016/0197-4580(91)90053-6.
11. Nelson, P. T., Head, E., Schmitt, F. A., Davis, P. R., Neltner, J. H., Jicha, G. A., Abner, E. L., Smith, C. D., Van Eldik, L. J., Kryscio, R. J., & Scheff, S. W. (2011). Alzheimer's disease is not "brain aging": Neuropathological, genetic, and epidemiological human studies. Acta Neuropathologica, 121(5), 571–587. https://doi.org/10.1007/s00401-011-0823-2.
12. Schneider, J. A., Arvanitakis, Z., Leurgans, S. E., & Bennett, D. A. (2009). The neuropathology of probable Alzheimer's disease and mild cognitive impairment. Annals of Neurology, 66(2), 200–208. https://doi.org/10.1002/ana.21705.
13. Spinney, L. (2014). Alzheimer's disease: The forgetting gene. Nature, 510(7503), 26–28. https://doi.org/10.1038/510026a.
14. Jackson, M., Pelone, F., Reeves, S., Hassenkamp, A. M., Emery, C., Titmarsh, K., & Greenwood, N. (2016). Interprofessional education in the care of people diagnosed with dementia and their carers: A systematic review. BMJ Open, 6(8), e010948. https://doi.org/10.1136/bmjopen-2015-010948.
15. Stojkovska, I., Krainc, D., & Mazzulli, J. R. (2018). Molecular mechanisms of α-synuclein and GBA1 in Parkinson's disease. Cell and Tissue Research, 373(1), 51–60. https://doi.org/10.1007/s00441-018-2833-7.
16. Holtzman, D. M., Herz, J., & Bu, G. (2012). Apolipoprotein E and apolipoprotein E receptors: Normal biology and roles in Alzheimer disease. Cold Spring Harbor Perspectives in Medicine, 2(3), a006312. https://doi.org/10.1101/cshperspect.a006312.
17. Voisin, T., & Vellas, B. (2009). Diagnosis and treatment of patients with severe Alzheimer's disease. Drugs & Aging, 26(2), 135–144. https://doi.org/10.2165/00002512-200926020-00002.
18. Wilson, R. S., Segawa, E., Boyle, P. A., Anagnos, S. E., Hizel, L. P., & Bennett, D. A. (2012). The natural history of cognitive decline in Alzheimer's disease. Psychology and Aging, 27(4), 1008–1017. https://doi.org/10.1037/a0029308.
19. Groot, C., Hooghiemstra, A. M., Raijmakers, P. G., van Berckel, B. N., Scheltens, P., Scherder, E. J., van der Flier, W. M., & Ossenkoppele, R. (2016). The effect of physical activity on cognitive function in patients with dementia: A meta-analysis of randomized control trials. Ageing Research Reviews, 25, 13–23. https://doi.org/10.1016/j.arr.2015.11.005.

20. Loy, C. T., Schofield, P. R., Turner, A. M., & Kwok, J. B. (2014). Genetics of dementia. Lancet (London, England), 383(9919), 828–840. https://doi.org/10.1016/S0140-6736(13)60714-3.
21. Petersen, R. C., Lopez, O., Armstrong, M. J., Getchius, T. S. D., Ganguli, M., Gloss, D., Gronseth, G. S., Marson, D., Pringsheim, T., Day, G. S., Sager, M., Stevens, J., & Rae-Grant, A. (2018). Practice guideline update summary: Mild cognitive impairment: Report of the guideline development, dissemination, and implementation subcommittee of the American Academy of Neurology. *Neurology, 90*(3), 126–135. https://doi.org/10.1212/WNL.0000000000004822.
22. Hebert, L. E., Bienias, J. L., Aggarwal, N. T., Wilson, R. S., Bennett, D. A., Shah, R. C., & Evans, D. A. (2010). Change in risk of Alzheimer's disease over time. *Neurology, 75*(9), 786–791. https://doi.org/10.1212/WNL.0b013e3181f53b7a.
23. Mayeux, R., Sano, M., Chen, J., Tatemichi, T., & Stern, Y. (1991). Risk of dementia in first-degree relatives of patients with Alzheimer's disease and related disorders. *Archives of Neurology, 48*(3), 269–273. https://doi.org/10.1001/archneur.1991.00530270069013.
24. Jellinger, K. A. (2007). The enigma of mixed dementia. *Alzheimer's & Dementia: The Journal of the Alzheimer's Association, 3*(1), 40–53. https://doi.org/10.1016/j.jalz.2006.11.006.
25. Lott, I. T., & Dierssen, M. (2010). Cognitive deficits and associated neurological complications in individuals with Down's syndrome. *The Lancet Neurology, 9*(6), 623–633. https://doi.org/10.1016/S1474-4422(10)70090-7.
26. Roberts, R., & Knopman, D. S. (2013). Classification and epidemiology of MCI. *Clinics in Geriatric Medicine, 29*(4), 753–772. https://doi.org/10.1016/j.cger.2013.07.004.
27. Schneider, J. A., Arvanitakis, Z., Bang, W., & Bennett, D. A. (2007). Mixed brain pathologies account for most dementia cases in community-dwelling older persons. *Neurology, 69*(24), 2197–2204. https://doi.org/10.1212/01.wnl.0000271090.28148.e4.
28. Michaelson, D. M. (2014). APOE ε4: The most prevalent yet understudied risk factor for Alzheimer's disease. *Alzheimer's & Dementia: The Journal of the Alzheimer's Association, 10*(6), 861–868. https://doi.org/10.1016/j.jalz.2014.03.003.
29. Saunders, A. M., Strittmatter, W. J., Schmechel, D., George-Hyslop, P. H., Pericak-Vance, M. A., Joo, S. H., Rosi, B. L., Gusella, J. F., Crapper-MacLachlan, D. R., Alberts, M. J., & et al. (1993). Association of apolipoprotein E allele epsilon 4 with late-onset familial and sporadic Alzheimer's disease. *Neurology, 43*(8), 1467–1472. https://doi.org/10.1212/WNL.43.8.1467.
30. Viswanathan, A., Rocca, W. A., & Tzourio, C. (2009). Vascular risk factors and dementia: How to move forward? *Neurology, 72*(4), 368–374. https://doi.org/10.1212/01.wnl.0000342758.40150.3e.
31. Ward, A., Tardiff, S., Dye, C., & Arrighi, H. M. (2013). Rate of conversion from prodromal Alzheimer's disease to Alzheimer's dementia: A systematic review of the literature. *Dementia and Geriatric Cognitive Disorders Extra, 3*(1), 320–332. https://doi.org/10.1159/000351513.
32. Jack, C. R., Jr., Lowe, V. J., Weigand, S. D., Wiste, H. J., Senjem, M. L., Knopman, D. S., Shiung, M. M., Gunter, J. L., Boeve, B. F., Kemp, B. J., Weiner, M., & Petersen, R. C. (2009). Serial PIB and MRI in normal, mild cognitive impairment and Alzheimer's disease: Implications for sequence of pathological events in Alzheimer's disease. *Brain: A Journal of Neurology, 132*(Pt 5), 1355–1365. https://doi.org/10.1093/brain/awp061.

33. Gilles, C., & Ertlé, S. (2000). Pharmacological models in Alzheimer's disease research. *Dialogues in Clinical Neuroscience, 2*(3), 247–255. https://doi.org/10.31887/DCNS.2000.2.3/cgilles.
34. Choi, J. H., Lee, E. B., Jang, H. H., Cha, Y. S., Park, Y. S., & Lee, S. H. (2021). Allium hookeri extracts improve scopolamine-induced cognitive impairment via activation of the cholinergic system and anti-neuroinflammation in mice. *Nutrients, 13*(8), 2718. https://doi.org/10.3390/nu13082718.
35. Jellinger, K. A., & Attems, J. (2007). Neuropathological evaluation of mixed dementia. *Journal of the Neurological Sciences, 257*(1–2), 80–87. https://doi.org/10.1016/j.jns.2007.01.039.
36. Kapasi, A., DeCarli, C., & Schneider, J. A. (2017). Impact of multiple pathologies on the threshold for clinically overt dementia. *Acta Neuropathologica, 134*(2), 171–186. https://doi.org/10.1007/s00401-017-1706-5.
37. Green, R. C., Cupples, L. A., Go, R., Benke, K. S., Edeki, T., Griffith, P. A., Williams, M., Hipps, Y., Graff-Radford, N., Bachman, D., & Farrer, L. A. (2002). Risk of dementia among white and African American relatives of patients with Alzheimer's disease. *JAMA, 287*(3), 329–336. https://doi.org/10.1001/jama.287.3.329.
38. Rajan, K. B., Barnes, L. L., Wilson, R. S., McAninch, E. A., Weuve, J., Sighoko, D., & Evans, D. A. (2017). Racial differences in the association between apolipoprotein E risk alleles and overall and total cardiovascular mortality over 18 years. *Journal of the American Geriatrics Society, 65*(11), 2425–2430. https://doi.org/10.1111/jgs.15043.
39. Kamat, P. K., Rai, S., Swarnkar, S., Shukla, R., Ali, S., Najmi, A. K., & Nath, C. (2013). Okadaic acid-induced tau phosphorylation in rat brain: Role of NMDA receptor. *Neuroscience, 238*, 97–113. https://doi.org/10.1016/j.neuroscience.2012.12.035.
40. Gordon, B. A., Blazey, T. M., Su, Y., Hari-Raj, A., Dincer, A., Flores, S., Christensen, J., McDade, E., Wang, G., Xiong, C., Cairns, N. J., Hassenstab, J., Marcus, D. S., Fagan, A. M., Jack, C. R., Jr., Hornbeck, R. C., Paumier, K. L., Ances, B. M., Berman, S. B., Brickman, A. M., Cash, D. M., Chhatwal, J. P., Correia, S., Förster, S., Fox, N. C., Graff-Radford, N. R., la Fougère, C., Levin, J., Masters, C. L., Rossor, M. N., Salloway, S., Saykin, A. J., Schofield, P. R., Thompson, P. M., Weiner, M. M., Holtzman, D. M., Raichle, M. E., Morris, J. C., & Bateman, R. J. (2018). Spatial patterns of neuroimaging biomarker change in individuals from families with autosomal dominant Alzheimer's disease: A longitudinal study. *The Lancet Neurology, 17*(3), 241–250. https://doi.org/10.1016/S1474-4422(17)30415-4.
41. Chen, Y., Liang, Z., Tian, Z., Blanchard, J., Dai, C. L., Chalbot, S., Iqbal, K., Liu, F., & Gong, C. X. (2014). Intracerebroventricular streptozotocin exacerbates Alzheimer-like changes of 3xTg-AD mice. *Molecular Neurobiology, 49*(1), 547–562. https://doi.org/10.1007/s12035-013-8464-6.
42. Reiman, E. M., Quiroz, Y. T., Fleisher, A. S., Chen, K., Velez-Pardo, C., Jimenez-Del-Rio, M., Fagan, A. M., Shah, A. R., Alvarez, S., Arbelaez, A., Giraldo, M., Acosta-Baena, N., Sperling, R. A., Dickerson, B., Stern, C. E., Tirado, V., Munoz, C., Reiman, R. A., Huentelman, M. J., Alexander, G. E., Langbaum, J. B., Kosik, K. S., Tariot, P. N., & Lopera, F. (2012). Brain imaging and fluid biomarker analysis in young adults at genetic risk for autosomal dominant Alzheimer's disease in the presenilin 1 E280A kindred: A case-control study. *The Lancet Neurology, 11*(12), 1048–1056. https://doi.org/10.1016/S1474-4422(12)70226-7.

43. Grieb, P. (2016). Intracerebroventricular streptozotocin injections as a model of Alzheimer's disease: In search of a relevant mechanism. *Molecular Neurobiology, 53*(3), 1741–1752. https://doi.org/10.1007/s12035-015-9185-6.
44. Sharma, M., Briyal, S., & Gupta, Y. K. (2005). Effect of alpha lipoic acid, melatonin, and trans-resveratrol on intracerebroventricular streptozotocin-induced spatial memory deficit in rats. *Indian Journal of Physiology and Pharmacology, 49*(4), 395–402.
45. Ye, M., Han, B. H., Kim, J. S., Kim, K., & Shim, I. (2020). Neuroprotective effect of bean phosphatidylserine on TMT-induced memory deficits in a rat model. *International Journal of Molecular Sciences, 21*(14), 4901. https://doi.org/10.3390/ijms21144901.
46. Fratiglioni, L., Ahlbom, A., Viitanen, M., & Winblad, B. (1993). Risk factors for late-onset Alzheimer's disease: A population-based, case-control study. *Annals of Neurology, 33*(3), 258–266. https://doi.org/10.1002/ana.410330308.
47. Golbidi, S., Botta, A., Gottfred, S., Nusrat, A., Laher, I., & Ghosh, S. (2014). Glutathione administration reduces mitochondrial damage and shifts cell death from necrosis to apoptosis in aging diabetic mice hearts during exercise. *British Journal of Pharmacology, 171*(23), 5345–5360. https://doi.org/10.1111/bph.12857.
48. Fukushima, R. L. M., do Carmo, E. G., Pedroso, R. D. V., Micali, P. N., Donadelli, P. S., Fuzaro, G. J., Venancio, R. C. P., Viola, J., & Costa, J. L. R. (2016). Effects of cognitive stimulation on neuropsychiatric symptoms in elderly with Alzheimer's disease: A systematic review. *Dementia & Neuropsychologia, 10*(3), 178–184. https://doi.org/10.1590/S1980-57642016DN10300004.
49. Marshall, S. A., Geil, C. R., & Nixon, K. (2016). Prior binge ethanol exposure potentiates the microglial response in a model of alcohol-induced neurodegeneration. *Brain Sciences, 6*(2), 16. https://doi.org/10.3390/brainsci6020016.
50. Tang, M. X., Stern, Y., Marder, K., Bell, K., Gurland, B., Lantigua, R., Andrews, H., Feng, L., Tycko, B., & Mayeux, R. (1998). The APOE-epsilon4 allele and the risk of Alzheimer's disease among African Americans, whites, and Hispanics. *JAMA, 279*(10), 751–755. https://doi.org/10.1001/jama.279.10.751.
51. Farrer, L. A., Cupples, L. A., Haines, J. L., Hyman, B., Kukull, W. A., Mayeux, R., Myers, R. H., Pericak-Vance, M. A., Risch, N., & van Duijn, C. M. (1997). Effects of age, sex, and ethnicity on the association between apolipoprotein E genotype and Alzheimer disease: A meta-analysis. *JAMA, 278*(16), 1349–1356. https://doi.org/10.1001/jama.278.16.1349.
52. Goldman, J. S., Hahn, S. E., Catania, J. W., LaRusse-Eckert, S., Butson, M. B., Rumbaugh, M., Strecker, M. N., Roberts, J. S., Burke, W., Mayeux, R., & Bird, T. (2011). Genetic counseling and testing for Alzheimer's disease: Joint practice guidelines of the American College of Medical Genetics and the National Society of Genetic Counselors. *Genetics in Medicine: Official Journal of the American College of Medical Genetics, 13*(6), 597–605. https://doi.org/10.1097/GIM.0b013e31821d6c5b.
53. Cherubini, M., & Wade-Martins, R. (2018). Convergent pathways in Parkinson's disease. *Cell and Tissue Research, 373*(1), 79–90. https://doi.org/10.1007/s00441-017-2728-6.
54. Evans, D. A., Bennett, D. A., Wilson, R. S., Bienias, J. L., Morris, M. C., Scherr, P. A., Hebert, L. E., Aggarwal, N., Beckett, L. A., Joglekar, R., Berry-Kravis, E., & Schneider, J. (2003). Incidence of Alzheimer disease in a biracial urban community: Relation to apolipoprotein E allele status. *Archives of Neurology, 60*(2), 185–189. https://doi.org/10.1001/archneur.60.2.185.

55. Farina, N., Rusted, J., & Tabet, N. (2014). The effect of exercise interventions on cognitive outcome in Alzheimer's disease: A systematic review. *International Psychogeriatrics, 26*(1), 9–18. https://doi.org/10.1017/S1041610213001683.
56. Rossor, M. N., Fox, N. C., Mummery, C. J., Schott, J. M., & Warren, J. D. (2010). The diagnosis of young-onset dementia. *The Lancet Neurology, 9*(8), 793–806. https://doi.org/10.1016/S1474-4422(10)70143-1.
57. Kelley, B. J., Boeve, B. F., & Josephs, K. A. (2009). Cognitive and noncognitive neurological features of young-onset dementia. *Dementia and Geriatric Cognitive Disorders, 27*(6), 564–571. https://doi.org/10.1159/000235939.

CHAPTER 5

The Road to Drug Discovery Targeting Abnormal Proteins: Taking a Glance at the Alzheimer's Treatments Through Rose-Colored Glasses

SHIVEENA BHATIA,[1] VARINDER SINGH,[2*] MOHIT KUMAR,[2] MANJINDER SINGH,[3] AMIT KUMAR,[3] KAVITA MUNJAL,[4] HASANDEEP SINGH,[5] and TANVEER SINGH[6]

[1]*Department of Pharmacology and Toxicology, Department of Pharmacy, Birla Institute of Technology and Science Pilani, Pilani Campus, Rajasthan, India*

[2]*Department of Pharmaceutical Sciences and Technology, Maharaja Ranjit Singh Punjab Technical University, Bathinda, Punjab, India*

[3]*Chitkara College of Pharmacy, Chitkara University, Punjab, India*

[4]*Amity Institute of Pharmacy, Amity University, Noida, Uttar Pradesh, India*

[5]*Department of Pharmaceutical Sciences, Guru Nanak Dev University, Amritsar, Punjab, India*

[6]*Department of Neuroscience and Experimental Therapeutics, College of Medicine, Texas A&M Health Science Center, TX, USA*

[*]Corresponding author.

ABSTRACT

Alzheimer's disease is a complex multifactorial neurodegenerative disorder that manifests as latent episodes of memory and cognitive impairment,

Neuro-Nutraceuticals and Drug Discovery and Delivery in Alzheimer's Disease, Volume 1: Targeting Key Pathological Pathways. Varinder Singh, Amit Kumar, Parul Sood (Eds.)

psychiatric symptoms, and behavioral disorders. The disease causes suffering for millions of patients worldwide. Despite extensive research, no effective treatment has been found yet. There are many underlying processes leading to the progression of this disorder, with the primary and major one being the formation and agglomeration of abnormal and misfolded proteins with neurotoxic activities. The accumulation of tau protein tangles intracellularly and β-amyloid plaques extracellularly serve as the primary pathological hallmarks and contributing factors of this deadly disorder. Many drugs and treatments have been designed to target these abnormally folded proteins, either to decrease their formation, promote their clearance, or minimize their cytotoxicity. The chapter explores various herbal therapies and phyto-constituents targeting various stages of formation and deposition of tau and β-amyloid proteins.

5.1 INTRODUCTION

According to the 2022 statistics, about 1 in 9 Americans aged 65 and older are suffering from Alzheimer's dementia. An estimated 6.5 million Americans aged 65 and older are living with Alzheimer's dementia in 2022 [1]. It is a progressive neurodegenerative disorder, first identified by Dr. Alois Alzheimer by observing the amyloid plaques and neurofibrillary tangles in the autopsied brains of the people who succumbed to the disorder. As of now, there are only a handful of therapies approved by the USFDA for the treatment of havoc caused by this disease, but it remains the cause of concern for neuropathologists all across the globe. Drug discovery efforts focus on drugs targeting various molecular pathways and clinical features of the disease in order to halt the disease progression [2]. The progressive disorder is characterized by severe cortical atrophy, leading to progressive loss of neurons. The communication link between neurons is impaired due to disrupted electrical impulses in the brain further causing dementia and cognitive impairments [3]. The major identifying feature of AD is the presence of amyloid plaques and neurofibrillary tangles. Amyloid plaques comprise extracellular deposits of Aβ plaque in the brain parenchyma and in the cerebral blood vessels. Other significant underlying pathogenic events comprise mitochondrial dysfunction, oxidative stress, impaired cellular clearance pathways like apoptosis causing excessive neuroinflammation, impaired acetylcholine neurotransmission, and many more [4]. However, even with the vast knowledge of the involved pathogenic pathways, not many treatment paradigms are available for its management and cure. With the emergence of herbals in all the arenas of healthcare, researchers have now started utilizing the immense potential harbored by nature's gifts for the management of this deadly disorder. Till now, there are multiple clinical trials evaluating the efficacy of herbal treatment in causing amelioration of symptoms and hallmarks of AD. One such Phase 2 clinical trial evaluated Curcumin formulation as a dietary supplement for patients suffering from mild to moderate AD [clinicaltrial.gov ID: NCT01001637]. Another retro-spective trial inspected the efficacy of GRAPE granules as a dietary supple-ment for the improvement of cognitive abilities in patients suffering from AD [clinicaltrial.gov ID: NCT03221894]. The traditional Chinese medicine preparations like Jia Wei Xiao Yao San granules and Gou Teng granules, Ba Ji Tian prepared in powdered formulation were also tested in AD patients for 12 weeks [clinicaltrial.gov ID: NCT03838952] [5]. The chapter explores the herbal drugs and phytoconstituents that have the potential to act on the formation, deposition, and accumulation of abnormal proteins in Alzheimer's disease.

5.2 ALZHEIMER'S DISEASE: A MAJOR PROTEINOPATHY

Aberrant and misfolded proteins with altered conformation are key identifying features of AD. This abnormal folding results in proteins turning neurotoxic from being physiological in nature initially. The abnormal proteins tend to agglomerate intracellularly in the case of tau proteins and extracellularly in synaptic spaces in the case of β-amyloid proteins, exhibiting abnormal protein-protein interactions. This whole mechanism has rendered Alzheimer's disease being termed as proteinopathy [6]. The folding of proteins in a normal or abnormal way is always influenced by multiple factors. The pathogenic processing of amyloid precursor protein (APP) leading to the formation of β-amyloid plaques results in synaptic dysfunction and also simultaneous phosphorylation of tau and activation of GSK-3β and cyclin-dependent kinase-5 (CDK5) [7]. The complete pathology of the formation of β-amyloid plaques and tau tangles has been covered in subsequent sections.

5.3 ORIGINATION OF PATHOGENIC AMYLOID PLAQUES

The APP is processed in 2 ways resulting in the generation of proteins that are non-amyloidogenic and that is amyloidogenic. The 3 secretase enzymes, i.e., α-secretase, β-secretase, and γ-secretase are responsible for cleaving APP. APP cleavage via α-secretase results in non-pathogenic non-amyloidogenic sAPPα and C-terminal fragment C83 which is further cleaved by γ-secretase leading to the generation of P3 and ACID domains which are cleared from neurons by cellular mechanisms. If the APP is cleaved by β-secretase, it results in amyloidogenic sAPPβ plaque formation and C-terminal C99. Further cleavage of results in Aβ [39, 40, 42, 43] and ACID fragments which instead of being cleared, pile up together in subcellular compartments like mitochondria, endoplasmic reticulum, and lysosomes [2, 7, 8].

5.4 HERBAL THERAPIES TARGETING AMYLOID BETA PLAQUES

β-amyloid is the major constituting part of the senile plaque, which is the signature hallmark of Alzheimer's disease and is regarded as the major driving force of the course of disease progression. Culminating their progression can be done using various pathways [3]. Various synthetic analogs have been designed that target β-amyloid plaque deposition and facilitate its clearance. With herbal therapies and complementary alternative treatment regimens making their way to every health arena, their potential is widely explored in the management of Alzheimer's disease. Herbal therapies targeting various stages of formation and deposition of Aβ are discussed in upcoming sections (Table 5.1 and Figure 5.1).

5.5 HERBALS HINDERING THE FORMATION OF AB

In the healthy human brain, the amyloid precursor protein (APP) is cleaved by α-secretase and γ-secretases, which does not result in the formation of toxic Aβ. However, when the APP is cleaved by the β-secretase enzyme, toxic Aβ production is increased, leading to accumulation in the neurons. Therefore, in order to hinder the progression of AD, drugs that promote the activity of α-secretases and dampen the activity of β-secretase are required. Many natural compounds have demonstrated this function.

The silymarin extract administered to Wistar rats expressing $A\beta_{1-42}$ at a dose of 70–140 mg/kg for 4 weeks led to a significant improvement in memory function, which resulted from the reduction in amyloid plaques in the brain and the dampening of APP expression [9]. APPV7171 Transgenic mice, when administered intragastrically with icariin (30 and 100 μmol/kg per day) for 6 months, showed a significant amelioration of Aβ burden and amyloid plaque deposition, with downregulation of APP and BACE1 expression, and remarkable improvement in memory and cognition [10]. Multiple studies have shown that Berberine is effective in modulating APP processing and BACE1 activity, along with decreasing gliosis and cognitive impairment. It has also been demonstrated to reduce Aβ-induced toxicity by attenuating the generation of Aβ-triggered monocyte chemotactic protein-1 and IL-6. Berberine also resulted in the inhibition of NOS (Nitric oxide synthase) and COX-2 by downregulating the PI3K/PKB and MAPK signaling pathway [11–14].

5.6 HERBALS HINDERING THE DEPOSITION OF AB

Uncaria rhynchophylla, which is one of the components of Kampo medicine "Yokukansan," has been shown to decrease the aggregation of $A\beta_{1-42}$. Uncarinic acid, which is one of its isolated constituents, was found to be the specific inhibitor of the nucleation phase of $A\beta_{42}$ aggregation, preventing the formation of oligomers which are mainly responsible for the synaptic dysfunction in AD [15]. Another traditional Chinese medicine formula, Shengmai Formula, consisting of *Panax ginseng, Ophiopogon japonicus*, and *Schisandra chinesis*, which has traditionally been implemented clinically in the treatment of heart failure and ischemic heart disease, was evaluated in *Caenorhabditis elegans* mice expressing $A\beta_{1-42}$. The Shengmai formula was found to reduce the number of Aβ deposits and downregulated the expression of various genes: hsp16–2, hsp16–41, ace-1, ace-2, and TNFA1PA homolog genes [16]. Treating Wistar rats expressing Aβ peptide with silymarin extract (70 and 140 mg/kg dose, once a day for 4 weeks) also showed efficacy in downregulating the Aβ plaque build-up and improving memory function when evaluated in a passive avoidance learning model.

(–)-Epigallocatechin-3-gallate was found to attenuate cognitive deterioration in AD mice models as it downregulated the APP expression. It was found to decrease the neurotoxic Aβ accumulation and upregulated the Neprilysin enzyme expression, which is associated with Aβ degradation, thus preventing the aggregation of Aβ plaques and halting the cognitive deterioration associated with the same [17, 18].

5.7 HERBALS ACCELERATING AB DEGRADATION

Onjisaponin B (1 mg/kg/day), isolated from *Polygala tenuifolia* Willd. (Family Polyagalaceae), was found to inhibit the Aβ generation by accelerating the APP breakdown without affecting β or γ-secretases [19]. Notoginsenoside R1, one of the chief ingredients present in the traditional Chinese herbal medicine Panax notoginseng, which is the root of Panax notoginseng (Burk.) Chen illustrated neuroprotective effects. It was found to cause a significant improvement in cognitive function and upregulation of acetyltransferase expression in 3-month-old mice fed with 5 mg/kg/day and 25 mg/kg/day NTR1. The mechanism behind the efficacy was found to inhibit the aggregation of Aβ and aggravate the insulin-degrading enzymes' expression in APP/PS1 mice and N2a-APP695sw cells, demonstrating its action through Aβ degradation [20, 21].

Another famous Chinese herbal decoction, Kai-Xin-San (KXS), used to treat amnesia, was evaluated, and it was found to cause Aβ degradation. The pretreatment of mice with a 1.08 g/kg/day decoction dose for 2 weeks prevented $A\beta_{42}$-induced cognitive impairment and diminished the hippocampal neuronal damage triggered by it. It was found that KXS initiated the $A\beta_{42}$ degradation and upregulated the NEP (Neprilysin) enzyme (an enzyme associated with $A\beta_{42}$ degradation) expression in the hippocampus, thus safeguarding the hippocampal neurons and enhancing cognitive ability in the rats expressing $A\beta_{42}$ [22].

Researchers found Dihydroartemisinin (DHA), the active metabolite of sesquiterpene trioxane lactone isolated from *Artemisia annua*, induces autophagy flux, ameliorates autophagy dysfunction in AD brains, and prevents abnormal neuronal death by assisting in the clearance of Aβ fibrils. This leads to a reduction in $A\beta_{40}$ and $A\beta_{42}$ levels in APP/PS1 mice brains and an improvement in the learning and memory function of mice [23].

The phyto-cannabinoids isolated from the plant *Cannabis sativa* L. (Family Cannabaceae), delta-9-tetrahydrocannabinol (THC)/cannabidiol (CBD), administered in APP/PS1 mice, led to a notable decrease in soluble Aβ fragments and a variation in plaque composition, thus reducing Aβ toxicity [24].

5.8 HERBAL DRUGS DAMPENING TOXICITY OF DEPOSITED AB

Many researchers have identified wine-related polyphenols to be effective in reducing the Aβ toxicity. Polyphenols like myricetin, morin, quercetin, kaempferol, (+)-catechin, and (–)-epicatechin were found to not only inhibit amyloid formation in a dose-dependent manner but some like myricetin and Rosemarinic acid were also found to inhibit the Aβ oligomerization and reduce the synaptic toxicity triggered by them [18, 25]. Resveratrol derived from red wine also shows a significant neuroprotective effect in patients with AD. Besides inhibiting the Aβ formation, it also inhibits the aggregation of IAPP and its amyloidogenic segment, and remodels soluble oligomers, fibrillar intermediates, and amyloid fibrils into non-toxic species, thus attenuating the cytotoxicity induced by Aβ [26, 27].

Naturally synthesized RRR-α-tocopherol quinone isolated from α-tocopherol was found to inhibit $A\beta_{42}$ fibril formation in a dose-dependent manner. It was also found to dampen the Aβ-induced neurotoxicity on SH-SY5Y neuroblastoma cells, disaggregate preformed fibrils, and disrupt the oligomer formation. Adding to its utility, it was also found to reduce the generation of reactive oxygen species and nitric oxide and regulate cytokine generation by reducing TNF-α and IL-1β [28].

Rhynchophylline, an active tetracyclic alkaloid derived from *Uncaria rhynchophylla* (Family Rubiaceae), demonstrated the inhibition of soluble $A\beta_{1-42}$ oligomer-induced increase in spontaneous discharges in the hippocampal CA1 region of rats in a concentration-dependent manner. It was also found to neutralize the harmful effects of $A\beta_{1-42}$ on the neural circuits [29].

Pretreatment of cells exposed to $A\beta_{25-35}$ with the Houttuynia Herba water extract was found to weaken the cell damage as it interfered with the elevation of intracellular calcium level, reactive oxygen species overproduction, mitochondrial membrane potential disruption, and Caspase 3 activation caused by the $A\beta_{25-35}$. Thus, it protected the neurons from the $A\beta_{25-35}$-triggered toxicity by modulating the calcium metabolism and mitochondria-mediated apoptosis [30].

Furthermore, the effect of ethyl extract from Persimmon leaves was evaluated, and it was found to be effective in exerting protective action against the cognitive defects induced by Aβ at doses of 200 mg/kg and 400 mg/kg by modulating the antioxidative defense system and mitochondria-mediated apoptosis.

5.9 HERBAL DRUGS TARGETING A-SECRETASES

A surrogate approach to minimize Aβ plaque generation and slow down the disease progression is modulating and upregulating the expression of α-secretases. α-secretase also cleaves the APP but in a non-toxic manner. It is done when the α-secretases (ADAM10, ADAM17, and ADAM9) cleave APP from the middle portion and result in the separation of large sAPPα fragments which is neuroprotective. Expression of ADAM10 can also be upregulated by activating nuclear retinoic acid receptor β, which results in non-amyloidogenic APP processing [7]. Some of the natural compounds triggering the increased expression of α-secretase comprise Huperzine A, an alkaloid isolated from Huperzia serrata which demonstrated improved cognitive action and daily activities as it activated Wnt signaling and reduced amyloidosis in AD brain by increasing α-secretase expression [31, 32].

Cryptotanshinone derived from *Salvia miltiorrhiza* was found to show improvement in learning and memory in various AD models. It was reported to attenuate the deposition of amyloid plaque in the brain of APP/PS1 transgenic mice and also reduce the formation of Aβ plaques in a concentration-dependent manner. Researchers found an increase in the concentration of N-terminal APP cleavage product, sAPPα, on treatment with Cryptotanshinone resulting in an overall improvement of spatial and learning memory [33].

The extract of *Caragana sinica* Rehder, consisting of alpha-viniferin, induces ADAM10 gene expression in peripheral tissue [34].

Curcumin compounds have also been implicated as activators of α-secretase. This includes curcumin-amino acid conjugates like curcumin-isoleucine, curcumin-phenylalanine, and curcumin-valine, which cause an elevation in ADAM10 immunoreactivity, upregulating the α-secretase activity [35].

Ligustilide, being a secondary metabolite extracted from *Ligusticum chuanxiong* Hort. (Family: Umbelliferae), possesses anti-inflammatory activity against TNF-α secretases. Studies have proved it to reduce Aβ neurotoxicity in APP/PS1 mice models at a dose of 10 or 40 mg/kg for 8 weeks [36]. It was found to target ADAM10, increasing the non-amyloidogenic processing of APP by enhancing the α-secretase activity [37, 38].

A vitamin A analog, Acitretin, upregulates ADAM10 expression and downregulates the Aβ concentration in APP/PS1 transgenic mice by acting on the retinoic acid receptor. Upregulation of α-secretase activity further leads to increased generation of sAPPα segments, which are neuroprotective [39].

Studies showed Bryostatin, a macrolide lactone derived from the bryozoan *Bugula neritina*, to decrease the mortality in AD mice models by stimulating the α-secretase activity and also enhancing the learning and memory functions [40, 41].

5.10 HERBAL DRUGS TARGETING Β-SECRETASES

BACE-1 (β-site amyloid precursor protein cleaving enzyme-1) has always been an attractive target for researchers working on designing treatments for the management of AD. BACE-1 is the rate-limiting enzyme in the process of formation of β-amyloid plaques, and inhibition of it can result in halting the most significant pathogenic factor, leading to an overall improvement in the memory and cognitive abilities of the individual. Many herbs do possess BACE-1 inhibitory effects. One of them is Curcumin, which was the first herb identified to inhibit BACE-1. It was also identified to downregulate Aβ40 and Aβ42 by inhibiting BACE-1 and inducing α-secretase [42]. Tryptoline was another herb found to act on the catalytic sites of BACE1 and inhibit it from cleaving the APP [43]. ε-viniferin, ampelosin A, vitisin A, and Vitisin B isolated from Vitis vinifera (Family: Vitaceae) resulted in dose-dependent inhibition of the BACE1 enzyme with an IC_{50} value of 0.8 μM and 0.4 μM for vitisin A and Vitisin B [44]. Another research study explored *Capsicum annuum* (Family: Solanaceae) to notably inhibit the BACE1 enzyme with an IC_{50} value of 2.17±0.17 μg/L exhibited by ripe fruits and 3.44±0.11 μg/L and also caused disintegration of preformed $A\beta_{40}$ fibrils [45]. Tannic acid also resulted in the reduction of $A\beta_{40}$ and $A\beta_{42}$ generation by causing inhibition of β-secretase [46].

5.11 HERBAL DRUGS TARGETING Γ-SECRETASES

γ-Secretases are also one of the enzymes involved in Alzheimer's physiology. They are known to cleave APP at the end of the Aβ domain in APP. Halting their action can shift the amyloidogenic process in a non-pathogenic direction by downregulating Aβ generation.

Although not many herbal γ-secretases have been explored, some of the herbal therapies targeting γ-secretases include Ginsenosides Rg1 derived from Radix Ginseng, which decreases the overall Aβ concentration generated. It exerts its inhibitory effect on the enzyme through the PKA/CREB signaling pathway, inducing neuroprotective action, enhancing neuron activity, reducing LDH release, and cytochrome C, and elevating the Bcl-2/Ba ratio [47].

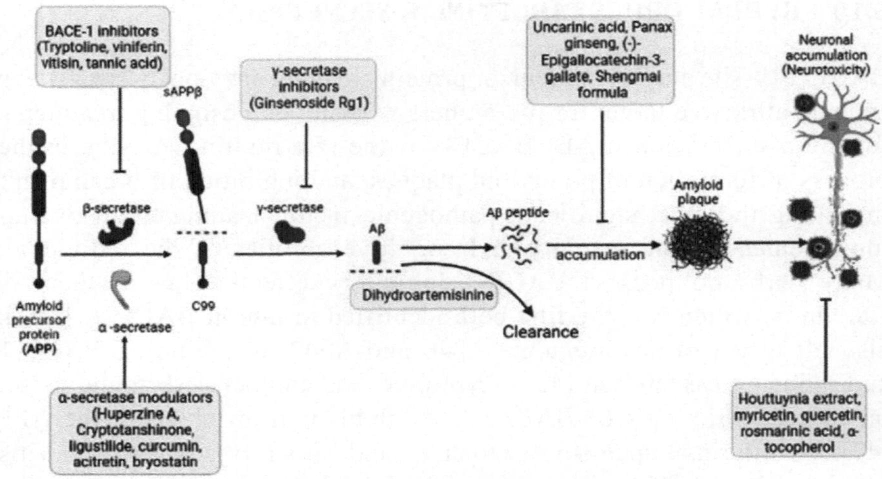

FIGURE 5.1 Herbals targeting various stages in the β-amyloid pathology.

TABLE 5.1 Herbal Phytoconstituents Targeting Aβ

Compound/Plant Species	Family	Dose	Mechanism	References
Teucrium polium	Lamiaceae	1 mg/ml	BACE-1 inhibitor and also acts on enzymes like AchE, and BchE.	[48]
Punica granatum	Lythraceae	IC50: 14.83±0.73 mg/l	–	[49]
Withania somnifera	Solanaceae	6.25–50 μg/ml	Target P13K/Akt signaling, toll-like receptors, neuro-trophins signaling, Glycogen synthase kinase-3β and β-secretase. Inhibits amyloid β fibril formation.	[50, 51]
Crocus sativus	Iridaceae	100 μg/ml	Inhibits aggregation and deposition of Aβ in the human brain.	[52]
Caesalpinia crista	Fabaceae	100 μg/ml	Inhibition of Aβ accumulation and disintegration of preformed fibrils.	[53]

TABLE 5.1 *(Continued)*

Compound/Plant Species	Family	Dose	Mechanism	References
Eleutherococcus senticosus (Siberian ginseng)	Araliaceae	1 and 10 μM	Preventing and modulating the Aβ induced axonal atrophy.	[54]
Cinnamomum zeylanicum	Lauraceae	–	Dose-dependent Inhibition of formation of fibrils and destabilization of pre-formed fibrils, decrease in deposition of Aβ.	[55]
Ficus macrophylla	Leguminosae	–	BACE inhibition and activation of insulin-degrading enzyme.	–
Houttuynia cordata	Saururaceae	0.1–100 μg/ml	Halted Aβ25–35 induced elevation of intracellular ROS, calcium ions, activation of caspase-3, and mitochondrial membrane disruption.	[30]
Zingiber officinale	Zingiberaceae	Dose-dependent inhibition with IC50 value of 52±2 μg/ml.	Prevented the oligomer formation and disintegrated the pre-formed fibrils.	[56]
Humulus japonicus	Cannabaceae	500 mg/kg/day	Reduced Aβ and tau tangles along with the downregulated expression of mRNA, TNF-α, IL-1β, and IL-6.	[57]
Pterocarpus erinaceus	Fabaceae	200 μg/ml	Inhibition of γ-secretase activity.	[58]
α-D-(1,4)-glucan derived from *Lonicera japonica*	Caprifoliaceae	200 μg/ml	Inhibited oligomerization of Aβ42 and also ameliorated the Aβ42 aggregate induced cytotoxicity.	[59]
Cochalinoside A, Polanoside A	Cactaceae	100 μg/ml	Inhibited aggregation of Aβ40 and Aβ42.	[60]
Chikusetsusaponin V derived from *Polaskia chichipe*				

TABLE 5.1 *(Continued)*

Compound/Plant Species	Family	Dose	Mechanism	References
α-Mangostin derived from *Garcinia mangostana*	Clusiaceae	25 nmol/L	Downregulation of Aβ generation by acting on β-secretase (IC50 value: 13.22 nmol/L) and γ-secretase (IC50 value: 16.98 nmol/L).	[61]
Silibinin isolated from *Silybum marianum*	Asteraceae	50 μM	Halting of oxidative damage in the hippocampus as well as inhibition of accumulation of Aβ (IC50 value: 2.36 μM) and dampening of the release of H2O2 triggered by Aβ.	[62]
Rutin derived from *Gingko Biloba*	Ginkgoaceae	200 μM	Inhibit fibrillization of Aβ and dampen the cytotoxicity induced by it in a dose-dependent manner.	[63]
Pomiferin derived from *Flemingia macrophylla*	Leguminosae	–	Altering the aggregation of Aβ by triggering the insulin-degrading enzymes.	[64]
Luteolin isolated from *Elsholtzia rugulosa*	Lamiaceae	1–10 μM	Suppression of APP (Aβ precursor protein) expression, downregulation of ROS.	[65]
Isofraxidin derived from *Eleutherococcus senticosus* (Siberian Ginseng)	Araliaceae	10 μM	Inhibition of Aβ25–35 triggered axonal and dendritic atrophy.	[54]
Z-ligustilide isolated from *Angelica Sinensis*	Apiaceae	0.1–30 μM	Safeguards against Aβ fibrils induced neurotoxicity via inhibition of p38 and triggering PI3-K/Akt signaling pathways.	[36]

5.12 HERBAL THERAPIES TARGETING TAU PROTEINS

Tau protein, serving as another key marker of AD, has been a widely researched target for scientists all across the globe. In normal human beings, tau protein supplies the microtubular framework and stability, thus aiding in the modulation of intracellular trafficking. However, in AD brains, the normal physiology of tau is hampered, leading to the development of neurofibrillary tangles or paired helical filaments [66]. In AD brains, the tau protein undergoes post-translational modifications including hyperphosphorylation, acetylation, N-glycosylation, and truncation, which serve as differentiating markers between normal tau and pathological tangles, stripping it of its normal physiological role of binding and stabilizing microtubules in the axon [2, 8]. The deposition begins in the entorhinal cortex and hippocampus and then proceeds to other regions. The tau protein in AD comprises monomers, small oligomeric species, paired helical filaments, and straight filaments. The phosphorylation of tau protein affects its ability to bind tubulin and promotes the organization of microtubules (Figure 5.2).

5.13 THERAPIES AIMED AT HALTING THE TAU PHOSPHORYLATION

Hyperphosphorylation of tau comprises one of the earliest events in the pathophysiology of AD, along with the extent of phosphorylation and changes in the level of kinases in the brains suffering from AD. This can occur as a result of an increase in kinase activity and disturbance in its regulation. Early phosphorylation events hamper the association of tau with microtubules and cause its relocation to somatodendritic compartments, resulting in an elevation in somatic tau concentration. Dysfunction in tau protein's association with microtubules affects the microtubule dynamics and transportation [66]. The AD brains demonstrate a reduction in the number and length of microtubules [67] and downregulated concentration of acetylated tubulin, which is a marker of stable microtubules along with axonal swellings [68].

Curcumin derived from *Curcuma longa* extracts was found to cause an elevation in IL-4 cytokine production and was found to decrease the Aβ and tau levels in the mice models that were found overexpressing them. Around a 40% decrease was observed in soluble fragments, a 20% decrease in insoluble fragments, and around an 80% reduction in tau protein concentration [69]. Other studies also reported turmeric to inhibit tau protein processing, and phosphorylation, and also halt the formation of neurofibrillary tangles [42].

5.14 THERAPIES WORKING AS TAU STABILIZERS AND AGGREGATION INHIBITORS

Loss of binding of tau to microtubules leads to elevated levels of tau in the cytosol, increasing the potential for tau-tau interactions and polymerization. In AD brains, the brain tissue is composed of tau multimer species like paired helical filaments, straight filaments, twisted ribbons, and small oligomeric aggregates. Larger fibrils cause cellular dysfunction and affect cellular metabolism [66, 70, 71].

Myrica cerifera (bayberry) was found to decrease endogenous and overexpressed tau protein levels in cells and murine brain slices. The flavonoids like myricetin, myricitrin, and (+)-aR, 11S-Myricanol were found to reduce the stability of tau tangles [72]. Aqueous extract of *Cinnamomum zeylanicum* (Fam. Lauraceae) at a dose of 0.11 mg/ml was found to significantly inhibit tau accumulation as well as trigger the separation of tau tangles and unravel the paired helical filaments by hampering the process of assembly of free tubulins in microtubules or filament formation in AD brain [73]. The crocin obtained from *Crocus sativus* L. (Iridaceae) was identified to halt the tau filament formation by hindering the tau protein nucleation (Table 5.2) [74]. Another study evaluated the effect of simple quinones (1,4-benzoquinone, 1,4-naphthoquinone, 9,10-anthraquinone, and 9,10-phenanthraquinone) and some anthraquinone derivatives (chrysophanol, emodin, aloe-emodin, and rhein) derived from *Rheum rhabarbarum* L. The results demonstrated that the quinones and anthraquinones led to a significant reduction in the generation of amyloid-mimicking insulin fibers and a decrease in hemolysis levels. It also impeded the generation of toxic insulin oligomers and thus halted the progression of protein misfolding [75]. Another study evaluated the efficacy of *Glycyrrhiza inflata* Batalin and *Panax ginseng* in lowering the tau protein concentration in the ΔK280tau$_{RD}$-DsRed SH-SY5Y cell model. Along with demonstrating the remarkable decrease in tau misfolding and reactive oxygen species generation, *G. inflata* further protected against the upregulation of ERN2 (pro-apoptotic factor) and lowered the concentration of unfolded protein response chaperones in these cells [76].

5.15 HERBAL THERAPIES TARGETING GSK-3B

Glycogen synthase kinase-3 is abundantly found in the central nervous system, mainly in the hippocampus region, and is reported to play a pivotal role in multiple pathways leading to the generation of lesions that signify the characteristic identifying features of AD pathology [89].

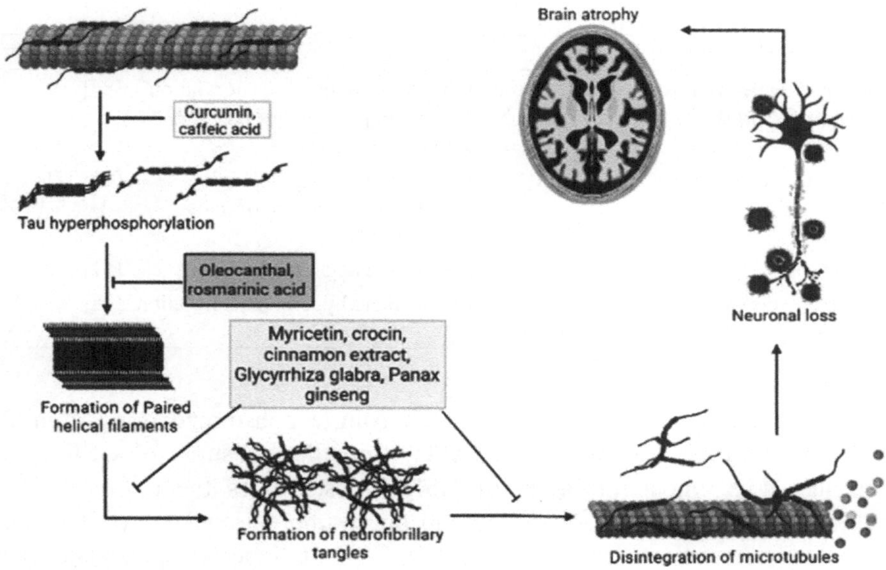

FIGURE 5.2 Herbals targeting various stages in the tau pathology.

TABLE 5.2 Herbal Phytoconstituents Targeting Tau Proteins

Compound/Plant Species	Dose	Mechanism	References
Allium sativum	3 g/mouse	Inhibits tau phosphorylation.	[41, 77]
Oleocanthal is derived from extra virgin olive oil.	100 μM	Alters the structure of tau protein, inhibits its aggregation AD prevents fibrillization.	[78, 79]
Caffeic acid	20 μg/ml	Reduced tau hyperphosphorylation.	[80]
Morin derived from *Maclura pomifera*	10 μM	Reduced tau hyperphosphorylation by inhibiting GSK-3β.	[81]
Rosmarininc acid derived from *Rosmarinus officinalis* L.	150 mg	Inhibited tau hyperphosphorylation and prevented fibrillization.	[82]
Asiatic acid derived from *Centella asiatica*	75 mg/kg body weight	Decreased phosphorylated tau by activating Akt/GSK-3β.	[83]
Fisetin	20 mg/kg/ day	Helps in the in vitro degradation of phosphorylated tau and decreases in vivo tau hyperphosphorylation.	[84]
Resveratrol	300 mg/kg	Inhibits phosphorylation via activation of PP2A and AMPK-induced activation of PI3K/Akt and inhibition of GSK-3β.	[85]

TABLE 5.2 *(Continued)*

Compound/Plant Species	Dose	Mechanism	References
Morroniside derived from *Cornus officinalis*	50–200 μM	Inhibits tau hyperphosphorylation by protein phosphatase-2A (PP2A) activation.	[86]
Epigallocatechin gallate	110 μM	Inhibits tau aggregation and elevates the clearance of phosphorylated tau.	[41, 77]
Tannic acid	30, 60 μM	Inhibits tau aggregation.	[87]
L-theanine derived from green tea	100 or 200 mg/kg/day	Inhibited tau hyperphosphorylation.	[88]

Microtubule-associated proteins like Collapsin response mediator protein-2 and Adenomatous polyposis coli (APC) form the substrate of GSK-3 in neurons; thus, phosphorylation of GSK-3 destabilizes the microtubules. Other substrates for GSK-3 are tau and microtubule-associated protein-1B (MAP-1B). In patients suffering from AD, GSK-3β hyperphosphorylates the microtubule-associated tau protein in an abnormal fashion, resulting in the separation of tau from the neuronal microtubules, leading to the generation of paired helical filaments and ultimately neurofibrillary tangles, which incapacitate the synapses and, ultimately, result in neuronal death [90]. Not only this, GSK-3 also plays a significant role in Aβ pathology by acting on the γ-secretase enzyme. Some studies also suggest that increased GSK-3 may be a cause for the increased PS1 mutations in AD brains, impairing kinesin-based motility. Given this intricate involvement of GSK-3 in Alzheimer's pathology, the inhibition of GSK-3 serves as an attractive target for halting its progression [90, 91].

Many of the marine sponge-derived phytoconstituents (sp. Porifera) are potent kinase inhibitors that act as potent inhibitors of GSK-3β. Manzamine A and other related derivatives derived from Indonesian sponges, *Acanthostrongongylophora,* showed non-competitive inhibition of GSK-3β and CDK-5, the two kinases majorly involved in tau hyperphosphorylation associated with the disease pathology. They also proved to be efficacious in downregulating the tau hyperphosphorylation in human neuroblastoma cell lines (SH-SY5Y cells) [92]. Another naturally derived marine sesquiterpene, Palinurin, also inhibits GSK-3β by an allosteric mechanism [93]. Indirubines, bis-indole compounds derived from multiple natural sources and recognized ingredients of Danggui Longhui Wan (Chinese medicine), also display potent inhibition of GSK-3 and

CDK-5 (dose: 50–100 nM) through an ATP-competitive mechanism [94]. *In-silico* studies have shown the compound to be poorly soluble, poorly absorbed, and toxic to the GIT, which has resulted in scientists investigating its substituted derivatives like indirubine-3-monoxime, which demonstrated an elevated inhibitory effect against GSK-3 and halted the *in-vivo* and *in-vitro* tau phosphorylation, as well as the phosphorylation of DARPP-32 by CDK-5 [94, 95].

Hymenialdisine extracted from marine sponges like Axinellidae, Agelasidae, and Halichondriidae also acts as an inhibitor of GSK-3β and CDK-1. It competes with ATP for binding to these kinases. It inhibits CDK5/p35 as evidenced by the downregulation of Pak1 kinase in E18 rat cortical neurons and GSK-3 *in vivo* as evidenced by the halting of MAP-1B phosphorylation. It also disrupts the *in vivo* phosphorylation of the microtubule-binding protein tau at sites that are hyperphosphorylated by GSK-3 and CDK-5/p35 in AD [96].

5.16 CONCLUSION AND FUTURE PROSPECTS

The chapter delves deep into the herbal therapies that have been explored for targeting abnormal protein accumulation in Alzheimer's disease. Various herbs and phytoconstituents have been mentioned which target various stages of formation, deposition, and cytotoxicity of the deposited plaques. However, these are only preclinical studies. The clinical efficacy of these mentioned herbs is yet to be evaluated before implicating them in clinical practice. Some drugs also exhibit the potential to cause multi-targeted degradation as they were able to target both Aβ and tau proteins, which can be a boon as AD is a combination of multiple factors. The therapeutic potential of these herbs can be further modulated artificially, and they can also be modified to target other contributing pathogenic markers. Furthermore, their mode of administration in humans remains a question as herbals, owing to their complex structure, would not be able to penetrate the blood-brain barrier to exert their function. For this issue too, researchers have started exploring nanoparticle formulations for enhancing their pharmacokinetic parameters as well as biocompatibility. The increased focus on herbal therapies also aims to minimize the adverse effects associated with synthetic therapies and enhance biocompatibility. So, while this is a positive step in the fog of uncertainty surrounding AD treatment, there remains a long way to go.

KEYWORDS

- **Alzheimer's disease**
- **amyloid precursor protein**
- **dementia**
- **neurofibrillary tangles**
- **tau tangles**
- **β-amyloid plaques**

REFERENCES

1. Alzheimer Association. (2022). 2022 Alzheimer's Disease Facts and Figures. Alzheimer's & Dementia, 15(3), 321–387. https://doi.org/10.1002/alz.12660.
2. Kumar, A., Singh, A., & Ekavali. (2015). A review on Alzheimer's disease pathophysiology and its management: An update. Pharmacological Reports, 67(2), 195–203. https://doi.org/10.1016/j.pharep.2014.09.004.
3. Behl, T., Kaur, I., Fratila, O., Brata, R., & Bungau, S. (2020). Exploring the potential of therapeutic agents targeted towards mitigating the events associated with amyloid-β cascade in Alzheimer's disease. International Journal of Molecular Sciences, 21(20), 7443. https://doi.org/10.3390/ijms21207443.
4. Bhatia, S., Rawal, R., Sharma, P., Singh, T., Singh, M., & Singh, V. (2021). Mitochondrial dysfunction in Alzheimer's disease: Opportunities for drug development. Current Neuropharmacology, 20(4), 675–692. https://doi.org/10.2174/1570159X19666210517114016.
5. Shri, R., Singh, V., Kaur, R., & Bhatia, S. (2021). Natural BACE1 inhibitors: Promising drugs for the management of Alzheimer's disease. In Alzheimer's Disease–A Comprehensive Review (pp. 137–171). https://doi.org/10.2174/978168108904112109 0007.
6. Bhatia, S., Singh, M., Singh, T., & Singh, V. (2022). Scrutinizing the therapeutic potential of PROTACs in the management of Alzheimer's disease. Neurochemical Research, 47(1), 1–13. https://doi.org/10.1007/s11064-021-03431-x.
7. Kuruva, C. S., & Reddy, P. H. (2017). Amyloid beta modulators and neuroprotection in Alzheimer's disease: A critical appraisal. Drug Discovery Today, 22(2), 223–233. https://doi.org/10.1016/j.drudis.2016.09.007.
8. DeTure, M. A., & Dickson, D. W. (2019). The neuropathological diagnosis of Alzheimer's disease. Molecular Neurodegeneration, 14(1), 32. https://doi.org/10.1186/s13024-019-0333-5.
9. Yaghmaei, P., Azarfar, K., Dezfulian, M., & Ebrahim-Habibi, A. (2014). Silymarin effect on amyloid-β plaque accumulation and gene expression of APP in an Alzheimer's disease rat model. DARU Journal of Pharmaceutical Sciences, 22(1), 24. https://doi.org/10.1186/2008-2231-22-24.

10. Zhang, L., Shen, C., Chu, J., Zhang, R., Li, Y., & Li, L. (2014). Icariin decreases the expression of APP and BACE-1 and reduces the β-amyloid burden in an APP transgenic mouse model of Alzheimer's disease. International Journal of Biological Sciences, 10(2), 181–191. https://doi.org/10.7150/ijbs.6232.
11. Haghani, M., Shabani, M., & Tondar, M. (2015). The therapeutic potential of berberine against the altered intrinsic properties of the CA1 neurons induced by Aβ neurotoxicity. European Journal of Pharmacology, 758, 82–88. https://doi.org/10.1016/j.ejphar.2015.03.016.
12. Yu, G., Li, Y., Tian, Q., Liu, R., Wang, Q., Wang, J. Z., & Wang, X. (2011). Berberine attenuates calyculin A-induced cytotoxicity and tau hyperphosphorylation in HEK293 cells. Journal of Alzheimer's Disease, 24(3), 525–535. https://doi.org/10.3233/JAD-2011-101779.
13. Jia, L., Liu, J., Song, Z., Pan, X., Chen, L., Cui, X., & Wang, M. (2012). Berberine suppresses amyloid-beta-induced inflammatory response in microglia by inhibiting nuclear factor-kappaB and mitogen-activated protein kinase signaling pathways. Journal of Pharmacy and Pharmacology, 64(10), 1510–1521. https://doi.org/10.1111/j.2042-7158.2012.01529.x.
14. Sadhukhan, P., Saha, S., Dutta, S., Mahalanobish, S., & Sil, P. C. (2018). Nutraceuticals: An emerging therapeutic approach against the pathogenesis of Alzheimer's disease. Pharmacological Research, 129, 100–114. https://doi.org/10.1016/j.phrs.2017.11.028.
15. Yoshioka, T., Murakami, K., Ido, K., Hanaki, M., Yamaguchi, K., Midorikawa, S., Taniwaki, S., Gunji, H., & Irie, K. (2016). Semisynthetic and structure-activity studies of uncarinic acid C isolated from Uncaria rhynchophylla as a specific inhibitor of the nucleation phase in amyloid β42 aggregation. Journal of Natural Products, 79(10), 2521–2529. https://doi.org/10.1021/acs.jnatprod.6b00392.
16. Zhang, W., Zhi, D., Ren, H., Wang, D., Wang, X., Zhang, Z., Fei, D., Zhu, H., & Li, H. (2016). Shengmai formula ameliorates pathological characteristics in AD C. elegans. Cellular and Molecular Neurobiology, 36(8), 1291–1302. https://doi.org/10.1007/s10571-015-0326-z.
17. Chang, X., Rong, C., Chen, Y., Yang, C., Hu, Q., Mo, Y., Zhang, C., Gu, X., Zhang, L., He, W., Cheng, S., Hou, X., Su, R., Liu, S., Dun, W., Wang, Q., & Fang, S. (2015). (−)-Epigallocatechin-3-gallate attenuates cognitive deterioration in Alzheimer's disease model mice by upregulating neprilysin expression. Experimental Cell Research, 334(1), 136–145. https://doi.org/10.1016/j.yexcr.2015.04.004.
18. Cheng, B., Gong, H., Xiao, H., Petersen, R. B., Zheng, L., & Huang, K. (2013). Inhibiting toxic aggregation of amyloidogenic proteins: A therapeutic strategy for protein misfolding diseases. Biochimica et Biophysica Acta–General Subjects, 1830(10), 4860–4871. https://doi.org/10.1016/j.bbagen.2013.06.029.
19. Li, X., Cui, J., Yu, Y., Li, W., Hou, Y., Wang, X., Qin, D., Zhao, C., Yao, X., Zhao, J., & Pei, G. (2016). Traditional Chinese nootropic medicine Radix Polygalae and its active constituent Onjisaponin B reduce β-amyloid production and improve cognitive impairments. PLoS One, 11(3), e0151147. https://doi.org/10.1371/journal.pone.0151147.
20. Ma, Y., Yang, M., Li, X., Yue, J., Chen, J., Yang, M., Huang, X., Zhu, L., Hong, F., & Yang, S. (2019). Therapeutic effects of natural drugs on Alzheimer's disease. Frontiers in Pharmacology. https://doi.org/10.3389/fphar.2019.00070.

21. Li, Z., Li, H., Zhao, C., Lv, C., Zhong, C., Xin, W., & Zhang, W. (2015). Protective effect of notoginsenoside R1 on an APP/PS1 mouse model of Alzheimer's disease by up-regulating insulin-degrading enzyme and inhibiting Aβ accumulation. *CNS & Neurological Disorders–Drug Targets, 14*(3), 360–369. https://doi.org/10.2174/18715 27314666150629124537.
22. Wang, N., Jia, Y., Zhang, B., Li, Y., Murtaza, G., Huang, S., & Liu, X. (2020). Kai-Xin-San, a Chinese herbal decoction, accelerates the degradation of β-amyloid by enhancing the expression of neprilysin in rats. *Evidence-Based Complementary and Alternative Medicine, 2020*, 3862342. https://doi.org/10.1155/2020/3862342.
23. Zhao, Y., Long, Z., Ding, Y., Jiang, T., Liu, J., Li, Y., Liu, Y., Peng, X., Wang, K., Feng, M., & He, G. (2020). Dihydroartemisinic ameliorates learning and memory in Alzheimer's disease by promoting autophagosome-lysosome fusion and autolysosomal degradation for Aβ clearance. *Frontiers in Aging Neuroscience*. https://doi.org/10.3389/fnagi.2020.00275.
24. Aso, E., Sánchez-Pla, A., Vegas-Lozano, E., Maldonado, R., & Ferrer, I. (2015). Cannabis-based medicine reduces multiple pathological processes in AβPP/PS1 mice. *Journal of Alzheimer's Disease, 43*(3), 977–991. https://doi.org/10.3233/JAD-141014.
25. Ono, K., Li, L., Takamura, Y., Yoshiike, Y., Zhu, L., Han, F., Mao, X., Ikeda, T., Takasaki, J., Nishijo, H., Takashima, A., Teplow, D. B., Zagorski, M. G., & Yamada, M. (2012). Phenolic compounds prevent amyloid β-protein oligomerization and synaptic dysfunction by site-specific binding. *Journal of Biological Chemistry, 287*(18), 14631–14643. https://doi.org/10.1074/jbc.M111.325456.
26. Jiang, P., Li, W., Shea, J. E., & Mu, Y. (2011). Resveratrol inhibits the formation of multiple-layered β-sheet oligomers of the human islet amyloid polypeptide segment 22–27. *Biophysical Journal, 100*(6), 1550–1558. https://doi.org/10.1016/j.bpj.2011.02.010.
27. Feng, Y., Wang, X., Yang, S., Wang, Y., Zhang, X., Du, X., Sun, X., Zhao, M., Huang, L., & Liu, R. (2009). Resveratrol inhibits beta-amyloid oligomeric cytotoxicity but does not prevent oligomer formation. *Neurotoxicology, 30*(6), 986–995. https://doi.org/10.1016/j.neuro.2009.08.013.
28. Yang, S., Wang, W., Ling, T., Feng, Y., Du, X., Zhang, X., Sun, X., Zhao, M., Xue, D., Yang, Y., & Liu, R. (2010). Alpha-tocopherol quinone inhibits beta-amyloid aggregation and cytotoxicity, disaggregates preformed fibrils, and decreases the production of reactive oxygen species, NO, and inflammatory cytokines. *Neurochemistry International, 57*(8), 914–922. https://doi.org/10.1016/j.neuint.2010.09.011.
29. Shao, H., Mi, Z., Ji, W., Zhang, C., Zhang, T., Ren, S., & Zhu, Z. (2015). Rhynchophylline protects against the amyloid β-induced increase of spontaneous discharges in the hippocampal CA1 region of rats. *Neurochemical Research, 40*(11), 2365–2373. https://doi.org/10.1007/s11064-015-1730-y.
30. Park, H., & Oh, M. S. (2012). Houttuyniae herbal protects rat primary cortical cells from Aβ25–35-induced neurotoxicity via regulation of calcium influx and mitochondria-mediated apoptosis. *Human & Experimental Toxicology, 31*(7), 698–709. https://doi.org/10.1177/0960327111433898.
31. Wang, C. Y., Zheng, W., Wang, T., Xie, J. W., Wang, S. L., Zhao, B. L., Teng, W. P., & Wang, Z. Y. (2011). Huperzine A activates Wnt/β-catenin signaling and enhances the nonamyloidogenic pathway in an Alzheimer transgenic mouse model. *Neuropsychopharmacology, 36*(5), 1073–1089. https://doi.org/10.1038/npp.2010.260.

32. Friedli, M. J., & Inestrosa, N. C. (2021). Huperzine A and its neuroprotective molecular signaling in Alzheimer's disease. *Molecules, 26(21), 6531.* https://doi.org/10.3390/molecules26216531.
33. Mei, Z., Zhang, F., Tao, L., Zheng, W., Cao, Y., Wang, Z., Tang, S., Le, K., Chen, S., Pi, R., & Liu, P. (2009). Cryptotanshinone, a compound from *Salvia miltiorrhiza*, modulates amyloid precursor protein metabolism and attenuates β-amyloid deposition through upregulating α-secretase in vivo and in vitro. *Neuroscience Letters, 452*(2), 90–95. https://doi.org/10.1016/j.neulet.2009.01.013.
34. Schuck, F., Schmitt, U., Reinhardt, S., Freese, C., Lee, I. S., Thines, E., Efferth, T., & Endres, K. (2015). Extract of *Caragana sinica* as a potential therapeutic option for increasing alpha-secretase gene expression. *Phytomedicine, 22*(11), 1027–1036. https://doi.org/10.1016/j.phymed.2015.08.001.
35. Narasingapa, R. B., Jargaval, M. R., Pullabhatla, S., Htoo, H. H., Rao, J. K. S., Hernandez, J. F., Govitrapong, P., & Vincent, B. (2012). Activation of α-secretase by curcumin-aminoacid conjugates. *Biochemical and Biophysical Research Communications, 424*(4), 691–696. https://doi.org/10.1016/j.bbrc.2012.07.010.
36. Xu, Y. J., Mei, Y., Qu, Z. L., Zhang, S. J., Zhao, W., Fang, J. S., Wu, J., Yang, C., Liu, S. J., Fang, Y. Q., Wang, Q., & Zhang, Y. B. (2018). Ligustilide ameliorates memory deficiency in APP/PS1 transgenic mice by restoring mitochondrial dysfunction. *Biomedical Research International, 2018*, 4606752. https://doi.org/10.1155/2018/4606752.
37. Lee, J. H., Ahn, N. H., Choi, S. B., Kwon, Y., & Yang, S. H. (2021). Natural products targeting amyloid beta in Alzheimer's disease. *International Journal of Molecular Sciences, 22(25), 2341.* https://doi.org/10.3390/ijms22052341.
38. Kuang, X., Zhou, H. J., Thorne, A. H., Chen, X. N., Li, L. J., & Du, J. R. (2017). Neuroprotective effect of ligustilide through induction of α-secretase processing of both APP and Klotho in a mouse model of Alzheimer's disease. *Frontiers in Aging Neuroscience, 9, 353.* https://doi.org/10.3389/fnagi.2017.00353.
39. Tippmann, F., Hundt, J., Schneider, A., Endres, K., & Fahrenholz, F. (2009). Up-regulation of the α-secretase ADAM10 by retinoic acid receptors and acitretin. *FASEB Journal, 23*(6), 1643–1654. https://doi.org/10.1096/fj.08-121664.
40. Schrott, L. M., Jackson, K., Yi, P., Dietz, F., Johnson, G. S., Basting, T. F., Purdum, G., Tyler, T., Rios, J. D., & Castor, T. P. (2015). Acute oral bryostatin-1 administration improves learning deficits in the APP/PS1 transgenic mouse model of Alzheimer's disease. *Current Alzheimer Research, 12*(1), 22–31. https://doi.org/10.2174/1567205012666151103112928.
41. Andrade, S., Ramalho, M. J., Loureiro, J. A., & Pereira, M. do C. (2019). Natural compounds for Alzheimer's disease therapy: A systematic review of preclinical and clinical studies. *International Journal of Molecular Sciences, 20*(9), 2313. https://doi.org/10.3390/ijms20092313.
42. Serafini, M. M., Catanzaro, M., Rosini, M., Racchi, M., & Lanni, C. (2017). Curcumin in Alzheimer's disease: Can we think of new strategies and perspectives for this molecule? *Pharmacological Research, 124*, 146–155. https://doi.org/10.1016/j.phrs.2017.08.004.
43. Oehlrich, D., Peschiulli, A., Tresadern, G., Van Gool, M., Vega, J. A., De Lucas, A. I., Alonso de Diego, S. A., Prokopcova, H., Austin, N., Van Brandt, S., Surkyn, M., De Cleyn, M., Vos, A., Rombouts, F. J. R., Macdonald, G., Moechars, D., Gijsen, H. J. M., & Trabanco, A. A. (2019). Evaluation of a series of β-secretase 1 inhibitors containing

novel heteroaryl-fused-piperazine amidine warheads. *ACS Medicinal Chemistry Letters, 10*(8), 1159–1165. https://doi.org/10.1021/acsmedchemlett.9b00181.

44. Choi, M., Choi, C., Cha, M. R., Yon, G. H., Kwon, D. Y., Kim, Y. S., Park, W. K., & Ryu, S. Y. (2009). A new specific BACE-1 inhibitor from the stembark extract of *Vitis vinifera*. *Planta Medica, 75*(5), 537–540. https://doi.org/10.1055/s-0029-1185311.
45. Ogunruku, O. O., Oboh, G., Passamonti, S., Tramer, F., & Boligon, A. A. (2017). *Capsicum annuum* var. grossum (bell pepper) inhibits β-secretase activity and β-amyloid 1–40 aggregation. *Journal of Medicinal Food, 20*(2), 124–130. https://doi.org/10.1089/jmf.2016.0077.
46. Braidy, N., Jugder, B. E., Poljak, A., Jayasena, T., Mohammad Nabavi, S., Sachdev, P., & Grant, R. (2017). Molecular targets of tannic acid in Alzheimer's disease. *Current Alzheimer Research, 14(8)*, 861–869.
47. Wang, Z. Y., Liu, J. G., Li, H., & Yang, H. M. (2016). Pharmacological effects of active components of Chinese herbal medicine in the treatment of Alzheimer's disease: A review. *American Journal of Chinese Medicine, 44*(8), 1525–1541. https://doi.org/10.1142/S0192415X16500853.
48. Benchikha, N., Messaoudi, M., Larkem, I., Ouakouak, H., Rebiai, A., Boubekeur, S., Ferhat, M. A., Benarfa, A., Begaa, S., Benmohamed, M., Almasri, D. M., Hareeri, R. H., & Youssef, F. S. (2022). Evaluation of possible antioxidant, anti-hyperglycaemic, anti-Alzheimer, and anti-inflammatory effects of *Teucrium polium* aerial parts (Lamiaceae). *Life, 12(10), 1579*. https://doi.org/10.3390/life12101579.
49. Bekir, J., Mars, M., Souchard, J. P., & Bouajila, J. (2013). Assessment of antioxidant, anti-inflammatory, anti-cholinesterase, and cytotoxic activities of pomegranate (*Punica granatum*) leaves. *Food and Chemical Toxicology, 55*, 470–475. https://doi.org/10.1016/j.fct.2013.01.036.
50. Hannan, M. A., Dash, R., Haque, M. N., Choi, S. M., & Moon, I. S. (2020). Integrated system pharmacology and in silico analysis elucidating neuropharmacological actions of *Withania somnifera* in the treatment of Alzheimer's disease. *CNS & Neurological Disorders–Drug Targets, 19*(7), 541–556. https://doi.org/10.2174/1871527319999200730214807.
51. Kumar, S., Harris, R. J., Seal, C. J., & Okello, E. J. (2012). An aqueous extract of *Withania somnifera* root inhibits amyloid β fibril formation in vitro. *Phytotherapy Research, 26*(1), 113–117. https://doi.org/10.1002/ptr.3512.
52. Papandreou, M. A., Kanakis, C. D., Polissiou, M. G., Efthimiopoulos, S., Cordopatis, P., Margarity, M., & Lamari, F. N. (2006). Inhibitory activity on amyloid-β aggregation and antioxidant properties of *Crocus sativus* stigmas extract and its crocin constituents. *Journal of Agricultural and Food Chemistry, 54*(23), 8762–8768. https://doi.org/10.1021/jf061932a.
53. Ramesh, B. N., Indi, S. S., & Rao, K. S. J. (2010). Anti-amyloidogenic property of leaf aqueous extract of *Caesalpinia cristia*. *Neuroscience Letters, 475*(2), 110–114. https://doi.org/10.1016/j.neulet.2010.03.062.
54. Bai, Y., Tohda, C., Zhu, S., Hattori, M., & Komatsu, K. (2011). Active components from Siberian ginseng (*Eleutherococcus senticosus*) for protection of amyloid β (25–35)-induced neuritic atrophy in cultured rat cortical neurons. *Journal of Natural Medicines, 65*(3), 417–423. https://doi.org/10.1007/s11418-011-0509-y.
55. Frydman-Marom, A., Levin, A., Farfara, D., Benromano, T., Scherzer-Attali, R., Peled, S., Vassar, R., Segal, D., Gazit, E., Frenkel, D., & Ovadia, M. (2011). Orally administrated

cinnamon extract reduces β-amyloid oligomerization and corrects cognitive impairment in Alzheimer's disease animal models. *PLoS One, 6*(1), e16564. https://doi.org/10.1371/journal.pone.0016564.

56. Mathew, M., & Subramanian, S. (2014). In vitro evaluation of anti-Alzheimer effects of dry ginger (Zingiber officinale Roscoe) extract. Indian Journal of Experimental Biology, 52(6), 606–612.
57. Park, T. S., Ryu, Y. K., Park, H. Y., Kim, J. Y., Go, J., Noh, J. R., Kim, Y. H., Hwang, J. H., Choi, D. H., & Oh, W. K. (2017). *Humulus japonicus* inhibits the progression of Alzheimer's disease in an APP/PS1 transgenic mouse model. *International Journal of Molecular Medicine, 39*(1), 21–30.
58. Hage, S., Kienlen-Campard, P., Octave, J. N., & Quetin-Leclercq, J. (2010). In vitro screening on β-amyloid peptide production of plants used in traditional medicine for cognitive disorders. *Journal of Ethnopharmacology, 131*(3), 585–591. https://doi.org/10.1016/j.jep.2010.07.044.
59. Zhou, L., Zhang, T., Lu, B., Yu, Z., Mei, X., Abulizi, P., & Ji, L. (2016). *Lonicerae japonicae* flos attenuates diabetic retinopathy by inhibiting retinal angiogenesis. *Journal of Ethnopharmacology, 189*, 117–125. https://doi.org/10.1016/j.jep.2016.05.039.
60. Fujihara, K., Koike, S., Ogasawara, Y., Takahashi, K., Koyama, K., & Kinoshita, K. (2017). Inhibition of amyloid β aggregation and protective effect on SH-SY5Y cells by triterpenoid saponins from the cactus *Polaskia chichipe*. *Bioorganic & Medicinal Chemistry, 25*(13), 3377–3383. https://doi.org/10.1016/j.bmc.2017.04.023.
61. Zhao, L. X., Wang, Y., Liu, T., Wang, Y. X., Chen, H. Z., Xu, J. R., & Qiu, Y. (2017). α-Mangostin decreases β-amyloid peptide production via modulation of the amyloidogenic pathway. *CNS Neuroscience & Therapeutics, 23*(6), 526–534. https://doi.org/10.1111/cns.12699.
62. Yin, F., Liu, J., Ji, X., Wang, Y., Zidichouski, J., & Zhang, J. (2011). Silibinin: A novel inhibitor of Aβ aggregation. *Neurochemistry International, 58*(3), 399–403. https://doi.org/10.1016/j.neuint.2010.12.017.
63. Wang, S., Wang, Y. J., Su, Y., Zhou, W., Yang, S., Zhang, R., Zhao, M., Li, Y., Zhang, Z., Zhan, D., & Liu, R. (2012). Rutin inhibits β-amyloid aggregation and cytotoxicity, attenuates oxidative stress, and decreases the production of nitric oxide and proinflammatory cytokines. *Neurotoxicology, 33*(3), 482–490. https://doi.org/10.1016/j.neuro.2012.03.003.
64. Lin, Y. L., Tsay, H. J., Liao, Y. F., Wu, M. F., Wang, C. N., & Shiao, Y. J. (2012). The components of *Flemingia macrophylla* attenuate amyloid β-protein accumulation by regulating the amyloid β-protein metabolic pathway. *Evidence-Based Complementary and Alternative Medicine, 2012, 795843*. https://doi.org/10.1155/2012/747930.
65. Liu, R., Meng, F., Zhang, L., Liu, A., Qin, H., Lan, X., Li, L., & Du, G. (2011). Luteolin isolated from the medicinal plant *Elsholtzia rugulosa* (Labiatae) prevents copper-mediated toxicity in β-amyloid precursor protein Swedish mutation overexpressing SH-SY5Y cells. *Molecules, 16*(3), 2084–2096. https://doi.org/10.3390/molecules16032084.
66. Congdon, E. E., & Sigurdsson, E. M. (2018). Tau-targeting therapies for Alzheimer's disease. *Nature Reviews Neurology, 14*(7), 399–415. https://doi.org/10.1038/s41582-018-0013-z.
67. Cash, A. D., Aliev, G., Siedlak, S. L., Nunomura, A., Fujioka, H., Zhu, X., Raina, A. K., Vinters, H. V., Tabaton, M., & Johnson, A. B. (2003). Microtubule reduction in

Alzheimer's disease and aging is independent of τ filament formation. *American Journal of Pathology, 162*(5), 1623–1627. https://doi.org/10.1016/S0002-9440(10)64008-1.

68. Stokin, G. B., Lillo, C., Falzone, T. L., Brusch, R. G., Rockenstein, E., Mount, S. L., Raman, R., Davies, P., Masliah, E., & Williams, D. S. (2005). Axonopathy and transport deficits early in the pathogenesis of Alzheimer's disease. *Science, 307*(5713), 1282–1288. https://doi.org/10.1126/science.1105681.
69. Shytle, R. D., Tan, J., Bickford, P. C., Rezai-zadeh, K., Hou, L., Zeng, J., & Sanberg, P. R. (2012). Optimized turmeric extract reduces β-amyloid and phosphorylated tau protein burden in Alzheimer's transgenic mice. *Current Alzheimer Research, 9*(4), 500–506. https://doi.org/10.2174/156720512800492459.
70. Kidd, M. (1963). Paired helical filaments in electron microscopy of Alzheimer's disease. *Nature, 197*, 192–193. https://doi.org/10.1038/197192a0.
71. Meraz-Ríos, M. A., Lira-De León, K. I., Campos-Peña, V., De Anda-Hernández, M. A., Mena-López, R. M., & López, J. (2010). Tau oligomers and aggregation in Alzheimer's disease. *Journal of Neurochemistry, 112*(6), 1353–1367. https://doi.org/10.1111/j.1471-4159.2009.06527.x.
72. Jones, J. R., Lebar, M. D., Jinwal, U. K., Abisambra, J. F., Koren, J. I., Blair, L., O'Leary, J. C., Davey, Z., Trotter, J., Johnson, A. G., Weeber, E., Eckman, C. B., Baker, B. J., & Dickey, C. A. (2011). The diarylheptanoid (+)-AR,11S-Myricanol, and two flavones from bayberry (*Myrica cerifera*) destabilize the microtubule-associated protein tau. *Journal of Natural Products, 74*(1), 38–44. https://doi.org/10.1021/np100572z.
73. Peterson, D. W., George, R. C., Scaramozzino, F., LaPointe, N. E., Anderson, R. A., Graves, D. J., & Lew, J. (2009). Cinnamon extract inhibits tau aggregation associated with Alzheimer's disease in vitro. *Journal of Alzheimer's Disease, 17*, 585–597. https://doi.org/10.3233/JAD-2009-1083.
74. Karakani, A. M., Riazi, G., Mahmood Ghaffari, S., Ahmadian, S., Mokhtari, F., Jalili Firuzi, M., & Zahra Bathaie, S. (2015). Inhibitory effect of corcin on aggregation of 1N/4R human tau protein in vitro. *Iranian Journal of Basic Medical Sciences, 18*(5), 485–492. https://doi.org/10.22038/IJBMS.2015.4781.
75. Gong, H., He, Z., Peng, A., Zhang, X., Cheng, B., Sun, Y., Zheng, L., & Huang, K. (2014). Effects of several quinones on insulin aggregation. *Scientific Reports, 4*, 5648. https://doi.org/10.1038/srep05648.
76. Lee-Chen, G. J., Chang, K. H., Chen, I. C., Lin, H. Y., Chen, H. C., Lin, C. H., Lin, T. H., Weng, Y. T., Chao, C. Y., Wu, Y. R., Lin, J. Y., & Chen, C. M. (2016). The aqueous extract of *Glycyrrhiza inflata* can upregulate unfolded protein response-mediated chaperones to reduce tau misfolding in cell models of Alzheimer's disease. *Drug Design, Development, and Therapy, 10*, 885–895. https://doi.org/10.2147/DDDT.S96454.
77. Armand, E. F., Shantaram, M., Nico, N. F., Simon, F. N., & Paul, M. F. (2019). Potential of medicinal plant compounds targeting tau protein in the therapy of Alzheimer's disease—A review. *Biomedicine, 39*(2), 217–227. https://doi.org/10.3892/br.2019.1144.
78. Monti, M. C., Margarucci, L., Riccio, R., & Casapullo, A. (2012). Modulation of tau protein fibrillization by oleocanthal. *Journal of Natural Products, 75*(9), 1584–1588. https://doi.org/10.1021/np300384h.
79. Li, W., Sperry, J. B., Crowe, A., Trojanowski, J. Q., Smith III, A. B., & Lee, V. M. (2009). Inhibition of tau fibrillization by oleocanthal via reaction with the amino groups of tau. *Journal of Neurochemistry, 110*(4), 1339–1351. https://doi.org/10.1111/j.1471-4159.2009.06333.x.

80. Sul, D., Kim, H. S., Lee, D., Joo, S. S., Hwang, K. W., & Park, S. Y. (2009). Protective effect of caffeic acid against beta-amyloid-induced neurotoxicity by the inhibition of calcium influx and tau phosphorylation. Life Sciences, 84(9), 257–262. https://doi.org/10.1016/j.lfs.2008.12.001.
81. Gong, E. J., Park, H. R., Kim, M. E., Piao, S., Lee, E., Jo, D. G., Chung, H. Y., Ha, N. C., Mattson, M. P., & Lee, J. (2011). Morin attenuates tau hyperphosphorylation by inhibiting GSK3β. *Neurobiology of Disease, 44*(2), 223–230. https://doi.org/10.1016/j.nbd.2011.07.005.
82. Cornejo, A., Aguilar Sandoval, F., Caballero, L., Machuca, L., Muñoz, P., Caballero, J., Perry, G., Ardiles, A., Areche, C., & Melo, F. (2017). Rosmarinic acid prevents fibrillization and diminishes vibrational modes associated with β sheet in tau protein linked to Alzheimer's disease. *Journal of Enzyme Inhibition and Medicinal Chemistry, 32*(1), 945–953. https://doi.org/10.1080/14756366.2017.1347783.
83. Ahmad Rather, M., Justin-Thenmozhi, A., Manivasagam, T., Saravanababu, C., Guillemin, G. J., & Essa, M. M. (2019). Asiatic acid attenuated aluminum chloride-induced tau pathology, oxidative stress, and apoptosis via AKT/GSK-3β signaling pathway in Wistar rats. *Neurotoxicity Research, 35*(4), 955–968. https://doi.org/10.1007/s12640-019-9999-2.
84. Ahmad, A., Ali, T., Park, H. Y., Badshah, H., Rehman, S. U., & Kim, M. O. (2017). Neuroprotective effect of fisetin against amyloid-beta-induced cognitive/synaptic dysfunction, neuroinflammation, and neurodegeneration in adult mice. *Molecular Neurobiology, 54*(3), 2269–2285. https://doi.org/10.1007/s12035-016-9795-4.
85. Shati, A. A., & Alfaifi, M. Y. (2019). Trans-resveratrol inhibits tau phosphorylation in the brains of control and cadmium chloride-treated rats by activating PP2A and PI3K/Akt induced-inhibition of GSK3β. *Neurochemical Research, 44*(2), 357–373. https://doi.org/10.1007/s11064-018-2683-8.
86. Yang, C., Kuai, X., Gao, W., Yu, J., Wang, Q., Li, L., & Zhang, L. (2016). Morroniside-induced PP2A activation antagonizes tau hyperphosphorylation in a cellular model of neurodegeneration. *Journal of Alzheimer's Disease, 51*, 33–44. https://doi.org/10.3233/JAD-150728.
87. Yao, J., Gao, X., Sun, W., Yao, T., Shi, S., & Ji, L. (2013). Molecular hairpin: A possible model for inhibition of tau aggregation by tannic acid. *Biochemistry, 52*(11), 1893–1902. https://doi.org/10.1021/bi400240c.
88. Ben, P., Zhang, Z., Zhu, Y., Xiong, A., Gao, Y., Mu, J., Yin, Z., & Luo, L. (2016). L-Theanine attenuates cadmium-induced neurotoxicity through the inhibition of oxidative damage and tau hyperphosphorylation. *Neurotoxicology, 57*, 95–103. https://doi.org/10.1016/j.neuro.2016.09.010.
89. Pandey, M. K., & DeGrado, T. R. (2016). Glycogen synthase kinase-3 (GSK-3)-targeted therapy and imaging. *Theranostics, 6*(4), 571.
90. Maqbool, M., Mobashir, M., & Hoda, N. (2016). Pivotal role of glycogen synthase kinase-3: A therapeutic target for Alzheimer's disease. *European Journal of Medicinal Chemistry, 107*, 63–81.
91. Huang, H. C., O'Brien, W. T., & Klein, P. S. (2006). Targeting glycogen synthase kinase-3 in Alzheimer's disease. *Drug Discovery Today: Therapeutic Strategies, 3*(4), 613–619.
92. Hamann, M., Alonso, D., Martín-Aparicio, E., Fuertes, A., Pérez-Puerto, M. J., Castro, A., Morales, S., Navarro, M. L., del Monte-Millán, M., & Medina, M. (2007). Glycogen

synthase kinase-3 (GSK-3) inhibitory activity and structure-activity relationship (SAR) studies of the manzamine alkaloids. *Journal of Natural Products, 70*(9), 1397–1405. https://doi.org/10.1021/np070087h.

93. Bidon-Chanal, A., Fuertes, A., Alonso, D., Pérez, D. I., Martínez, A., Luque, F. J., & Medina, M. (2013). Evidence for a new binding mode to GSK-3: Allosteric regulation by the marine compound palinurin. *European Journal of Medicinal Chemistry, 60*, 479–489. https://doi.org/10.1016/j.ejmech.2012.12.001.
94. Leclerc, S., Garnier, M., Hoessel, R., Marko, D., Bibb, J. A., Snyder, G. L., Greengard, P., Biernat, J., Wu, Y. Z., & Mandelkow, E. M. (2001). Indirubins inhibit glycogen synthase kinase-3β and CDK5/P25, two protein kinases involved in abnormal tau phosphorylation in Alzheimer's disease: A property common to most cyclin-dependent kinase inhibitors? *Journal of Biological Chemistry, 276*(1), 251–260. https://doi.org/10.1074/jbc.M004686200.
95. Silva, T., Reis, J., Teixeira, J., & Borges, F. (2014). Alzheimer's disease, enzyme targets, and drug discovery struggle: From natural products to drug prototype. *Ageing Research Reviews, 15*, 116–145. https://doi.org/10.1016/j.arr.2014.03.008.
96. Meijer, L., Thunnissen, A. M., White, A. W., Garnier, M., Nikolic, M., Tsai, L. H., Walter, J., Cleverley, K. E., Salinas, P. C., Wu, Y. Z., Biernat, J., Mandelkow, E. M., Kim, S. H., & Pettit, G. R. (2000). Inhibition of cyclin-dependent kinases, GSK-3β and CK1 by hymenialdisine, a marine sponge constituent. *Chemistry & Biology, 7*(1), 51–63. https://doi.org/10.1016/S1074-5521(00)00063-6.

CHAPTER 6

Preclinical Testing Methods for Evaluation of Potential Anti-Alzheimer's Drugs

MINTU MATHEW,[1] VAISHNAVI R. UNNITHAN,[1] RAJAN SWAMI,[2] JAYA THOMAS,[1] and MANISH KUMAR JEENGAR[1*]

[1]Department of Pharmacology, Amrita School of Pharmacy, Amrita Vishwa Vidyapeetham, AIMS Health Sciences Campus, Kochi, Ernakulam, Kerala, India

[2]Chitkara College of Pharmacy, Chitkara University, Punjab, India

*Corresponding author.

ABSTRACT

Alzheimer's disease (AD) is the most common form of dementia, characterized by a gradual decline in cognitive abilities, functional capacity, mood, and behavior. To better understand the etiology and pathology of AD, numerous preclinical models have been developed in recent years, including *in vivo* animal models, and *in vitro* 2D and 3D models. However, despite promising preclinical data, several neuroprotective drugs have failed in human clinical trials, highlighting the limitations of conventional preclinical models in replicating human pathophysiology. Nevertheless, careful characterization of animal models and parallel *in vitro* and *ex vivo* studies using human or relevant animal cell lines/tissues can overcome some limitations. This chapter provides an overview of the most relevant and commonly used preclinical testing methods, both *in vitro* and *in vivo*, for screening anti-Alzheimer drugs. Among the *in vitro* cell culture models, 3D models are considered promising because they closely replicate some aspects of the brain environment, mimic neuronal and glial cell interactions, and incorporate the impact of blood flow.

Neuro-Nutraceuticals and Drug Discovery and Delivery in Alzheimer's Disease, Volume 1: Targeting Key Pathological Pathways. Varinder Singh, Amit Kumar, Parul Sood (Eds.)

Additionally, this chapter discusses the animals used in AD research and the potential mechanisms of different chemical agents in AD induction. Transgenic animals have been particularly useful in identifying drug targets and designing novel therapeutic strategies. Although each animal model has its limitations and strengths, using them together in a complementary fashion is beneficial for the development of effective treatments for AD and improving the patient's quality of life.

6.1 INTRODUCTION

Alzheimer's disease (AD) is a debilitating degenerative brain ailment that primarily affects the elderly. It is a kind of dementia characterized by a gradual deterioration in cognitive processes that affect visuospatial and language skills, memory, and behavioral abnormalities such as heightened mood swings, aggressiveness, and depression, eventually impairing quality of life [1–3]. The prevalence of Alzheimer's dementia is rising globally, accounting for about 12.7 million people aged 65 and older who are at risk of developing AD by 2050. According to US statistics, about 6.5 million elderly Americans are living with AD, of which the majority are females [4, 5].

6.2 PATHOPHYSIOLOGY OF AD

Numerous contributing factors are attributed to the pathophysiology of this neurodegenerative AD, of which the key elements are the beta-amyloid plaque (Aβ) hypothesis and the neurofibrillary tangles (NFTs) formation [6, 7].

6.2.1 BETA-AMYLOID (AB) CASCADE HYPOTHESIS

The most widely accepted and researched theory, with a significant role in AD's pathophysiology. Beta-amyloid peptides are derived from amyloid precursor protein (APP), a transmembrane protein initially cleaved by beta-site APP cleaving enzyme 1 (BACE1). Then, the enzymatic action of proteases is called alpha, beta, and gamma-secretase. The APP plaque, when cleaved by α-secretase followed by γ-secretase, results in a soluble or non-amyloidogenic form of Aβ. In contrast, the successive breakdown by beta and then gamma-secretase leads to increased production of insoluble or amyloidogenic Aβ plaques. Excess production, release, and impaired clearance of these insoluble polypeptides (about 4 kDa) lead to the accumulation of amyloid plaques in the brain parenchyma, ultimately leading to neuronal toxicity [6–8]. The coalesce and multifocal grey matter deposits will form microscopic spherical lesions called plaques, but the presence of plaques in the brain scan is not reliable evidence of dementia [7].

Depending upon the amount and presence of the Aβ species, the toxic Aβ level varies. $A\beta_{1-40}$ and $A\beta_{1-42}$ are the most abundant isoforms, followed by $A\beta_{1-38}$, $A\beta_{1-43}$, as well as the post-translationally modified pAβ (Aβ with phosphorylated serine at position 8 or 26), AβN3pE (N-terminally truncated Aβ with a pyroglutamate modification), and Aβ5-x (N-terminally truncated Aβ) are seen in the cerebral vessels, meningeal, and grey matter region [7].

Previous studies report that the abnormal functioning of APP produces neurotoxic irregular insoluble Aβ isoforms, which assemble and aggregate in the form of oligomers and protofibrils [9]. The amyloid bodies, which are densely packed structures containing fibrillogenic proteins and non-fibril components, lead to the extracellular accumulation of Aβ protein and form senile plaques (SP). These are responsible for the abnormal accumulation of amyloid in the organs, a condition called amyloidosis [9].

6.2.2 NEUROFIBRILLARY TANGLES (NFTS)

The intracytoplasmic paired twisted helical fibrillary structures in the neurons called neurofibrillary tangles (NFTs) are formed by the protein tau, which first appears in the hippocampus and extends to the cerebral cortex. The presence of microtubules in the neuronal axon helps in the smooth intracellular transport, which is assembled and stabilized by the tau protein [6, 7]. The accumulation of extracellular beta-amyloid in AD increases the risk of tau hyperphosphorylation and leads to the formation of tau aggregates. The topographical staging system developed by Braak, which explains the 6 stages of neurofibrillary tangles formation from the tau aggregates, is considered a more reliable diagnostic criteria for AD than the plaque hypothesis by the National Institute on Aging and Reagan Institute [6, 10].

6.2.3 GENETICS

Genetics plays a prominent role in AD in which the autosomal dominant mutation in any of the three genes such as Amyloid Beta a4 precursor protein

(APP), Presenilin1 (PSEN1), and Presenilin2 (PSEN2) located on chromosomes 21, 14, and 1, respectively may lead to the increased processing of gamma-secretase, thereby increasing the beta-amyloid protein accumulation. Mutations in these genes increase the risk of occurrence of the most common type of AD called sporadic Alzheimer's disease (sAD) [11]. Polymorphisms in various genetic loci have been linked to both sAD and early-onset Alzheimer's disease (EOAD), such as Isoform e4 of Apolipoprotein E (APOE) gene on chromosome 19, which is a lipid metabolism regulator with high affinity for amyloid protein. Similarly, the genetic variants of the sortilin receptor, SORT1, are necessary for transporting APP from the cell surface of Golgi-ERC (endoplasmic reticulum complex) [7, 12].

6.2.4 CHOLINERGIC HYPOTHESIS

One of the most popular theories for the etiology of AD states that a decrease in acetylcholine-containing neurons leads to a decrease in acetylcholine (ACh) neurotransmitter levels, which leads to cognitive decline in AD patients. The damage to these cholinergic neurons will affect memory, attention, stress response, learning, sensory responses, wakefulness, and sleep. Based on this hypothesis, the first-line drug therapy for AD with acetylcholinesterase inhibitors such as memantine, rivastigmine, donepezil, and galantamine came into practice, providing palliative care and continuing even after decades [9].

6.2.5 INFLAMMATION AND OXIDATIVE STRESS HYPOTHESIS

Over the past decades, the inflammation hypothesis highlights the crucial role of elevated inflammatory markers, microglia activation, and immune cells in CNS-related pathways, which increases the risk of neuroinflammation and aberrant gliosis. In a healthy brain, the microglia are inactive or in a resting state. They get activated and enlarged by triggering factors, leading to the disruption of the pro- and anti-inflammatory signaling equilibrium and promoting acute inflammation. Later, this progresses to chronic inflammatory changes, where Aβ is not able to be processed and accumulates along with pro-inflammatory cytokines, leading to neuronal damage [13, 14]. However, the intake of non-steroidal anti-inflammatory drugs (NSAIDs) in regulation is found to be controversial. The mutation in a protein called Triggering Receptor Expressed on Myeloid Cells 2 (TREM2) affects synaptic reduction and plasticity, affecting the process of learning and memory. PD-1 immune crossing point barrier and CX3CL1 (fractalkine), an inhibitory factor released by the neurons, decrease the expression of inflammatory mediators in a dose-dependent manner. Currently, research is focused on newer strategies for regulating microglial homeostasis [9, 13].

Oxidative stress plays a momentous part in AD. During mitochondrial respiration, the brain is likely to consume more energy, increasing the risk of exposure to reactive oxygen species (ROS). The aggregation of Aβ exacerbates oxidative stress, similarly, increasing protein oxidation, glycoxidation, protein nitration, and glycoxidation, which increases the risk of AD. Combination therapy with antioxidants is found to be effective in managing AD [9, 15].

6.2.6 VASCULAR HYPOTHESIS

The vascular contribution of AD is not fully understood, but it is stated that amyloid angiopathy causes degeneration of hippocampal pyramidal cells. Hypertension, hyperhomocysteinemia, and diabetes play an important role in cardiovascular disease, acting as vascular risk factors for AD. Decreased cerebral blood flow leading to cerebral hypoperfusion acts as a major contributing factor for AD. The degree of dementia and cognitive impairment depends on the presence of subcortical infarcts, cerebrovascular disease, associated hypoxia, mild and severe ischemia, CCH, low acetylcholine levels, increased inflammation, oxidative stress, and decreased density of pyramidal neurons' presynaptic boutons [7, 16].

6.2.7 BRAIN AND AD

Brain imaging studies reveal a significant correlation of brain anatomical changes as AD progresses. The macroscopic examination of the AD brain lateral view shows the spreading of sulcal space and gyri narrowing compared to the normal brain, clearly evident in the coronal sections. Sometimes, it is accompanied by enlargement of the lateral ventricles of the frontal and temporal horns, as well as the loss of pigmented neurons in the locus coeruleus [17]. The major difference between a normal brain and an AD brain is that, as a part of aging, the healthy brain shrinks without exhibiting a large number of neuronal changes or loss, while in AD, the neuronal damage is very severe, adversely affecting the overall functioning of the normal brain.

Among the different brain regions, the alteration in the cortex and hippocampus exacerbates the symptoms of AD. Based on functional connectivity, the hippocampal region is divided into three regions which play a key role in the changes in episodic memory [18, 19]. Initially, it destroys the neurons in the entorhinal cortex and hippocampus, affecting memory, especially verbal and visual memory. Later, it affects the cerebral cortex area leading to cognitive dysfunction, including difficulties in reasoning, language, and social behavior [19–21]. Depending on the side of the brain (left or right) that is affected, the changes will differ. The other brain regions affected by AD include:

1. **Limbic System:** Controls emotions and memory. AD patients exhibit difficulty in remembering and finding objects; they may also show signs of suspicion, along with comorbid depression and anxiety.
2. **Frontal Lobe:** Controls overall activity and is responsible for inhibition and behavior regulation. AD patients usually lose interest in hobbies and activities they previously enjoyed. Social withdrawal, repetition, and disorganized actions are commonly observed.
3. **Temporal Lobes:** Control short-term memory and learning ability. AD patients have difficulty recalling familiar faces, places, and objects, and may experience vocabulary loss.
4. **Parietal Lobes:** Control coordination, organization, logical thinking, and spatial information. AD patients may have difficulty writing, speaking, and understanding.
5. **Occipital Lobes:** Control vision, and recognition of shapes and colors. While this lobe is not directly linked to AD, patients may experience difficulty with identification and perception [18, 20, 22].

6.3 EXPERIMENTAL MODELS IN AD

The heart of drug discovery lies in the appropriate selection of the animal model, which should be capable enough to exhibit the pathogenesis of diseases, as well as to evaluate novel drug development strategies. Alzheimer's disease (AD) was described in 1906 by Alois Alzheimer. Soon after that, experimental model research of AD began, but it took several decades for the discovery of the first drug named Tacrine for AD. Later, within a decade, with the aid of well-established and promising AD models that imply a pathology-driven mechanism of AD, especially Aβ deposits and tau phosphorylation, paved the way for landmark discoveries and approvals of AD drugs by the US FDA as follows: Donepezil in 1996, Rivastigmine in 2000, Galantamine in 2001, Memantine in 2003, and Aducanumab in 2021 [14, 23].

The complexity in the pathophysiology and clinical presentation of AD always acts as a gap in the advancement of drug discovery, as none of the animal models so far replicate the exact human pathophysiology of AD. Therefore, advancing research is focusing on newer models to decode the deeper mechanistic approaches of AD and to facilitate the discovery of newer classes of anti-Alzheimer drugs. Currently, there are numerous cell, animal, and computational models for Alzheimer's research [14, 23]. The majority of the literature has explained AD models based on the mechanism and type of species used. Through this chapter, we mainly focus on the method of induction in both *in vivo* and *in vitro* models (Figure 6.1).

6.3.1 IN-VITRO MODELS

In *in vitro* 2D cell models, different kinds of brain cells are grown at high cell densities on 2D culture plates, where they spontaneously self-organize. They are frequently employed in preclinical testing because they are easier to operate, repeatable, and less expensive than *in vivo* models. However, 2D monolayer platforms cannot capture the intricate 3D structure of the brain because they lack tissue-specific spatial and morphological cellular organization, cell-cell interactions, immune system cells, and waste accumulation and clearance dynamics [24, 25]. The building of 3D human brain models (Table 6.1) poses a significant challenge for improving *in vitro* replication of the complex human brain architecture and functionality due to the constraints of *in vivo*, *ex vivo*, and *in vitro* 2D models that have been previously discussed. Between 2D cell cultures and animal models, *in vitro* 3D models of brain tissue cover the knowledge gap by enabling the investigation of cell-ECM interactions, cell-cell communication, and electrical network features. In addition to recreating the 3D cellular environment, 3D models need to simulate different brain region architectural components and neural networks in order to reproduce brain activities. Due to these factors, 3D brain models may serve as more effective tools for the *in vitro* investigation of brain illness pathophysiology and effective medication treatments [26, 27].

6.3.1.1 2D MODELS

Cell lines used:

- Induced pluripotent stem cells;
- Embryonic stem cells;
- Neural stem cells;
- Mesenchymal stem cells;
- Neuroblastoma cells;
- Fibroblasts;
- Human brain microvascular endothelial cells;
- Brain capillary endothelial cells;
- Brain microvascular endothelial cells;
- Human cerebro microvascular endothelial cells.

TABLE 6.1 Different 3D *In Vitro* Brain Models for AD

In Vitro 3D Models	Advantages	Disadvantages	References
Spheroids	• It gives an overview of the basic characteristics of brain tissue. • Cell–cell, and cell–ECM interactions are optimal.	• Necrotic core formation.	[28]
Organoids	• Brain mimetic characteristics. • Self-organization of cells. • Long-term culture.	• Reproducibility low. • Inter batch instability.	[28]
Organs on chip	• Effective modeling of brain states and functions. • Dynamic culture.	• The technical side is challenging. • Media renewal methods are challenging.	[25]
Tissue engineering	• There is a possibility of dynamic cultures in bioreactors.	• Large model size. • Expensive.	[25]

6.3.1.2 SPHEROIDS

Cells are produced in clusters, on 3D tissue engineering platforms, or drowned in gels in 3D culturing techniques. There are other names for aggregates, including mammosphere micro-mass, spheroids, and microfabricated tissues. Spheroids are clusters of cells that don't attach to any kind of growing medium (e.g., polystyrene) [29]. An immortalized line of human neural progenitor cells called ReN cells can easily develop into neurons and glial cells. These immortalized ReN cells give rise to FAD neurospheroids, which mimic the main symptoms of Alzheimer's disease, like the buildup of extracellular Aβ amyloid deposits and intracellular Tau proteins and plaques [30]. Spheroids are mainly fabricated by the hanging drop method, static liquid overlay technique, and centrifugation. Embryoid bodies can be developed using this technique. Spinner flasks are used for aggregating cells spontaneously as an alternative technique. In the static liquid overlay technique (LOT), suspended cells are cultured on a nonadherent substrate which results in cell aggregation instead of adhering to a surface. Centrifugation is another method for creating spheroids. In microfabricated devices, cells have been seeded on non-adherent surfaces recently [29].

6.3.1.3 PREPARATION OF SPHEROIDS

6.3.1.3.1 Hanging Drop Method

These can be done in two steps. A single-cell suspension is prepared, followed by the formation of hanging drops.

- Steps in Preparation:

Harvesting cultured cells

↓

Generating a single cell suspension

↓

Drops of suspension deposited onto the underside of the inverted lid from a tissue culture dish.

↓

The lid is inverted the into hydration chamber.

↓

Incubate hanging drops for 24 to 48 hours.

↓

Allow aggregates to form.

↓

She was transferred to a shaking water bath.

↓

Incubate up to five more days.

↓

The stereomicroscope is used to assess the formation of aggregates.

Concentration may have to be modified either upwards or downwards depending on cell size. Prior to the production of hanging drops, cells can be labeled with membrane-intercalating fluorescent dyes. Prior to the creation of hanging drops, two separate cell types can be differently labeled and combined in a 1:1 (or other) ratio [31]. An immortalized line of human neural progenitor cells called ReNcell can easily develop into neurons and glial cells. These immortalized ReN cells give rise to FAD neurospheroids, which mimic the main symptoms of Alzheimer's disease, like the buildup of extracellular Aβ amyloid deposits and intracellular Tau proteins and plaques [30]. There are protein markers for mature neurons and astrocyte cells in the brain. Park et al. developed a three-dimensional spheroid model derived from iPSCs-NPCs of AD as models expressing marker proteins [32]. Pomeshchik et al. developed a chemical method to generate free-floating hippocampal spheroids (HSs) from human iPSCs. Both APP and atypical PS1 variant HSs revealed elevated Ab42/Ab40 peptide ratios and lower amounts of synaptic protein when employed to simulate AD [33]. Many genes, including those involved in synaptic transmission, had their expression altered as a result of NeuroD1-mediated gene therapy in HS-derived progenitors. Consequently, by using these free-floating HSs, early pathogenic alterations in the hippocampus of patients with AD can be uncovered, and they offer a strong basis for the development of treatment approaches that specifically target the early stages of AD [34]. Developed iPSCs-derived 3D spheroid model from AD patients' blood. Their findings showed that a 3D human spheroid model might be a useful tool for evaluating the effectiveness of AD medications.

6.3.1.3.2 Static Liquid Overlay Technique

This method forms cellular aggregates in suspension by stirring large volumes of culture medium. This is an attractive solution for mass production that mainly benefited from the development of bioreactors. It currently does not allow for precise control of the size of aggregates [29, 35].

6.3.1.4 ORGANOIDS

Brain organoids are artificially grown *in vitro* miniature organs resembling the brain. Pluripotent stem cells are cultured in a 3D rotational bioreactor to develop these organoids. These organoids contain different types of nerve cells and possess certain features that resemble regions of the cortex seen in the brain, mostly the choroid plexus and cortex.

Preparation of organoids:

- Embryos grown from natural stem cells are used.
- Since this embryo has three layers and the nervous system is grown from the ectoderm, to prepare the brain organoids, ectodermal cells are placed in a nutrient broth in a rotating bioreactor. Organoids develop into neurons after 10 days. Approximately 30 days are needed to display regions like brain parts.

➢ **Steps to Generate Organoids:**

- Culturing pluripotent stem cells;
- Formation of the embryoid body;
- Formation of neuroectoderm;
- Neuroectoderm grown in a Matrigel droplet;
- Spin cerebral organoids in a bioreactor;
- Self-organization.

One of the major limitations in organoid development is the lack of vasculature that limits the size the organoid can grow. Brain organoids provide a means to understand brain development and comprehend the specific causes of neurodegenerative diseases since they closely mimic the characteristics of different brain areas [36]. Cerebral organoids may represent an excellent model of genetic forms of AD that may enable studying pathology at more physiological levels of gene expression in cortical tissue derived from stem cells with the same genetic background as the patients [37]. So far, there have been no *in vitro* studies that simulate the complexity of neurodegenerative disorders. However, Human induced pluripotent stem cell models allow studying aspects of the electrical properties of AD neurons in a human context in both 2D cultures and 3D cerebral organoids and compare them to known *in vivo* phenotypic studies in AD transgenic mouse models and human AD brain [38]. This opens a golden door to understanding the complexity of AD pathophysiology.

6.3.1.5 ORGANS ON CHIP MODEL

Systems called "Organs-on-Chip" (OoCs) incorporate artificial or real tiny tissues developed within microfluidic chips. Several single or multiple microchambers coupled with microchannels make up the system [39]. This technique enables tiny simulations of human physiology. The objective is to rebuild a functional unit of this organ. In this method, cells are seeded in a modern tissue engineering platform called a 3D scaffold, which provides a 3D environment and promotes cell survival, proliferation, and differentiation [40].

In some investigations, this 3D technology might replace the usage of animals. They are inexpensive too in comparison with *in vivo* models for Alzheimer's. Isolation of an exact organ (or a functional unit) is not tedious when compared to animal use. Additionally, using organs on a chip in combination with patient-derived cells might prevent the need to employ transgenic animals. The advantages are great control overseeding and cell organization, as well as the chemical, mechanical, or physical microenvironment. Compared to 2D, organs-on-chips are more complex systems. These organs-on-chip models are used to study cell–cell or cell–ECM interactions and to study the response to stimuli. An automated system uses a tiny quantity of culture media and can be made to use widefield fluorescence microscopy to view cells instantaneously. Spheroids or organoids may also be generated in these platforms without the use of hydrogel, which could be useful for toxicity research or drug screening. Organs-on-chips, though, are a difficult-to-use technology that is more sophisticated and automated, and even a minor technological issue can cause the experiment to be halted. As they make it possible to investigate extremely sophisticated and complicated structures, organ-on-chip technology is commonly employed [39]. Organ-on-chip models can be used to explore the pathophysiological characteristics of Alzheimer's disease, such as reduced cell viability, increased neuronal degeneration and synaptic dysfunction, and neurotoxic effects of amyloid beta. This 3D scaffold model provides an *in vivo*-like microenvironment that has promising importance as an *in vitro* brain model [41].

6.3.2 IN VIVO MODELS/ANIMAL MODELS

The selection of a valid animal model for AD research is challenging since it is difficult to replicate AD's complex pathophysiology as well as to mimic the classical signs and symptoms of the disease, including cognitive decline and neuronal loss. Moreover, every animal model has its merits and demerits, and none of the models exhibit the exact disease pathology. The clinical translation of drug therapy from animal models might yield poor efficacy

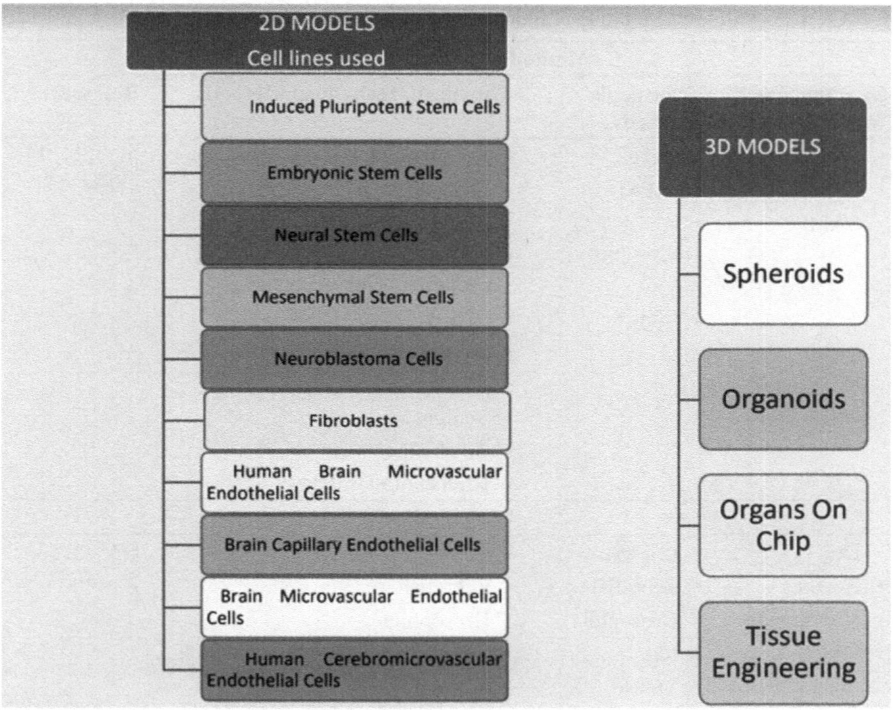

FIGURE 6.1 *In vitro* 2D and 3D models in AD.

and tolerability in the clinical population [6, 14, 42]. Despite the limitations, utilizing both transgenic and non-transgenic models (Table 6.2) in a complementary manner leads to the milestone discovery of AD drugs which have contributed tremendously to global healthcare. The non-transgenic models mainly involve natural AD animal models or spontaneous models, chemically induced models, lesion models, and high-fat diet-induced models. Different species of organisms have been explored efficiently for milestone findings in AD research [43].

6.3.2.1 SPONTANEOUS MODELS

One of the promising models mainly involves non-human primates (NHP), dogs, and rodents of which NHP and dogs are relatively large animals hence it is difficult to handle them. These species exhibit AD pathology naturally in an age-dependent manner, representing amyloid neuropathology like

TABLE 6.2 Different Methods of Induction of AD Along with the Species of Animal Used

Method of Induction of AD			
Spontaneous Method	**Transgenic Methods**	**Chemical/Mechanical Methods**	**References**
• Age • KKAy • SAMP8	• 3xTg • 5xFAD • APOE-KO • APP/PSI • J20 • Tg2576	• Scopolamine • D-galactose • Ethanol/Alcohol • Heavy metals – aluminum, cadmium, lead, manganese • LPS • Streptozotocin (STZ) • Okadaic Acid (OKA) • Sodium azide • Colchicine • High cholesterol diet	[6, 9, 11, 14, 28, 44–57]
Animals Used			
• Dog • Rodents • Non-human primates	• *C. elegans* • Zebrafish • Drosophila • Rat • Mouse	• C. elegans • Zebrafish • Drosophila • Rhesus macaque • Marmoset • Vervet monkey • Cat • Dog • Rodents • Rabbit • Guinea pig • Sheep	[11, 43, 53, 58–60]

humans. However this model alone is not sufficient to carry out efficacy analysis of the AD therapies due to several reasons such as ethical considerations, housing costs, and maintenance, only able to evaluate the late onset of AD, and longevity of lifespan [53].

6.3.2.2 NON-HUMAN PRIMATES (NHP)

Mammalian models are the most appropriate models that exhibit similar pathology to human AD. Mammals with ancestral resemblance to humans, especially non-human primates (NHP) including chimpanzees, orangutans, rhesus monkeys, and baboons, develop pathological and clinical features similar to human AD during natural aging without any techniques of neuro-chemical exposure or non-invasive methods. Among NHP, chimpanzees, the great apes, show senile plaques, tau hyperphosphorylation, neurofibrillary tangles formation, and cerebral amyloidosis in aged brains, closely resembling human AD condition, although the distribution pattern of plaques and NFT varies [55, 59]. In aged rhesus monkeys, dense neuritic amyloid plaques are observed more, along with APOE similar to humans, but the type of Aβ species deposition may vary drastically. For example, in human brains, Aβ42 is more observed in early AD stages, followed by Aβ40 protein deposition, while in old orangutans, rhesus monkeys, and chimpanzees, Aβ40 species is more common. This variation might be due to changes in metabolic genes involved in APOE-Aβ [11]. In baboons aged between 26 and 30 years old, 91% of amyloid and Tau hyperphosphorylation is observed in glial and neuronal cells. However, the use of NHP in laboratories is restricted due to ethical concerns, limitations in evaluating AD drugs, limited availability and difficulty in obtaining them, long aging time for AD pathology formation, and high maintenance costs (housing) [11, 55].

The lower primates including grey mouse lemurs and tree shrews serve as a reliable model for AD. Grey mouse lemurs have a short lifespan of 8–10 years, and after the age of 5 years, the majority of them exhibit cholinergic neuronal loss, NFTs, amyloid plaque deposition, and brain atrophy with cognitive and cytoskeletal abnormalities [53]. However, the distribution of Aβ accumulation varies, as in humans it starts in the hippocampus, whereas in lemurs it is observed in the neocortex. The tree shrew, which has a similar body size to rats and a longer lifespan than rodents, has Aβ deposition in the brains of the aged ones [59, 61].

6.3.2.3 DOGS

Dogs that share a phylogenetic relationship with humans can be used as a suitable model for AD research, wherein older dogs especially canines (beagles) with a lifespan of 12–14 years, have the deposition of Aβ amyloids in the brain that correlates with cortical atrophy. Even in the absence of NFTs, they exhibit similar age-dependent cognitive dysfunction [11, 53, 60]. The most affected brain regions initially include the prefrontal cortex, including the gyrus proteus and hippocampus. The majority of aged dogs resemble the pathology of sporadic AD and can be used as an effective model for evaluating non-pharmacological therapies, including dietary approaches, behavioral therapy, and assessing the efficacy of AD drugs such as antioxidants, cholinesterase inhibitors, and mitochondrial enzymatic cofactors. Despite the positive efficacy outcome in drug trials, such as a reduction in the Aβ plaque load, the cognitive domains show no improvement, while significant changes were observed in rodent models. Compared to other primates, dogs are widely available and cheaper, but due to their long lifespan, relatively large body size, housing costs, and ethical constraints, the use of dog models is restricted in AD research [11, 55, 60].

6.3.2.4 SHEEP

Sheep exhibit a similar human pathology of AD based on the NFTs formation by tau hyperphosphorylation and involvement of apolipoprotein (APOE). The polymorphism in the genes contributes a lot to disease pathology, but in sheep, it is not evident. The neuritic plaques in the brain can be easily detected by ELISA. The resemblance in metabolism and reproduction patterns, including breeding, oestrus periodicity, and metabolic rate between sheep and humans, paves an opportunity to investigate the involvement of sex hormones, especially estrogen, which plays a key role in oxidative stress and Aβ accumulation in sheep brain [11].

6.3.2.5 GUINEA PIGS

The most amenable models than large-sized mammals are small-sized mammalian models including rabbits and guinea pigs, which have more genes related to AD than rats and mice. A lesser-studied Dunkin-Hartley (DH) strain and standard Pigmented (PET) strain of non-transgenic guinea pig models mimic the features of the human aging brain. Reports show that the APP is 97% similar to human APP and exhibits a similar transcriptional splicing pattern. Both models exhibit a high risk of neuroinflammation as the aging process, due to the increased amount of neurofilament light chain (NFL), increased amount of calcium-binding protein S100β, ionized calcium-binding adapter molecule 1 (Iba1), age-independent limited hyperphosphorylation of tau, and amyloid deposition [62]. Moreover, they share many similar factors in human AD such as sequential AD risk genes like presenilin's, formation of PSEN2 truncation, PS2V, and the capacity to form large oligomers which are all responsible for neurotoxicity [11, 62]. Guinea pig models are considered an ideal model for investigating the cardiovascular complications associated with AD by inducing high-cholesterol diets since they can resemble the metabolism of human cholesterol and lipoproteins, whereas rabbits have VLDL as they are deficient in hepatic lipase, and in rats and mice, HDL is more since they lack cholesterol ester transfer protein in plasma [11]. However, this model is not suitable for carrying out memory and learning tasks.

6.3.2.6 RABBITS

Rabbits are considered one of the economical mammalian models that share a mostly similar age-independent amino acid sequence for amyloid compared to the mice models. The method of induction of AD is a determining factor in rabbits exhibiting AD-like pathology, especially with the combination of copper and a high-cholesterol diet. It shows neuronal loss at the hippocampus, frontal cortex, and cerebellar cortex, NFT, Aβ deposition, and learning impairment, which can be ameliorated if the triggering factor is removed. Studies prove that plasma tau levels and NFT are increased in cholesterol-fed rabbits (1% for 7 months). Interestingly, depending on the type of diluent used, whether distilled water or water containing copper (0.12 ppm), the intensification of NFT formation varies. This model is very effective for evaluating the diet-based risk factors of AD [58, 63].

Apart from these mammals, recent studies report that dolphins and polar bears have an identical sequence similar to Aβ of humans but require extensive research for consideration as an animal model for AD [55].

6.3.2.7 TRANSGENIC MODELS

6.3.2.7.1 Zebrafish

Zebrafish (*Danio rerio*), which belongs to the class of teleost fishes, is an excellent transitional non-mammalian model used efficiently for understanding disease pathology and drug screening. This futuristic model with vast research opportunities was introduced by Streisinger et al. in the late 1960s [64]. It has an average lifespan of about 2–5 years, requires an adequate temperature range of 27–29°C, and can produce around 200–250 eggs. The nucleotide sequence of zebrafish resembles about 70% of the human genome and is a viable model with a unique ability for tissue regeneration, visualizing genotypic effects, and carrying out genetic manipulations [65, 66]. Zebrafish's brain biochemically resembles the human brain; although they have no cortex or hippocampus, they are used extensively as a promising model in AD research since they have similar cognitive domains and can carry out essential learning and memory tasks [67, 68]. Oxidative stress and mutations in the presenilin genes 1 and 2 and apolipoprotein E associated with FAD and SAD, respectively, will lead to insoluble amyloid beta accumulation [69, 70].

6.3.2.7.2 Drosophila Melanogaster

Drosophila melanogaster is a member of the family Drosophilidae of the biological order Diptera. Fruit flies are very small oval flies with adults growing only to be 1/8th of an inch in length. The main advantages of this model are they have a very short lifespan of about 2 to 3 months, are relatively cheap to maintain in large quantities, and have rapid reproducibility. Moreover, it is the first organism with complete genome sequencing, so it has been used as a genetic model for decades [6, 11].

The Drosophila model has wide applications in the field of biomedical research as well as for studying the pathophysiological characteristics of neurodegenerative diseases such as AD, as it possesses a more complex nervous system like that of humans. Drosophila's quickness, sensitivity, and reliability in results make these models ideal as the first in vivo tests for determining medication effectiveness and toxicity. Numerous drosophila models have been generated by a mutation in equivalent homologous genes associated with Aβ pathology by transgene analysis including BACE1, BACE2, PS1, PS2, APP, MEGF10, CD2AP, SNRPN, PTPRD, XYLT1, FERMT2, CELF1, MAST4, ITGAM, and ITGA9 [71]. Alyce Finelli et al. developed a model for studying Alzheimer's Aβ-induced toxicity in Drosophila. In their fly model, they showed that the Aβ42 peptide is more stable than Aβ40 in photoreceptor cells. However, Aβ40 expression led to the production of significant quantities of intact peptides in S2 cells, indicating that cell type selectivity may be important for Aβ40 stability [72]. Drosophila homologs of AD-associated genes have shed light on the human genes involved in the progression of AD as well as the disease-causing pathways. Glial cells protect against AD by engulfing the amyloid peptides. In a Drosophila model, they showed that Draper (a highly conserved engulfment receptor) homologous to MEGF10 in humans offered neuroprotection by ameliorating the Aβ peptide level and extending lifespan [73]. Crowther et al., by developing a Drosophila model, showed that non-amyloid Aβ aggregates and intracellular accumulation are enough to produce the neurodegeneration of AD. They demonstrated that the glutamate receptor antagonist MK-801 notably redeemed the phenotypical features of AD and reproduced the beneficial effect of the NMDA receptor antagonist memantine, hence proving the promising features of that particular model for future drug discovery [74]. Moreover, these flies' central nervous systems can mimic some of the clinical, neuroanatomical, and behavioral abnormalities found in AD patients because of the presence of Aβ [75].

6.3.2.7.3 Caenorhabditis Elegans

Caenorhabditis elegans is a non-parasitic nematode, introduced by Sydney Brenner in 1963. They have an average lifespan of about 3 days from egg to adult at a temperature of 25°C, and their length is about 1 mm. They belong to the class Chromadorea of the kingdom Animalia [76]. Genome sequencing of *C. elegans* was completed in 1998, which showed a genetic homology of about 38% with human amyloid precursor protein and tau protein, making it a promising model for studying the pathophysiological features of AD [77]. The amyloid precursor protein-related gene in *C. elegans* is APL-1. This gene consists of extracellular domains that possess a similar sequence pattern when compared with human APP. In both FAD and SAD, cleavage of APP results in insoluble Aβ aggregates, which is the main pathophysiological feature of AD but is not present in the APL-1 gene [78]. Additionally, *C. elegans* does not have any β-secretase activity to produce insoluble Aβ. However, effective transgene analysis can make this *C. elegans* model a highly promising *in vivo* genetic model for studying the neurotoxic effects of Aβ. Many transgenic strains have been developed, which consist of a main signal sequence followed by the human amyloid β sequence that is expressed in various cells, including muscle and neuronal cells, capable of producing $A\beta_{1-42}$ and $A\beta_{3-42}$. This *in vivo* model mainly provides an inexpensive platform for finding new compounds, validating new targets, etc. There were so many Aβ models of *C. elegans* which possess aggregates of $A\beta_{3-42}$ instead of $A\beta_{1-42}$ [79]. Compared to $A\beta_{1-42}$, $A\beta_{3-42}$ is more hydrophobic in nature, and it showed a rapid aggregation profile *in vitro*. Since $A\beta_{1-42}$ is the predominant form in human AD, new transgenic models of *C. elegans* were developed which involve the accumulation of $A\beta_{1-42}$ peptides. For this, the insertion of additional amino acids in between synthetic signal peptide and amyloid β peptide was performed, resulting in the expression of full-length $A\beta_{1-42}$ [80]. GMC101 and CL2122 were some of the strains of *C. elegans* in which GMC 101 expresses full-length human $A\beta_{1-42}$ whereas CL2122 did not express transgene $A\beta_{1-42}$. Compared to the human nervous system, the nervous system of *C. elegans* is less complex. However, *C. elegans* does not have the same intricate network of connections and cell interactions that humans have, and this complexity may be a contributing factor to some of the pathophysiology of neurodegenerative illnesses. This can be considered a disadvantage of this model.

6.3.2.7.4 Rodents

Rodents (mice and rats) are the most promising and extensively studied models, both transgenic and non-transgenic models, in AD research due to the low cost of maintenance, easy availability and breeding, ease of handling, well-characterized behavior, and ease of genetic modification. Moreover, the nervous system functioning of rodents shares many similarities with the human brain, making them an appropriate model for elucidating AD brain pathology, including cognitive functions [6, 14]. The cognitive domains, especially the major AD symptom, memory impairment, can be easily evaluated using different behavioral tests, even though none of the models can completely represent the complex pathology of human AD.

Research conducted reveals the underlying pathology of APP processing in rats, where Aβ degradation was implicated by the two primary proteases, insulin-degrading enzyme and neprilysin. Even though the structure and profile of rat's Aβ peptide generated from APP processing differ from humans, rat models have been used to evaluate the effect of newer therapeutics on the short-term effects of APP, analyze the expression of APP isoforms in temporal and spatial regions, the influence of diet and age on the intracerebral injections of Aβ peptides, and the cognitive dysfunction in AD [59].

The term "Transgenic" indicates that the artificial introduction of the genetic material of an organism is inserted into the DNA of an unrelated organism. Transgenic rodents, especially mice models, contribute tremendously to AD research [57]. The 3 amino acids, such as H13R, R5G, and Y10F, in the Aβ sequence differ drastically between humans and mice, which disrupts the Aβ deposition and prevents the formation of amyloid plaques in wild-type mice. This indicates the necessity of incorporating human APP expression in transgenic mice models. When wild human APP was expressed in transgenic mice models, it increased the production of APP but failed to demonstrate the clinical presentation and pathology of AD. However, FAD-associated mutations in the expression of human APP show steady plaque formation with AD-related features. The promoter, FAD mutation, and the type of mouse strain used determine the actual phenotype of every transgenic strain. Prion protein (PrP), platelet-derived growth factor-b (PDGF-b), and Thy1 were the frequently used promoters [6, 59, 81].

In 1981, the senescence-accelerated mouse (SAM) model was developed from the mutual genetic pool of AKP/J strain of mice, including 9 sub-strains of senescence-accelerated mouse-prone (SAMP) undergoing accelerated aging whereas 3 SAM resistant with the normal aging process. SAMP8 strains are considered an ideal non-transgenic model for dementia since they can develop memory and learning deficits at an early age [43]. While the OXYS rats have AD pathology resemblance by the tau and Aβ accumulation as well as the APP overexpression. These organisms are widely used to explore the mechanistic approach of age-dependent cognitive domains, by observing the alteration in the genes and protein levels responsible for signal conduction, immune reactions, neuroprotection, and immune reaction [59].

The 3xTg and the 5xFAD models of transgenic mouse models are the most popular models which develop Aβ plaques at 6 months and 2 months as well as exhibit behavioral symptoms at 4 months and 2–4 months, respectively. Transgenic APP and tau are overexpressed in 3xTg mice, which shows the progressive onset of AD symptoms considered an apt model to study the SAD, while the overexpressed APP in 5xFAD model develops significant amyloid pathology with rapid and severe onset of disease used to study FAD [14].

1st generation models consist of presenilin-1 and 2 (PSEN1& PSEN2) and APP mutations with more than 300 and 50 AD-associated mutations, respectively, which have been widely used for drug screening and elucidating AD pathology. The 2nd generation models, which mainly focused on the process of APP knock-in, will reproduce the pathogenesis of AD without APP overexpression. Currently, 2nd generation models are widely used due to the limitations of 1st generation models, such as the mislocalization of APP and overproduction of APP, which might lead to changes in transgenic models. The majority of the models are dependent on the FAD mutations, which will hinder translatability since the clinical trials of AD are focusing on SAD patients, where the pathogenesis is different [6, 81].

6.4 CHEMICAL/MECHANICAL METHODS OF AD INDUCTION

Chemicals play a prominent role in the induction of AD-like symptoms in various animal models. Scopolamine, D-galactose, Ethanol/Alcohol, LPS, Streptozotocin (STZ), Okadaic Acid, Sodium azide, Colchicine, and heavy metals such as Aluminum, lead, cadmium, and manganese are the most used chemicals. The selection of the chemical is decisive since every chemical has a different mechanism of inducing AD pathogenesis in different animal models depending on the dosage, route, duration, as well as gender and age of the animal species used [9].

6.4.1 METALS AS INDUCING AGENTS IN AD

6.4.1.1 LEAD

Natural heavy metals are the agents known to cause neurotoxicity, of which lead, and cadmium are two of the potent neurotoxic metals, even at modest exposure levels. Although manganese is a vital trace element needed for many physiological processes, including the functioning of neurons, it is hazardous when present in low or excessive amounts. It is crucial to understand how heavy metals contribute to the genesis of dementia and AD [44]. Lead can cause non-specific brain disruption through various processes including oxidative stress, endoplasmic reticulum stress, neuroinflammation, lipid peroxidation, apoptosis, epigenetic alterations (DNA damage), and excito-toxicity in the brain. It is widely utilized for research on neurotoxicity and neurodegeneration and acts as an excellent toxin for inducing dementia in the popular zebrafish model [44, 82]. Research shows that when larvae of zebrafish are exposed to a combination of lead with decabromodiphenyl ether (BDE-209) in various proportions, it reports growth inhibition of axons of secondary motor neurons as well as genes related to CNS development [83].

6.4.1.2 ALUMINUM

Aluminum is the most widely used heavy metal, which is scattered universally as an industrial and environmental toxin that causes osteomalacia, anemia, and hepatic, and neurological disorders. In Alzheimer's disease (AD) brain, a high amount of aluminum is found, which causes deleterious effects in the brain [44]. Aluminum chloride ($AlCl_3$) is a compound highly susceptible to inducing AD-associated cognitive impairments through cholinergic dysfunction and oxidative stress by increasing the activity or expression of acetylcholinesterase (AChE), malondialdehyde (MDA), and decreasing the activity and expression of glutathione peroxidase (GPX), glutathione reductase (GR), and glutathione S-transferase (GST). Histopathological examination reveals drastic changes in brain histology, including pericellular edema with diffuse gliosis, neuronal loss, and neuronophagia [9, 44]. In rat models, when $AlCl_3$ is administered orally and intraperitoneally, it induces the deposition of Aβ and NFTs in the brain with oxidative stress and cholinergic deficiency, ultimately promoting cognitive impairment. Different behavioral tests such as the Morris water maze, object recognition test, and dipping hole test are used to evaluate various cognitive domains [14].

6.4.1.3 DRUGS AND CHEMICALS AS INDUCING AGENTS IN AD

6.4.1.3.1 Streptozotocin

Streptozotocin (STZ) is found in Streptomyces achromogenes strain derived from glucosamine nitrosourea, used as an antibiotic and an anticancer agent. STZ is proven to induce severe and long-term effects in the brain mainly through its diabetogenic property, which is characterized by decreased glucose uptake and energy consumption [45]. STZ increases the release of reactive nitrogen species (RNS) and ROS, leading to the stimulation of hyperphosphorylation of tau and neuronal damage. Simultaneously, by destructing the glycolytic enzyme, it will decrease the concentration of creatine phosphate and ATP, interrupting the energy cycle [9].

When administered in animals, especially in rats, STZ will exhibit decreased acetylcholine due to the increased activity of AChE. It will also increase the gene expression of neurotrophic factors such as BDNF, GDNF, and integrin-alpha-M, while the expression of genes for metallothionein 1/2 and NGE-IB are downregulated, leading to changes in apoptosis and cell survival processes. The route of administration determines the intensity of neuronal damage and associated symptoms. When STZ is administered via intracerebroventricular injection, it can intensify the loss of learning and memory skills. The long-term impairment of these skills can mimic the sporadic dementia of AD [9, 14, 45].

6.4.1.3.2 Scopolamine

Scopolamine is a potent anticholinergic drug used widely in studies to induce memory loss along with various visuospatial impairments. At the cerebral cortex, it can non-selectively block the binding site of ACh muscarinic receptors, resulting in unequal ACh discharge and ultimately leading to learning and memory deficits along with hippocampal neuronal loss in a dose-dependent manner [46]. Scopolamine can induce Alzheimer's disease-associated pathology involving memory and spatial learning deficiencies in animal models through different mechanisms such as increased oxidative damage, mitochondrial and cholinergic dysfunction, apoptosis, neuroinflammation, suppression of trophic factors, insufficient spine maturation, excitation of glycogen synthase kinase-3 beta (GSK-3β), arborization of dendrites, involvement of N-methyl-D-aspartate (NMDA) receptor, and amyloid and tau deposition [54]. One of the major limitations of this drug is that sometimes, even at normal doses, it can induce hallucinations, confusion, agitation, confused speech, paranoid behaviors, and delusions [9, 54].

6.4.1.3.3 Colchicine

Colchicine is an alkaloid drug extracted from plants, initially used for the treatment of gouty arthritis. It is a neurotoxin capable of inducing dementia through cholinergic dysfunction (inhibiting the cholinergic pathway and reducing the number of cholinergic neurons). Microtubule interruption causes hippocampal lesions due to granule cell destruction [9, 48]. Reduction in neurotransmitter levels such as dopamine, serotonin, and norepinephrine within the hippocampus, caudate nucleus, and cerebral cortex can contribute to memory decline. Intracerebroventricular (ICV) administration of colchicine (7.5 μg in 10 μL) in rats and mice exhibits cognitive and spatial memory impairment after two weeks of induction. This sudden drop in cognitive function can be due to dysregulations such as an increased ratio of glutamate and GABA in the cortex, which triggers the NMDA receptors causing a sudden influx of Ca^{2+}, increased expression of iNOS, cyclooxygenase-1 and 2 (COX-1 and COX-2) generating ROS, and decreased activities of AChE and ChAT enzymes, ultimately precipitating similar human symptoms of sporadic Alzheimer's type of dementia in animals [9, 47].

6.4.1.3.4 Okadaic Acid

Okadaic acid, $C_{44}H_{68}O_{13}$, is a polyether toxin produced by several species of dinoflagellates, which accumulate in both marine sponges and shellfish. It is one of the primary causes of diarrhetic shellfish poisoning. Okadaic acid is a potent inhibitor of specific protein serine/threonine phosphatases

1 and 2A which are associated with long- and short-term memory and potentiates the hyperphosphorylation of tau. It acts as a selective inhibitor of protein synthesis through hyperphosphorylation of elongation factor EF2 [48, 84]. Clinical observation showed that OKA causes memory impairment in human subjects who consumed seafood contaminated with dinoflagellate (*Helicondria okadai*) [85].

Similarly, in animal models such as rats and zebrafish, OKA is used effectively for the screening of anti-dementia drugs due to its property of inducing memory loss. Different mechanistic pathways have been attributed to OKA-induced memory decline, which includes decreased basal synaptic transmission and hindering the initiation of synaptic plasticity, mitochondrial abnormalities in the brain due to the increased production of ROS in the hippocampus, and decreased mitochondrial activity. Also, the proinflammatory mediators such as IL-1 and TNF-α with increased total nitrate and iNOS expression in the cortex and hippocampus exacerbate memory loss [9, 86]. Hyperphosphorylation of proteins due to inhibition of phosphatases as well as ionotropic excitatory amino acid receptors causes increased calcium in the cultured hippocampal cells leading to neuronal stress. Decreased GSH, increased expression of GFAP, higher protein carbonylation, and mitogen-activated protein kinase 38 (p38MAPK) precipitate the spatial cognitive deficit. Hyper-phosphorylated tau is a crucial feature of AD pathology exhibited through this method of induction by the presence of different kinases like MAPK, GSK-3β, and cyclin-dependent kinase 5 (Cdk5) [9]. Phosphatase PP2A enzyme will aid in the dephosphorylation of tau or slow down the hyperphosphorylation. Moreover, OKA induces AD's similar neuropathological changes in test animals' brains such as hippocampal neurodegeneration, formation of NFT, and Aβ peptide-like structures [9, 87, 88].

In a study by Koehler et al., they evaluated OKA-induced pathophysiological changes of AD, including Aβ amyloid deposits, intracellular tau protein accumulation, and pGSK3α/β. They tested various doses ranging from 10 nM to 1 μM OKA (with the inclusion of a control group). OKA is dissolved in a suitable solvent and administered to zebrafish by adding it directly to the water. Upon comparison with the control group, there was a significant increase in the pathophysiological features, indicating okadaic acid-induced AD-like pathological changes with cognitive decline in the zebrafish model. Immunohistochemistry showed the formation of phosphorylated glycogen synthase-3α/β, Aβ, p-tau, tau protein, and senile plaque in the zebrafish brain, all significantly increased with increasing exposure to

OKA [86]. These zebrafish models have been extensively used to evaluate the neurotrophic or neuroprotective effects of several natural compounds used for AD [89].

6.4.1.3.5 Sodium Azide

Sodium azide (NaN_3) is a mitochondrial toxin that appears as a crystalline white solid used for the production of lead azide explosives. It inhibits the mitochondrial enzyme cytochrome oxidase (CoX), which maintains the respiratory chain and leads to the dysfunction of mitochondria, including ROS generation and metabolic impairment by hindering mitochondrial complex-IV and reducing ATP levels. It also induces neuronal loss in the hippocampal CA3 regions, highlighting the role of NaN_3 in AD induction [9]. The administration of NaN_3 by minipumps requires a long duration of exposure with one-time use only and is highly costly. Meanwhile, the intraperitoneal administration of NaN_3 in a dose-dependent manner will induce AD-like dementia early and adversely affect cognitive functions such as learning and memory by selectively inhibiting the cytochrome C complex and increasing AChE levels [9, 49].

6.4.1.3.6 Ethanol/Alcohol

Ethanol is an organic compound, which gets rapidly absorbed from the gastrointestinal tract and is well known for its bactericidal properties. It is widely used as a solvent. For years, the deleterious effects of alcohol on health have been well-known and considered a significant risk factor for cognitive impairment. Acute alcohol intoxication can lead to the alteration of neurochemicals like Gamma-aminobutyric acid (GABA), opiate, dopamine, and glutamine. Alcohol increases the effects of the inhibitory GABA in the brain, causing sluggish movements and slurred speech, while also inhibiting the excitatory neurotransmitter glutamate. Excessive alcohol consumption might generate sufficient acetaldehyde in the brain to condense with biogenic amines including dopamine, serotonin, and norepinephrine to produce psychoactive alkaloids such as salsolinol. This results in the alteration of brain signals and damages hippocampal and cholinergic neurons [90, 91]. It elevates the level of nitric oxide (NO) and adenosine, and decreases the expression of BDNF, altering the mitochondrial morphology in a dose-dependent manner, eventually leading to a drastic decline in learning and memory [9, 93].

6.4.1.3.7 Lipopolysaccharide (LPS)

LPS is well known for inducing amyloidosis and neuroinflammation in models studying neurodegenerative disease. It is an endotoxin obtained from the outer membrane of bacteria (gram-negative) capable of degrading mammalian enzymes. It activates intracellular molecules that stimulate inflammatory processes, leading to increased expression and production of proinflammatory cytokines IL-1β and IL-6, resulting in changes in the expression of isoforms of APP in the cerebellum. AD pathology can be attributed to inflammation, as elevated levels of IL-6 and C-reactive protein (CRP) are observed years before the occurrence of dementia. This is followed by an increase in mRNAs and changes in the expression of APP isoforms in the cerebellum [9, 93].

6.4.1.3.8 Cigarette Smoke Extract

The two components of cigarette smoke are vapor and a particulate phase, which contain almost a thousand unidentified compounds and 4,500 molecules that have been identified. These chemicals have a history of inducing pro-inflammatory and cancerous responses, as well as oxidative damage [88]. They can harm tight junction proteins like ZO-1 and occludin, leading to oxidative stress and vascular inflammation, which affect the pathophysiology of the BBB [94]. The risk of Alzheimer's disease is increased by smoking. A study looked at the impact of ambrisentan, a selective endothelin-A receptor antagonist, on the cognitive impairment caused by cigarette smoke in Danio rerio [95]. Tests using light and dark chambers, color identification, partition preferences, horizontal compartments, and T-Mazes were used to evaluate cognitive abilities. In addition, evaluations of the biomarker alterations caused by CSE in zebrafish brain samples were obtained. Ambrisentan therapy showed a possible ameliorative impact against CSE-induced cognitive functions as well as a reduction in metabolic alterations [96].

6.4.1.3.9 Stereotaxic Surgery

The introduction of stereotaxic surgery brings a breakthrough in AD research. Since most of the *in vivo* models only partially mimic the AD features, it was very difficult to rule out the main pathological hallmarks of AD. In this method, the soluble infusion of highly neurotoxic amyloid-beta peptide (1–42) ($A\beta_{(1-42)}$) is injected stereotaxically into the mice brain by a well-trained expert to study the Aβ peptide's short-term effects on specific regions of the brain [97]. Usually, the infusion is targeted toward the hippocampal dentate gyrus, which is closely connected to the cholinergic pathway. The results highlight that prominent cholinergic neuronal loss and cell death occur within 1 week, and the effects last for 2 weeks, suggesting that this can be used as a promising model for studying region-specific neuronal damage in a short span of time [52, 97] (Figure 6.2).

The boxes represented under the 10 individual chemical agents represent specific mechanisms and the outer circle implies the general mechanisms by which chemical agents cause AD induction. Finally, these agents will increase the amyloid plaques and neurofibrillary tangles formation leading to AD.

6.5 LIMITATIONS

Despite the advances in AD research, including the breakthrough discovery of the AD transgenic models from 1995 onwards, various possibilities are being explored. Still, none of the studies could establish a hopeful model that would replicate the exact human AD pathology mainly due to the complexity of the brain. Even though the *in vitro* study requires proper maintenance of cell lines and high investment cost, it has very low reproducibility and inter-batch instability.

Moreover, the longer developmental period of AD features, the high cost of maintenance, and the controversies in various AD hypotheses, especially the beta-amyloid hypothesis, exacerbate the challenges in the development of an ideal animal model for AD. The failure of the anti-Alzheimer's drugs to prove their clinical effect, even after successful preclinical results, highlights the glaring gaps in AD research.

6.6 FUTURE DIRECTIONS

Incorporating the possibilities of artificial intelligence (AI) and machine learning into animal models for anti-Alzheimer's drug development may bring milestone discoveries. Researchers have explored the potential of AI in decoding the individual risk factors and mechanisms behind AD by processing huge datasets and reproducing high-quality output with more accuracy. Upgrading the 2D models to 3D models will help understand the more complex characteristics of brain tissue, thereby ruling out the in-depth AD pathophysiology. Developing advanced organoid models and tissue engineering can replace the use of animal models for preclinical research.

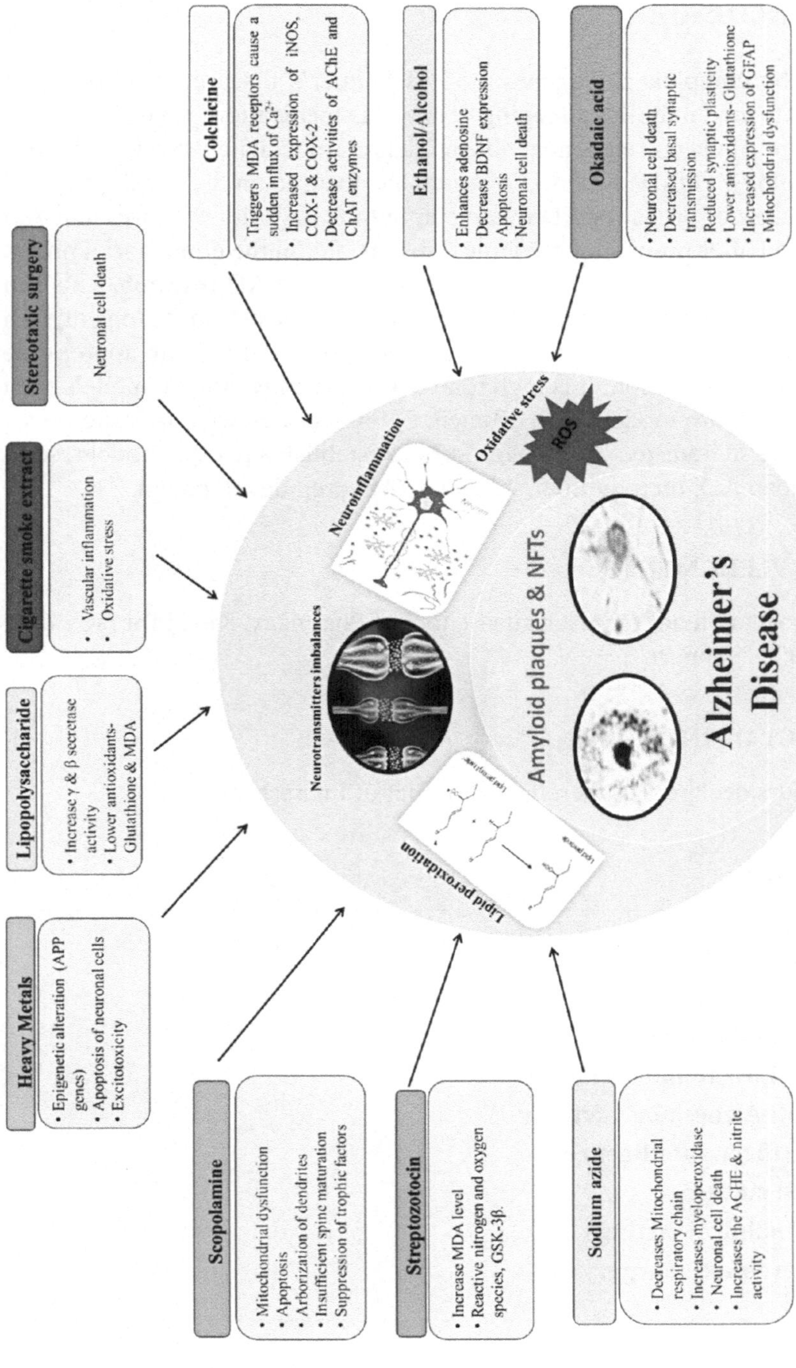

FIGURE 6.2 Potential mechanisms implicated in chemical-induced AD.

6.7 CONCLUSION

Due to the complex pathogenesis of Alzheimer's disease, identifying an appropriate model for the screening of anti-AD medications is always a challenge; none of the currently available models can adequately replicate human AD pathology. For decades, AD research has focused on the development of a newer class of drugs for AD treatment, but the majority of newer anti-AD drugs, even after promising preclinical results, fail in the clinical trial phase, highlighting the glaring gap in the current system of AD research. This can be overcome to a certain extent by addressing the current limitations of each model and selecting an ideal *in vitro* and *in vivo* model with an appropriate method of AD induction. It is high time to replace conventional models such as 2D cell culture models with efficient 3D models, as well as explore vast possibilities in transgenic animal models to establish a perfect model resembling human AD, thereby flourishing anti-AD drug development.

ACKNOWLEDGMENTS

The authors are thankful to Amrita School of Pharmacy, Kochi for providing the technical support.

CONFLICT OF INTEREST

The authors declare that there is no conflict of interest.

KEYWORDS

- **Alzheimer's disease**
- **amyloid β**
- **animal models**
- **anti-Alzheimer drugs**
- **anti-Alzheimer's activity**
- **artificial intelligence**
- **cell culture**
- **preclinical testing**
- **stereotaxic surgery**

REFERENCES

1. Silva, M. V. F., Loures, C. D. M. G., Alves, L. C. V., De Souza, L. C., Borges, K. B. G., & Carvalho, M. D. G. (2019). Alzheimer's disease: Risk factors and potentially protective measures. Journal of Biomedical Science, 26(1), 1–11. https://doi.org/10.1186/s12929-019-0524-y.
2. Neugroschl, J., & Wang, S. (2011). Alzheimer's disease: Diagnosis and treatment across the spectrum of disease severity. Mount Sinai Journal of Medicine, 78(4), 596–612. https://pubmed.ncbi.nlm.nih.gov/21748748/ (accessed on 22 July 2024).
3. Benny, A., & Thomas, J. (2019). Essential oils as a treatment strategy for Alzheimer's disease: Current and future perspectives. Planta Medica, 85(3), 239–248. https://pubmed.ncbi.nlm.nih.gov/30360002/.
4. Alzheimer's Association. (2022). Alzheimer's facts and figures report. Retrieved from: https://www.alz.org/alzheimers-dementia/facts-figures (accessed on 22 July 2024).
5. Arya, M. A., Manoj Kumar, M. K., Sabitha, M., Krishnakumar Menon, K., & Nair, S. C. (2019). Nanotechnology approaches for enhanced CNS delivery in treating Alzheimer's disease. Journal of Drug Delivery Science and Technology, 51, 297–309.
6. Drummond, E., & Wisniewski, T. (2017). Alzheimer's disease: Experimental models and reality. Acta Neuropathologica, 133(2), 155–175.
7. Kumar, A., Sidhu, J., Goyal, A., & Tsao, J. W. (2022). Alzheimer disease. StatPearls. Retrieved from: https://www.ncbi.nlm.nih.gov/books/NBK499922/ (accessed on 22 July 2024).
8. Sun, X., Chen, W. D., & Wang, Y. D. (2015). β-Amyloid: The key peptide in the pathogenesis of Alzheimer's disease. Frontiers in Pharmacology, 6, 221.
9. Tunku Abdul Rahman, U., Aris Mohd Moklas, M., Mahdi, O., Taufik Hidayat Baharuldin, M., Huda Mohd Nor, N., Musa Chiroma, S., et al. (2019). Chemicals used for the induction of Alzheimer's disease-like cognitive dysfunctions in rodents. Biomedical Research and Therapy, 6(11), 3460–3484. http://www.bmrat.org/index.php/BMRAT/article/view/575 (accessed on 22 July 2024).
10. Braak, H., Alafuzoff, I., Arzberger, T., Kretzschmar, H., & Tredici, K. D. (2006). Staging of Alzheimer's disease-associated neurofibrillary pathology using paraffin sections and immunocytochemistry. Acta Neuropathologica, 112(4), 389–404. https://pubmed.ncbi.nlm.nih.gov/16906426/ (accessed on 22 July 2024).
11. Newman, M., Kretzschmar, D., Khan, I., Chen, M., Verdile, G., & Lardelli, M. (2017). Chapter 40 – Animal models of Alzheimer's disease. In Animal Models for the Study of Human Disease.
12. Bekris, L. M., Yu, C. E., Bird, T. D., & Tsuang, D. W. (2010). Genetics of Alzheimer's disease. Journal of Geriatric Psychiatry and Neurology, 23(4), 213. https://doi.org/10.1177/0891988710383527.
13. Kinney, J. W., Bemiller, S. M., Murtishaw, A. S., Leisgang, A. M., Salazar, A. M., & Lamb, B. T. (2018). Inflammation is a central mechanism in Alzheimer's disease. Alzheimer's & Dementia: Translational Research & Clinical Interventions, 4, 575–590. https://doi.org/10.1002/trc2.12088.
14. Blaikie, L., Kay, G., Maciel, P., & Kong Thoo Lin, P. (2022). Experimental modeling of Alzheimer's disease for therapeutic screening. European Journal of Medicinal Chemistry Reports, 5, 100044.

15. Gella, A., & Durany, N. (2009). Oxidative stress in Alzheimer's disease. Cell Adhesion & Migration, 3(1), 88–93. https://doi.org/10.4161/cam.3.1.7271.
16. Scheffer, S., Hermkens, D. M. A., Van Der Weerd, L., De Vries, H. E., & Daemen, M. J. A. P. (2021). Vascular hypothesis of Alzheimer's disease. Arteriosclerosis, Thrombosis, and Vascular Biology, 41(4), 1265–1283. https://doi.org/10.1161/ATVBAHA.120.311911.
17. Deture, M. A., & Dickson, D. W. (2019). The neuropathological diagnosis of Alzheimer's disease. Molecular Neurodegeneration, 14(1), 1–18. https://doi.org/10.1186/s13024-019-0333-5.
18. Coupé, P., Manjón, J. V., Lanuza, E., & Catheline, G. (2019). Lifespan changes of the human brain in Alzheimer's disease. Scientific Reports, 9(1), 1–12. https://doi.org/10.1038/s41598-019-39809-8.
19. Zarei, M., Beckmann, C. F., Binnewijzend, M. A. A., Schoonheim, M. M., Oghabian, M. A., Sanz-Arigita, E. J., et al. (2013). Functional segmentation of the hippocampus in the healthy human brain and Alzheimer's disease. NeuroImage, 66, 28–35. https://doi.org/10.1016/j.neuroimage.2012.10.077.
20. National Institute on Aging. (2017). What happens to the brain in Alzheimer's disease? Retrieved from: https://www.nia.nih.gov/health/what-happens-brain-alzheimers-disease (accessed on 22 July 2024).
21. Jahn, H. (2022). Memory loss in Alzheimer's disease. *Dementia and Cognitive Disorders, 15*(4), 445–454. https://doi.org/10.31887/DCNS.2013.15.4/hjahn.
22. Mostafavi, S., Gaiteri, C., Sullivan, S. E., White, C. C., Tasaki, S., Xu, J., et al. (2018). A molecular network of the aging human brain provides insights into the pathology and cognitive decline of Alzheimer's disease. *Nature Neuroscience, 21*(6), 811–819. https://doi.org/10.1038/s41593-018-0154-9.
23. Casadesus, G., Arendash, G., Laferla, F., & McDonald, M. (2010). Animal models of Alzheimer's disease. *International Journal of Alzheimer's Disease, 2(11), a006320.* https://doi.org/10.1155/2010/a006320.
24. Anton, D., Burckel, H., Josset, E., & Noel, G. (2015). Three-dimensional cell culture: A breakthrough in vivo. *International Journal of Molecular Sciences, 16*(16), 5517–5527. https://doi.org/10.3390/ijms16075517.
25. Centeno, E. G. Z., Cimarosti, H., & Bithell, A. (2018). 2D versus 3D human induced pluripotent stem cell-derived cultures for neurodegenerative disease modeling. *Molecular Neurodegeneration, 13*(1), 27. https://doi.org/10.1186/s13024-018-0347-0.
26. Gopalakrishnan, A., Shankarappa, S. A., & Rajanikant, G. K. (2019). Hydrogel scaffolds: Towards restitution of ischemic stroke-injured brain. *Translational Stroke Research, 10*(1), 1–18. https://doi.org/10.1007/s12975-018-0693-7.
27. Madhusudanan, P., Raju, G., & Shankarappa, S. (2020). Hydrogel systems and their role in neural tissue engineering. *Journal of the Royal Society Interface, 17*(162). https://doi.org/10.1098/rsif.2019.0675.
28. Cenini, G., Hebisch, M., Iefremova, V., Flitsch, L. J., Breitkreuz, Y., Tanzi, R. E., et al. (2021). Dissecting Alzheimer's disease pathogenesis in human 2D and 3D models. *Molecular and Cellular Neuroscience, 110, 103568*. https://doi.org/10.1016/j.mcn.2021.103568.
29. Fennema, E., Rivron, N., Rouwkema, J., van Blitterswijk, C., & De Boer, J. (2013). Spheroid culture as a tool for creating 3D complex tissues. *Trends in Biotechnology, 31*(8), 108–115. https://doi.org/10.1016/j.tibtech.2013.01.007.

30. Jorfi, M., D'Avanzo, C., Tanzi, R. E., Kim, D. Y., & Irimia, D. (2018). Human neurospheroid arrays for in vitro studies of Alzheimer's disease. *Scientific Reports, 8*(1), 2450.
31. Foty, R. (2011). A simple hanging drop cell culture protocol for generation of 3D spheroids. *Journal of Visualized Experiments, (51)*. https://doi.org/10.3791/2516.
32. Park, H. J., Kim, J., & Ryou, C. (2023). A three-dimensional spheroid co-culture system of neurons and astrocytes derived from Alzheimer's disease patients for drug efficacy testing. *Cell Proliferation, 56(6), e13399.*
33. Pomeshchik, Y., Klementieva, O., Gil, J., & Reports, I. M. S. C. (2020). Human iPSC-derived hippocampal spheroids: An innovative tool for stratifying Alzheimer disease patient-specific cellular phenotypes and developing treatments. *Elsevier, 15(1), 80–94.* https://doi.org/10.1016/j.stemcr.2020.06.004.
34. Lee, H. K., Velazquez Sanchez, C., Chen, M., Morin, P. J., Wells, J. M., Hanlon, E. B., et al. (2016). Three-dimensional human neuro-spheroid model of Alzheimer's disease based on differentiated induced pluripotent stem cells. *PLoS ONE, 11*(9), e0163072. https://doi.org/10.1371/journal.pone.0163072.
35. Want, A. J., Nienow, A. W., Hewitt, C. J., & Coopman, K. (2012). Large-scale expansion and exploitation of pluripotent stem cells for regenerative medicine purposes: Beyond the T flask. *Regenerative Medicine, 7*(1), 71–84. https://doi.org/10.2217/rme.11.73.
36. Lee, S. E., Choi, H., Shin, N., Kong, D., Kim, N. G., Kim, H. Y., et al. (2022). Zika virus infection accelerates Alzheimer's disease phenotypes in brain organoids. *Cell Death Discovery, 8*(1), 1–10. https://doi.org/10.1038/s41420-022-00814-7.
37. Chatterjee, N., Walker, G., Lucia, M. S., & Ahn, H. (2017). HHS Public Access. *Physiology & Behavior, 176*(10), 139–148. https://doi.org/10.1016/j.physbeh.2017.03.024.
38. Ghatak, S., Dolatabadi, N., Trudler, D., Zhang, X., Wu, Y., Mohata, M., et al. (2019). Mechanisms of hyperexcitability in Alzheimer's disease hiPSC-derived neurons and cerebral organoids versus isogenic control. *eLife, 8, e50333.* https://doi.org/10.7554/eLife.50333.
39. Galbraith, T., & Berthod, F. (2023). In vitro 3D modeling of neurodegenerative diseases. *Neurobiological Reviews, 10(1), 93.*
40. Doyle, A. D., Carvajal, N., Jin, A., Matsumoto, K., & Yamada, K. M. (2015). Local 3D matrix microenvironment regulates cell migration through spatiotemporal dynamics of contractility-dependent adhesions. *Nature Communications, 6*, 8720. https://doi.org/10.1038/ncomms9720.
41. Park, J., Lee, B. K., Jeong, G. S., Hyun, J. K., Lee, C. J., & Lee, S. H. (2015). Three-dimensional brain-on-a-chip with an interstitial level of flow and its application as an in vitro model of Alzheimer's disease. *Lab on a Chip, 15*(1), 141–150. https://doi.org/10.1039/C4LC00762G.
42. Sukoff Rizzo, S. J., Masters, A., Onos, K. D., Quinney, S., Sasner, M., Oblak, A., et al. (2020). Improving preclinical to clinical translation in Alzheimer's disease research. *Alzheimer's & Dementia: Translational Research & Clinical Interventions, 6*(1), e12038. https://doi.org/10.1002/trc2.12038.
43. Woodruff-Pak, D. S. (2008). Animal models of Alzheimer's disease: Therapeutic implications. *Journal of Alzheimer's Disease, 15*(4), 507–521. https://doi.org/10.3233/JAD-2008-15404.

44. Bakulski, K. M., Seo, Y. A., Hickman, R. C., Brandt, D., Vadari, H. S., Hu, H., et al. (2020). Heavy metals exposure and Alzheimer's disease and related dementias. *Journal of Alzheimer's Disease, 76*(4), 1215–1229. https://doi.org/10.3233/JAD-190982.
45. Park, J., Won, J., Seo, J., Yeo, H. G., Kim, K., Kim, Y. G., et al. (2020). Streptozotocin induces Alzheimer's disease-like pathology in hippocampal neuronal cells via CDK5/Drp1-mediated mitochondrial fragmentation. *Frontiers in Cellular Neuroscience, 14*, 235. https://doi.org/10.3389/fncel.2020.00235.
46. Yadang, F. S. A., Nguezeye, Y., Kom, C. W., Betote, P. H. D., Mamat, A., Tchokouaha, L. R. Y., et al. (2020). Scopolamine-induced memory impairment in mice: Neuroprotective effects of *Carissa edulis* (Forssk.) Valh (Apocynaceae) aqueous extract. *International Journal of Alzheimer's Disease, 2020(3), 1–10*. https://doi.org/10.1155/2020/6372059.
47. Kumar, A., Seghal, N., Naidu, P. S. V., Padi, S. S. V., & Goyal, R. (2007). Colchicines-induced neurotoxicity as an animal model of sporadic dementia of Alzheimer's type. *Journal of Alzheimer's Disease, 11*(4), 343–351. https://doi.org/10.3233/JAD-2007-11403.
48. Malekzadeh, S., Amin, M., Mehrabani, D., & Shariati, M. (2017). Drugs induced Alzheimer's disease in animal models. *Galen Medical Journal, 6*(3), 185–196. https://doi.org/10.22086/gmj.v6i3.820.
49. Nöldner, M. (2017). Oral treatment with the Ginkgo biloba extract EGb 761® prevents sodium azide-induced memory deficits in rats. *Planta Medica International Open, 4*(S 01), Tu-PO-78. https://doi.org/10.1055/s-0037-1608413
50. Batista, C. R. A., Gomes, G. F., Candelario-Jalil, E., Fiebich, B. L., & de Oliveira, A. C. P. (2019). Lipopolysaccharide-induced neuroinflammation as a bridge to understand neurodegeneration. *International Journal of Molecular Sciences, 20*(9), 2293. https://doi.org/10.3390/ijms20092293.
51. Aedo, G., Miranda, M., Chávez, M. N., Allende, M. L., & Egaña, J. T. (2019). A reliable preclinical model to study the impact of cigarette smoke in development and disease. *Current Protocols in Toxicology, 80*(1). https://doi.org/10.1002/cptx.80.
52. Jean, Y. Y., Baleriola, J., Fà, M., Hengst, U., & Troy, C. M. (2015). Stereotaxic infusion of oligomeric amyloid-beta into the mouse hippocampus. *Journal of Visualized Experiments, (100)*, 52805. https://doi.org/10.3791/52805.
53. Zeiss, C. J. (2020). Utility of spontaneous animal models of Alzheimer's disease in preclinical efficacy studies. *Cell and Tissue Research, 380*(2), 273–286. https://doi.org/10.1007/s00441-020-03198-6.
54. Tang, K. S. (2019). The cellular and molecular processes associated with scopolamine-induced memory deficit: A model of Alzheimer's biomarkers. *Life Sciences, 233*, 116695. https://doi.org/10.1016/j.lfs.2019.116695.
55. Li, Y. (2013). Establishment of experimental models for Alzheimer's disease research. *International Journal of Neuroscience, 123*(12), 823–831. https://doi.org/10.3109/00207454.2013.838206.
56. Ros-Cucurull, E., Palma-Álvarez, R. F., Cardona-Rubira, C., García-Raboso, E., Jacas, C., & Grau-López, L. (2017). Outpatient unit in Barcelona. *Psychiatry Research, 261, 361–366*. https://doi.org/10.1016/j.psychres.2017.12.069.
57. Sasaguri, H., Hashimoto, S., Watamura, N., Sato, K., Takamura, R., Nagata, K., et al. (2022). Recent advances in the modeling of Alzheimer's disease. *Frontiers in Neuroscience, 16*(March), 1–16. https://doi.org/10.3389/fnins.2022.746946.

58. Woodruff-Pak, D. S., Agelan, A., & Del Valle, L. (2007). A rabbit model of Alzheimer's disease: Valid at neuropathological, cognitive, and therapeutic levels. *Journal of Alzheimer's Disease, 11*(3), 371–383. https://doi.org/10.3233/JAD-2007-11303.
59. Li, X., Bao, X., & Wang, R. (2016). Experimental models of Alzheimer's disease for deciphering the pathogenesis and therapeutic screening (Review). *International Journal of Molecular Medicine, 37*(2), 271–283. https://doi.org/10.3892/ijmm.2015.2424.
60. Schütt, T., Pedersen, J. T., & Berendt, M. (2018). The domestic dog as a model for human brain aging and Alzheimer's disease. In *Conn's Handbook of Models for Human Aging* (pp. 177–194). Academic Press. https://doi.org/10.1016/B978-0-12-809873-4.00009-7.
61. Fan, Y., Luo, R., Su, L. Y., Xiang, Q., Yu, D., Xu, L., et al. (2018). Does the genetic feature of the Chinese tree shrew (*Tupaia belangeri chinensis*) support its potential as a viable model for Alzheimer's disease research? *Journal of Alzheimer's Disease, 61*(3), 1015–1028. https://doi.org/10.3233/JAD-171188.
62. Wahl, D., Moreno, J. A., Santangelo, K. S., Zhang, Q., Afzali, M. F., Walsh, M. A., et al. (2022). Nontransgenic guinea pig strains exhibit hallmarks of human brain aging and Alzheimer's disease. *The Journals of Gerontology: Series A, 77*(9), 1766–1774. https://doi.org/10.1093/gerona/glac082.
63. Weiss, C., Bertolino, N., Procissi, D., Aleppo, G., Smith, Q. C., Viola, K. L., et al. (2022). Diet-induced Alzheimer's-like syndrome in the rabbit. *Alzheimer's & Dementia: Translational Research & Clinical Interventions, 8*(1), e12241. https://doi.org/10.1002/trc2.12241.
64. Stewart, M. A., & Kalueff, A. V. (2012). The developing utility of zebrafish models for cognitive enhancers research. *Current Neuropharmacology, 10*(3), 263–271. https://doi.org/10.2174/157015912800014398.
65. Bhattarai, P., Turgutalp, B., & Kizil, C. (2022). Zebrafish as an experimental and preclinical model for Alzheimer's disease. *ACS Chemical Neuroscience, 13*(20), 2939–2941. https://doi.org/10.1021/acschemneuro.2c00583.
66. Koster, R., & Sassen, W. A. (2015). A molecular toolbox for genetic manipulation of zebrafish. *Advances in Genomics and Genetics, 5*, 151–164. https://doi.org/10.2147/AGG.S67585.
67. Shenoy, A., Banerjee, M., Upadhya, A., Bagwe-Parab, S., & Kaur, G. (2022). The brilliance of the zebrafish model: Perception on behavior and Alzheimer's disease. *Frontiers in Behavioral Neuroscience, 16*(June), 1–17. https://doi.org/10.3389/fnbeh.2022.788224.
68. Panula, P., Sallinen, V., Sundvik, M., Kolehmainen, J., Torkko, V., Tiittula, A., et al. (2006). Modulatory neurotransmitter systems and behavior: Towards zebrafish models of neurodegenerative diseases. *Zebrafish, 3*(2), 235–247. https://doi.org/10.1089/zeb.2006.3.235.
69. Parker, M. O., Brock, A. J., Walton, R. T., & Brennan, C. H. (2013). The role of zebrafish (*Danio rerio*) in dissecting the genetics and neural circuits of executive function. *Frontiers in Neural Circuits, 7*, 33. https://doi.org/10.3389/fncir.2013.00033.
70. Newman, M., Ebrahimie, E., & Lardelli, M. (2014). Using the zebrafish model for Alzheimer's disease research. *Frontiers in Genetics, 5*(June), 1–10. https://doi.org/10.3389/fgene.2014.00105.
71. Shulman, J. M., Imboywa, S., Giagtzoglou, N., Powers, M. P., Hu, Y., Devenport, D., et al. (2014). Functional screening in *Drosophila* identifies Alzheimer's disease

susceptibility genes and implicates tau-mediated mechanisms. *Human Molecular Genetics, 23*(4), 870–877. https://doi.org/10.1093/hmg/ddt488.

72. Finelli, A., Kelkar, A., Song, H. J., Yang, H., & Konsolaki, M. (2004). A model for studying Alzheimer's Aβ42-induced toxicity in *Drosophila melanogaster*. *Molecular and Cellular Neurosciences, 26*(3), 365–375. https://doi.org/10.1016/j.mcn.2004.05.003.
73. Ray, A., Speese, S. D., & Logan, M. A. (2017). Glial draper rescues Aβ toxicity in a *Drosophila* model of Alzheimer's disease. *The Journal of Neuroscience, 37*(49), 11881–11893. https://doi.org/10.1523/JNEUROSCI.2234-17.2017.
74. Crowther, D. C., Kinghorn, K. J., Miranda, E., Page, R., Curry, J. A., Duthie, F. A. I., et al. (2005). Intraneuronal Aβ, non-amyloid aggregates and neurodegeneration in a *Drosophila* model of Alzheimer's disease. *Neuroscience, 132*(1), 123–135. https://doi.org/10.1016/j.neuroscience.2004.11.048.
75. Chakraborty, R., Vepuri, V., Mhatre, S. D., Paddock, B. E., Miller, S., Michelson, S. J., et al. (2011). Characterization of a *Drosophila* Alzheimer's disease model: Pharmacological rescue of cognitive defects. *PLoS ONE, 6*(6), e21160. https://doi.org/10.1371/journal.pone.0021160.
76. Cheon, Y. J., Hwang, H., & Kim, K. (2020). Plasticity of pheromone-mediated avoidance behavior in *C. elegans*. *Journal of Neurogenetics, 34*(3–4), 420–426. https://doi.org/10.1080/01677063.2020.1792133.
77. Shaye, D. D., & Greenwald, I. (2011). Ortholist: A compendium of *C. elegans* genes with human orthologs. *PLoS ONE, 6*(5), e20085. https://doi.org/10.1371/journal.pone.0020085.
78. Daigle, I., & Li, C. (1993). apl-1, a *Caenorhabditis elegans* gene encoding a protein related to the human β-amyloid protein precursor. *Proceedings of the National Academy of Sciences U S A, 90*(24), 12045–12049. https://doi.org/10.1073/pnas.90.24.12045.
79. McColl, G., Roberts, B. R., Gunn, A. P., Perez, K. A., Tew, D. J., Masters, C. L., et al. (2009). The *Caenorhabditis elegans* Aβ1–42 model of Alzheimer disease predominantly expresses Aβ3–42. *Journal of Biological Chemistry, 284*(34), 22697–22702. https://doi.org/10.1074/jbc.M109.029825.
80. McColl, G., Roberts, B. R., Pukala, T. L., Kenche, V. B., Roberts, C. M., Link, C. D., et al. (2012). Utility of an improved model of amyloid-beta (Aβ1–42) toxicity in *Caenorhabditis elegans* for drug screening for Alzheimer's disease. *Molecular Neurodegeneration, 7*(1), 57. https://doi.org/10.1186/1750-1326-7-57.
81. Sasaguri, H., Nilsson, P., Hashimoto, S., Nagata, K., Saito, T., De Strooper, B., et al. (2017). APP mouse models for Alzheimer's disease preclinical studies. *EMBO Journal, 36*(17), 2473–2487. https://doi.org/10.15252/embj.201696182.
82. Lee, J., & Freeman, J. L. (2014). Zebrafish as a model for investigating developmental lead (Pb) neurotoxicity as a risk factor in adult neurodegenerative disease: A mini-review. *Neurotoxicology, 43*, 57–64. https://doi.org/10.1016/j.neuro.2014.01.008.
83. Zhu, B., Wang, Q., Shi, X., Guo, Y., Xu, T., & Zhou, B. (2016). Effect of combined exposure to lead and decabromodiphenyl ether on neurodevelopment of zebrafish larvae. *Chemosphere, 144*, 1646–1654. https://doi.org/10.1016/j.chemosphere.2015.10.078.
84. Bialojan, C., & Takai, A. (1988). Inhibitory effect of a marine-sponge toxin, okadaic acid, on protein phosphatases: Specificity and kinetics. *Biochemical Journal, 256*(1), 283–290. https://doi.org/10.1042/bj2560283.
85. Baier, C. (2007). Biotoxins—The first responder. *Aristatek*. Retrieved from: https://www.aristatek.com/Newsletter/DEC07/DEC07ts.aspx (accessed on 22 July 2024).

86. Nada, S. E., Williams, F., & Shah, Z. (2016). Development of a novel and robust pharmacological model of okadaic acid-induced Alzheimer's disease in zebrafish. *CNS & Neurological Disorders–Drug Targets, 15*(1), 86–94. https://doi.org/10.2174/187152 7315666151228123026.
87. Billingsley, M., Van A, Michael, O., Trojanowski, J. Q., & Lee, V. M. (1994). Biopsy-derived adult human brain tau is phosphorylated at many of the same sites as Alzheimer's disease paired helical filament tau. *The Journal of Neuroscience, 13*(3), 989–1002. https://doi.org/10.1523/JNEUROSCI.13-03-00989.1994.
88. Thawkar, B. S., & Kaur, G. (2021). Zebrafish as a promising tool for modeling neurotoxin-induced Alzheimer's disease. *Neurotoxicity Research, 39*(3), 949–965. https://doi.org/10.1007/s12640-021-00310-x.
89. Koehler, D., Shah, Z. A., Hensley, K., & Williams, F. E. (2018). Lanthionine ketimine-5-ethyl ester provides neuroprotection in a zebrafish model of okadaic acid-induced Alzheimer's disease. *Neurochemistry International, 115*, 61–68. https://doi.org/10.1016/j.neuint.2018.03.009.
90. Sullivan, E. V., Harris, R. A., & Pfefferbaum, A. (2010). Alcohol's effects on brain and behavior. *Alcohol Research & Health, 33*(2), 127–142.
91. Bernardin, F., Maheut-Bosser, A., & Paille, F. (2014). Cognitive impairments in alcohol-dependent subjects. *Frontiers in Psychiatry, 5*(July), 1–6. https://doi.org/10.3389/fpsyt.2014.00074.
92. Koch, M., Fitzpatrick, A. L., Rapp, S. R., Nahin, R. L., Williamson, J. D., Lopez, O. L., et al. (2019). Alcohol consumption and risk of dementia and cognitive decline among older adults with or without mild cognitive impairment. *Journal of the American Geriatrics Society, 67*(9), 1954–1963. https://doi.org/10.1111/jgs.16008.
93. Hou, Y., Xie, G., Miao, F., Ding, L., Mou, Y., Wang, L., et al. (2014). Pterostilbene attenuates lipopolysaccharide-induced learning and memory impairment possibly via inhibiting microglia activation and protecting neuronal injury in mice. *Progress in Neuro-Psychopharmacology & Biological Psychiatry, 54*, 92–102. https://doi.org/10.1016/j.pnpbp.2014.06.013.
94. Naik, P., Fofaria, N., Prasad, S., Sajja, R. K., Weksler, B., Couraud, P. O., et al. (2014). Oxidative and pro-inflammatory impact of regular and denicotinized cigarettes on blood-brain barrier endothelial cells: Is smoking reduced or nicotine-free products really safe? *BMC Neuroscience, 15*, 51. https://doi.org/10.1186/1471-2202-15-51.
95. Muthuraman, A., Na, K., & Srinivasmurthy, K. (2019). Role of ambrisentan (selective endothelin-A receptor antagonist) on cigarette smoke exposure-induced cognitive impairment in *Danio rerio*. *Journal of Biochemical and Molecular Toxicology, 33*(12), e22328. https://doi.org/10.1002/jbt.22328.
96. Aedo, G., Miranda, M., & Ch, M. N. (2019). A reliable preclinical model to study the impact of cigarette smoke in development and disease. *Current Protocols in Toxicology, 99(2), 224–234*. https://doi.org/10.1002/cpt.206.
97. Facchinetti, R., Bronzuoli, M. R., & Scuderi, C. (2018). An animal model of Alzheimer's disease based on the intrahippocampal injection of amyloid β-peptide (1–42). In *Methods in Molecular Biology* (Vol. 1785, pp. 343–352). Humana Press Inc. https://doi.org/10.1007/978-1-4939-7880-0_20.

PART II

Nutraceutical for the Management of Alzheimer's Disease

CHAPTER 7

Medhya Rasayanas for the Management of Alzheimer's Disease

NIKITA NAIN,[1] KAVITA MUNJAL,[2*] VINOD KUMAR GAUTTAM,[3] SUMEET GUPTA,[1] VARINDER SINGH,[4] and SHREYA KAUL[2]

[1]*Department of Pharmacy, M.M. College of Pharmacy, M.M. (Deemed to be University), Mullana, Ambala, Haryana, India*

[2]*Amity Institute of Pharmacy, Amity University, Noida, Uttar Pradesh, India*

[3]*Department of Pharmacognosy, Shiva Institute of Pharmacy, Bilaspur, Himachal Pradesh, India*

[4]*Department of Pharmaceutical Sciences and Technology, Maharaja Ranjit Singh Punjab Technical University, Bathinda, Punjab, India*

*Corresponding author.

ABSTRACT

Alzheimer's disease (AD), which accounts for 60 to 80% of dementia cases in older persons (>65 years), is the main cause of dementia. This neurodegenerative brain condition causes memory loss and a gradual decline of mental ability. The hallmarks of AD, which frequently cause behavioral abnormalities and cognitive decline, are extracellular amyloid-beta (Aβ) plaques and neurofibrillary tangles. Alternative therapeutic approaches are needed because current medications merely treat the symptoms and do not address the underlying neuronal deterioration. There has recently been a strong desire to study medicinal plants worldwide to boost cognitive function. "Medhya Rasayanas" (memory enhancing and rejuvenating) are a group of medicinal herbs that have been specially identified by Prabhava (specific action) as having multiple benefits, including enhancing memory

Neuro-Nutraceuticals and Drug Discovery and Delivery in Alzheimer's Disease, Volume 1: Targeting Key Pathological Pathways. Varinder Singh, Amit Kumar, Parul Sood (Eds.)

and intellect. The Medhya Rasayanas are used to restore mental and cognitive function. These ayurvedic remedies act by modulating the neuroendocrine-immune system through antioxidant and anti-inflammatory characteristics, improving memory and reviving cognitive functioning. Regular intake of such Rasayanas will help to prevent the onset of degenerative changes in the brain prematurely. In this chapter, the focus will be given to the protective role of some of the commonly used herbs from the Medhya Rasayana group, along with their phytoconstituents and mechanisms in clinical prospects in AD.

7.1 INTRODUCTION

Alzheimer's disease (AD) is a progressive neurological condition that affects the medial temporal lobe and associative neocortical regions. Its pathological features include amyloid-beta (Aβ) peptide accumulation and neurofibrillary tangles, as well as cytoskeletal changes brought on by tau protein hyperphosphory castration in neurons [1, 2]. It leads to clinical manifestations such as disturbances in memory and language tone, visual problems, and higher executive function. Moreover, it also causes psychosis, mood instability, agitation, and sleep abnormalities [3]. Previous approaches to treating AD have emphasized the use of cholinesterase inhibitors like Donepezil, Rivastigmine, and Galantamine as well as NMDA receptor antagonists (memantine). Only temporary relief from behavioral problems is provided by AChE inhibitors [4]. Although cognitive improvement in persons with mild to severe AD has been seen, their effectiveness for neuro-psychiatric symptoms remains controversial. Further, it is reported for some negative effects including nausea, vomiting, diarrhea, and dizziness [5]. A number of Ayurvedic drugs that are said to enhance memory and revitalize cognitive capacities can be used to treat acute and chronic neurological illnesses. Ayurvedic medicinal herbs are abundant in antioxidants and anti-inflammatory chemicals, and they also influence the neuroendocrine and immunological systems [6, 7].

The ancient discipline of Ayurveda investigates the therapeutic potential of naturally occurring plant products and how they might be used to cure a variety of illnesses [8, 9]. Ayurveda has been practiced since antiquity through its eight specific branches, including [10].

- Kayachikitsa or internal medicine;
- Salya or surgery;

- Salakya or ophthalmology and ENT;
- Kaumarabhritya or pediatrics;
- Aagada tantra or toxicology;
- Bhuta vidya or psychiatry;
- Rasayana or rejuvenation;
- Vajikarana or sexology.

In the present era, modern science has taken a keen interest in Ayurveda since a number of its extracts have demonstrated neuroprotective potential against a variety of neurological illnesses [11]. The pathogenesis of AD may be targeted by herbal medications on a variety of levels, including cellular and molecular ones. Some herbs may protect against cognitive decline by acting specifically on AChE, the production of amyloid fibrils, and tau aggregation, in addition to having general antioxidant and anti-inflammatory properties [12]. This chapter compiles the role of some of the commonly used herbs from the Medhya Rasayana group, with a brief knowledge about the Ayurvedic prospects of AD regarding neuroprotection.

7.2 ALZHEIMER'S DISEASE – AYURVEDA PERSPECTIVE

According to Ayurveda, the human body is affected by the "*Vata*," "*Pitta*," and "Kapha" energies or "doshas." Diseases would be produced if these components were out of balance [13]. Memory loss, poor blood circulation, anxiety, and other neurological diseases are caused by the preponderance of "*Vata*" dosha [14]. To stabilize the "*Vata*" component of the body, which is affected by imbalanced "*Vata*," herbal formulations are administered to patients with neurodegenerative illnesses [15].

Vata's subdosha, Prana *Vata*, is located and moves principally in the brain, head, throat, and. It is responsible for maintaining a state of physiological balance in everything associated with brain function [16]. *Vibhramsa* (perversion) of *mana, buddhi, Sanja* (awareness), *smriti, bhakti* (desire), *sheela* (manner), *chesta* (behavior), and *achara* are characteristics of *unmada* (conduct). Memory loss, or *smriti bhramsa*, is the primary symptom of AD in its early stages. As the illness worsens, *vibhramsa* causes the cognitive function to interact with daily tasks [17].

Symptoms of AD according to Ayurveda are:

1. ***Smriti bhramsa*:** Loss of memory, decreased language skills, and trouble finding words (aphasia).

2. ***Sheela vibhramsa*:** Some patients with anosognosia experience frustration and distress.
3. ***Cheshta vibhramsa*:** Difficulty with sequential motor actions including eating, dressing, and other activities, as well as slowness and awkwardness of movement (apraxia).
4. ***Budhi vibhramsa*:** Delusions and hallucinations, such as failing to recognize an old acquaintance or believing a visitor to be a burglar.
5. ***Cheshta vibhramsa*:** Even basic chores like eating, dressing, and using the restroom require assistance.
6. ***Budhi vibhramsa*:** Complete mental disarray, loss of insight, and other symptoms.
7. **Age and *Akalaj Jara*:** These are the key *Hetu* (etiological parameters) taken into account (early aging). The main causes of *Vata* vitiation are "margavarodh" (obstruction of the nourishment channel) and "dhatukshay" (tissue degeneration). This ailment is regarded in Ayurveda as a kind of *Vataj Manas vyadhi* (age-related *smriti vibhransh*), which manifests in late middle age (around 40–60 years). A combination of "shodhan" (purification through panchakarma), "shaman" (pacification through palliative drugs), and "rasayan chikitsa" can be used to treat *Manas vyadhi*, particularly Dementia/disease. Alzheimer's (tissue rejuvenating therapy) [18].

7.3 CONCEPT OF RASAYANS AND MEDHYA RASAYANAS

The literal meaning of the word "Rasayana" is "the route that takes" (Rasa: plasma; Ayana: path). According to Ayurveda, the health of the body's various dhatus (tissues) is influenced by the characteristics of the "rasadhatu." Therefore, any medication that enhances the quality of "rasa" ("Rasayana") should strengthen or advance all body tissues [19].

Ayurveda's *Rasayana* branch focuses on ways to lengthen life and improve quality of life. In order to postpone aging and improve well-being, it mentions plants, animal products, metals, and minerals: minerals that can be employed as *Rasayana* ingredients. It also discusses non-materialistic approaches to well-being, such as meditation, positive thinking, appropriate behavior, and a healthy lifestyle [20]. *Rasayanas* are effective for promoting, maintaining, and curing health [10, 21].

They primarily behave in one of three ways [22]:

1. ***Agnivyapara*:** Through enhancing "Agnivyapara," or digestion and metabolism, to promote nutrition. Such *Rasayana* medications, such as haritaki, bhallataka, etc., increase nutritional status at the level of "dhatus" by promoting the digestion of food and energizing metabolic activity.
2. ***Srotosodhana*:** By opening up the macro- and micro-channels and boosting tissue perfusion. This procedure enhances the capability of srotas, or tissue perfusion and microcirculation. These *Rasayana* medicines increase the body's microcirculatory channels, which promote tissue perfusion and the bioavailability of nutrients to the tissues, both of which contribute to an improvement in nutritional status, such as Guggulu [23].
3. ***Posana*:** By directly enhancing the nutritional value of rasa (*poshaka* rasa), or the plasma's nutrient content. Such Rasayana agents, such as ghrita, dugdha, satavari, etc., include in their bulk good quality nutrients and as such, when provided, they directly add to the pool of nutrition and afterward help in improved tissue nourishing leading to future Rasayana effects.
4. ***Rasayana Tantra*:** This promotes an energetic way of living, a nutritious diet, and a variety of herbal and mineral medicines that are said to support nourishing medicinal foods, boost immunity, and foster memory and cognitive abilities [24, 25].

7.4 THE AYURVEDIC NOTION OF RASAYANA

It refers to a group of specific medications that boost immunity, prevent aging, lengthen life expectancy, promote lifespan, and give energy and vitality to the body. In India, herbs have been utilized for thousands of years to treat cognitive decline. The Indian school of medicine known as Ayurveda mentions the use of medications known as "Medhya Rasayana" (meaning "rejuvenating and intellect-promoting") in the treatment of neurological illnesses [26].

7.5 CLASSIFICATION OF RASAYANA (FIGURE 7.1)

i. As per method of use [27]:

a. *Kuti praveshika* meaning in-door use;

b. *Vatatapika* meaning outdoor use.

ii. As per Scope of use [28]:

a. *Kamya Rasayana* as a promoter of normal health:
- *Prana Kamya* as a promoter of longevity;
- *Medha Kamya* is an improver of mental faculties;
- *Shri Kamya* is an improver of the luster of the body.

b. *Naimittika Rasayana*;
c. *Ajasrika Rasayana*.

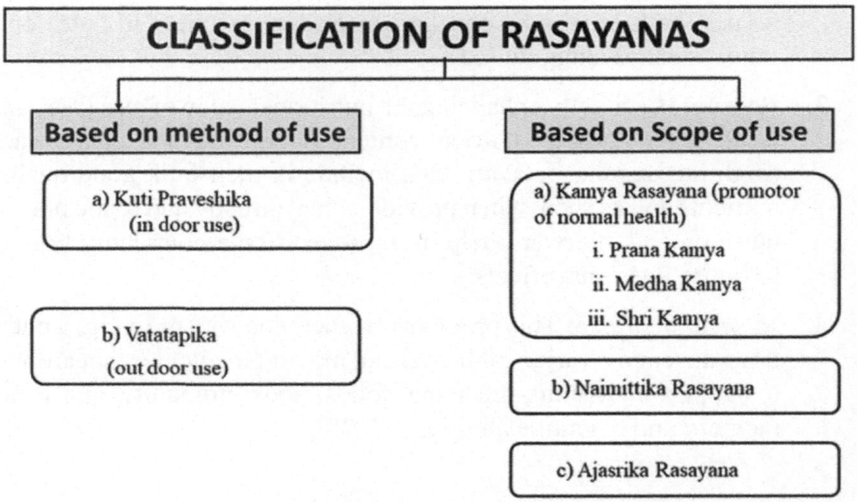

FIGURE 7.1 Classification of *Rasayanas*.

7.6 ROLE OF MEDHYA RASAYANAS IN NEUROPROTECTION

The Sanskrit terms "Rasayana," which implies rejuvenation, and "medhya," which indicates intellect or insight, are combined to form the phrase "Medhya Rasayanas." Therapeutic herbs are categorized as brain tonics or rejuvenators in the Ayurvedic medical system. These plants are reportedly used in both herbal and conventional medicine, and they have benefits that pharmaceutical medications do not [29].

Ayurveda, an ancient Indian medical system, lists a group of medicinal herbs called *Medhya Rasayanas* as having numerous advantages, including the capacity to improve memory and cognition. *Rasayana* is a medicinal method or preparation that, when used regularly, can enhance nutrient intake, health, memory, intelligence, immunity, and consequently lifetime. Medha denotes intellect and/or retention. *Medhya Rasayana* is used alone or in mixtures with other herbs [6, 30, 31].

Medha needs to be able to properly correlate and comprehend her knowledge of existing objects. Because of medha, a person will be able to learn about existent objects and so become knowledgeable. The majority of Medhya Rasayana medications have a variety of qualities. They can help with stress and anxiety, as well as improve cognition and memory [32].

There are two types of *Medhya Rasayana*: *Kutipraveshika* and *Vatatapika*. *Kutipraveshika* is a *Rasayana* intake used as an indoor management approach in which the person remains in a specially constructed cottage for a predetermined period. *Vata*tapika, which is made from the words "air" and "heat" or "sun," is primarily advantageous to people who engage in outdoor activities [33]. Figure 7.2 represents the role of Medhya Rasayanas in Neuroprotection.

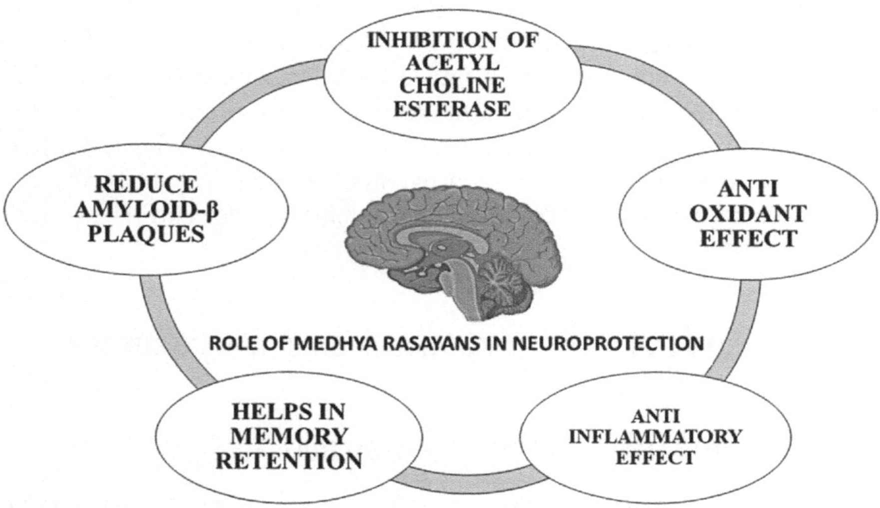

FIGURE 7.2 Role of Medhya Rasayanas in neuroprotection.

Medhya Rasayana is a class of medications that have been utilized in Ayurveda from antiquity to strengthen memory and intelligence through its prabhava (specific effect), notably medhya (nootropic). Figure 7.2 illustrates the application of the four herbal medicines that make up Medhya Rasayana, which include *mandukaparni* (*Centella asiatica*), *yastimadhu* (*Glycyrrhiza glabra*), *Guduchi* (*Tinospora cordifolia*), and *shankhapushpi* (*Convolvulus pleuricaulis* or *Evolvulus alsinoides*) [34–36]. These processes lead to neurodegenerative illnesses like Parkinson's, Alzheimer's, and Huntington's. The rejuvenation techniques described in Ayurvedic scriptures provide biological nourishment for the body's tissues. Some *Rasayanas* are only appropriate for certain… organs and tissues. *Medhya Rasayana*, or brain tonics, targets brain tissue specifically. *Rasayanas* have anti-stress, adaptogenic, and memory-improving qualities, as well as the ability to slow brain aging and promote neural tissue regeneration [21].

Medhya Rasayana drugs are used to treat mental problems in persons of all ages. They boost cognition (dhi), memory (smriti), and retention power (dhriti), and have a neuronutrient effect via increasing cerebral metabolism. Medhya Rasayana system drugs are known to improve mental performance by enhancing "buddhi" and "*Manas*" functioning and addressing disruptions in "rajas" and "tamas." This alleviates stress, anxiety, and depression in patients with mental health issues. This could help patients with challenging medical conditions including tissues affected by diseases like osteoarthritis, age-related macular degeneration (AMD), Alzheimer's, and Parkinson's disease (PD), among others [37]. *In vitro*, higher doses of Medhya Rasayanas offered neuroprotection, and in animal experiments, the improved antioxidant defense provided neuroprotection against doxorubicin-induced neuronal injury [38]. A pre-clinical study has revealed that Medhya Rasayana (ayurvedic nootropics) such as *ashwagandha*, turmeric, and *Brahmi* can eliminate amyloid plaques from neurons, which are seen in Alzheimer's disease [9, 39].

7.7 MEDICINAL PLANTS AS MEDHYA DRUGS IN ALZHEIMER'S DISEASE

7.7.1 MANDUKAPARNI (CENTELLA ASIATICA)

Centella asiatica, commonly known as *Gotu kola*, is a plant used in traditional Chinese medicine to cure a range of ailments in China and Southeast Asian nations [40]. This tiny, herbaceous annual plant of the subfamily Mackinlaya lives in marshy regions of India, Sri Lanka, Madagascar, Africa, Australia, China, Indonesia, Malaysia, and Southern and Central Africa. It is a perennial creeper that thrives in moist settings [41].

The leaves of *C. asiatica* are a popular vegetable and have found their way into dietary supplements due to their high levels of carotenoids, vitamins B and C, and other nutrients like phenols, terpenoids, carbohydrates, and amino acids. The major chemical constituents, Asiatic acid, Asiaticoside, and Madecassic acid are responsible for the neuroprotective activity of this plant. An alkaloid called hydrocotylin is among the other components of *C. asiatica*. Phenolic compounds such as quercitrin and glycosides like glycoside D, asiaticoside A, and asiaticoside B, as well as centelloside, madecassoside, and caffeoylquinic acids. Other phytochemicals include glycerides of oleic, palmitic, stearic, lignoceric, and linolenic acids, pectic acid, tannins, sugars, resins, campesterol, polyacetylenes, carotenoids, and vitamins B and C [20, 42]. According to reports, *C. asiatica* has a variety of biological qualities that are beneficial to human health, such as those that can be used to treat venous deficiency as well as those for wound healing, anti-inflammatory, anti-psoriatic, anti-ulcer, hepatoprotective, anticonvulsant, sedative, immunostimulant, cardioprotective, and antitumor properties [43]. The usage of *C. asiatica* for its cognitive benefits as a brain tonic, in the treatment of mental diseases, and as a memory-improving agent are all significant indications in Ayurveda. In animal studies, *C. asiatica* was found to increase neuronal morphology, learning capacity, and memory retention. *C. asiatica* has antioxidant, as well as Smritiprada (memory-enhancing), effects [45]. Additionally, there were non-significant improvements in general cognitive performance when *C. asiatica* was combined with other herbs. However, some research on combination products has shown that they may have an impact on attention and concentration [46]. According to previous research on the nervous system, *C. asiatica* and its triterpenes can treat several neurological disorders, but AD has received the most attention. Neuroinflammatory processes, oxidative stress, mitochondrial dysfunction, and brain-derived neurotrophic factor malfunctions all play a role in the etiology of AD [40]. Since its antioxidant activity has been discovered to be equivalent to that of Rosemary and sage, *C. asiatica* has a great deal of promise to be a natural source of antioxidants. *C. asiatica* demonstrated a comparably high amount of natural antioxidant components, including vitamin C, vitamin E, carotenes, tannins, and total phenolics, in comparative research encompassing 43 edible plants in Thailand [47]. In a concentration-dependent manner, treatment with the raw extract of *C. asiatica* dramatically reduced the levels of oxidative stress and pro-inflammatory cytokines/mediators produced in the Sprague Dawley rat model. The *C. asiatica* crude extract is capable of suppressing oxidative stress, inflammation, and high levels of acetylcholinesterase (AChE) both *in vitro* and *in vivo* [48]. It has been demonstrated that the triterpenes asiatic acid, asiaticoside, and madecassoside, as well as caffeoylquinic acids, aid in the herb's neurological effects. Increased dendritic arborization and synaptogenesis are two examples of *C. asiatica's* neurotropic effects, which may be brought on by modifications to signal transduction pathways like ERK1/2 and Akt. With the ability to strengthen the Nrf_2-antioxidant response pathway, caffeoylquinic acids are now becoming a second significant category of active chemicals in *C. asiatica* [49]. Araliadiol, a component of *C. asiatica*, exhibited neuroprotective properties against ER stress and oxidative damage. Ar her studies, *C. asiatica* extract can lessen the cytotoxicity of Aβ, enhance scopolamine-induced amnesia, and lower Aβ levels in the hippocampus of PS/APP mice [50].

7.7.1.1 CLINICAL DATA

The safety and tolerability assessment showed that oral administration of *Centella asiatica* (ECa 233) capsules in single and multiple doses at 250 and 500 mg was well tolerated [51]. A randomized, placebo-controlled, double-blind research was run to see how *C. asiatica* affected the cognitive function of healthy elderly volunteers. Around 28 healthy senior volunteers received the plant extract once daily for two months in doses of 250, 500, and 750 mg. A large dose of the plant extract improved mood and working memory, according to the results [52]. Another study examined the impact of *C. asiatica* on healthy middle-aged volunteers' cognitive function. The *C. asiatica* capsules were given to 41 healthy middle-aged individuals (22 females and 19 males) once daily for two months at varied doses ranging from 3 g to 4 g (according to body weight). The findings demonstrated that numerous cognitive tests measured at various times in both males and females were improved by *C. asiatica*. Another study looked at how healthy middle-aged volunteers' cognitive performance was affected by *C. asiatica*. The *C. asiatica* capsules were given to 41 healthy middle-aged individuals (22 females and 19 males) once daily for two months at varied dosages ranging from 3 g to 4 g (according to body weight). The outcomes demonstrated that *C. asiatica* improved several of the cognitive tests taken at various times in both males and females. A six-month study was conducted to determine the efficacy of *C. asiatica* for treating moderate cognitive impairment (MCI) in older adults aged 65 to 69 years old, as well as other clinical concerns related to aging. A dosage of 500 mg twice daily (1,000 mg daily) of *C.*

asiatica aqueous extract was advised. The research showed that *C. asiatica* can be therapeutically beneficial for those with mild cognitive impairment. Additionally, this medication is useful for diastolic blood pressure, peripheral neuritis, sleeplessness, appetite loss, etc. [52, 53].

7.7.2 SHANKHAPUSHPI (CONVOLVULUS PLURICAULIS)

A perennial herb known as *Convolvulus pluricaulis* resembles morning glory. It is recognized that the herb's entire plant is medicinal [54]. *C. pluricaulis* is a Rasayana medicine primarily recommended for use in rejuvenation and treatment to stimulate the mind. Ayurvedic practitioners called it *Shankhpushpi*, and it was a well-known memory-improving drug, a psychostimulant, and a tranquilizer in conventional Indian medicine [55]. The chemical constituents of *C. pluricaulis* include a variety of substances, including sugars, proteins, amino acids, alkaloids, fatty acids, volatile acids, fixed oils, phenolic compounds, glycosides, triterpenoids, palmitic acids, linoleic acids, myristic acids, flavonoids, D-glucose, maltose, sucrose, starch, rhamnose, cinnamic acid, vitamin E, ascorbic acid, and steroids [56]. *C. pluricaulis* has a number of medical applications. It is used to treat hypertension, ulcers, high blood pressure, epilepsy, vomiting, diabetes, sunstroke, and bleeding. It is also used to treat neurological illnesses. Additionally, it is said to be a well-known memory enhancer, a psychostimulant, and a tranquilizer, also reportedly lowers mental strain [57]. The herb produces a considerable reduction in the amount of anxiety and neuroticism that develops due to varied levels of stress, promotes restful sleep, and relieves stress, anxiety, and mental exhaustion. It helps to balance and vitiate the *Kapha*, *Vata*, and *Pitta* doshas and is astringent and bitter [58]. Preclinical (*in-vivo* and *in-vitro*) studies have demonstrated nootropic, antidepressant, anti-stress, neurodegenerative, antioxidant, hypolipidemic, immunomodulatory, antimicrobial, antidiabetic, antiulcer, and cardiovascular activity [55].

Convolvulus pluricaulis, also known as *sankhpushpi*, is believed to enhance memory and regenerate nerves. Triterpenoids, flavonol glycosides, anthocyanins, and steroids namely Ayapin, Scopolin, and Convolamine are the main chemical components, giving nootropic and memory-improving effects [59]. The plant has also been shown to reduce the human microtubule-associated protein tau-induced neurotoxicity in the Alzheimer's disease Drosophila model [60]. In the cerebral cortex of rats, *C. pluricaulis* reversed the impairment of cholinergic and antioxidant activities brought on by aluminum [61]. Its aqueous extract is known to decrease levels of APP, tau, and Aβ [62]. The high antioxidant status of *C. pluricaulis* is demonstrated by its capacity to scavenge free radicals. *C. pluricaulis* reduces H_2O_2-induced neuronal injury by reducing oxidative stress and promoting apoptosis [63]. Amnesia in mice induced from scopolamine was found to be reduced by *C. pluricaulis* [64]. Similar to this, administering its extract to young and old mice increased acetylcholine esterase activity in the CA1 and CA3 areas linked to learning and memory, but memory retention was greater in the former [65].

There are already several medications on the market in India that are created by combining a variety of plant powders or two or three Medhya plant extracts, including *C. pluricaulis*. Remem (Zydus Industries, India), Tirukati, Ayumemo (Welexlabs, India), Abana (The Himalaya Drug & Co, India), Tejras (Sandu Brothers, India), and Shankhapushpi are the most recent Ayurvedic treatments for *C. pluricaulis* [54].

7.7.2.1 CLINICAL DATA

A clinical investigation was carried out to investigate the nootropic (medhya) impact of *shankhapushpi* pills. The treatment was administered to 30 physically fit participants (18 men and 12 women). For a period of 60 days, four tablets of śaṅkhapuṣpī (each 500 mg) were administered at *udānakala* (2 hours after a meal) with milk. Results demonstrate that the "śaṅkhapuṣpī" tablet has improved memory, notably in younger age groups where long-term memory loss is more prevalent [66]. A yoga intervention was compared to a 2-month supplementation of *shankhpushpi* (500 mg tablets, twice a day after meals with milk) in open-label clinical research of 102 young, healthy volunteers (ages 16 to 25): *Satvavajaya Chikitsa* was included in yogic practices like chanting, pranayama (controlling breath), and asana (sitting position with breathing methods) [67]. An open-label trial with 90 schoolchildren compared an Ayurvedic treatment regimen consisting of *Mandukaparni, yashtimadhu, Guduchi,* and *shankhpushpi* (dose of 2 g twice daily with milk) to a control group or a group that practiced yoga (*Asanas Pranayama*) [68].

7.7.3 YASHTIMADHU (GLYCYRRHIZA GLABRA)

One of the most well-known members of the Fabaceae family of medicinal plants is *Glycyrrhiza glabra* (also known as Leguminosae). Liquorice, glycyrrhiza, sweet wood, and *Liquiritiae radix* are further names for *Glycyrrhiza glabra* (in English) [69].

G. glabra is found in Central Asia, the northwestern region of China, Spain, Italy, Turkey, and Iraq, and also in Iran [70]. Polysaccharides, flavonoids, triterpenes, saponins, pectins, simple sugars, mineral salts, amino acids, isoliquiritin, isoflavones, and several other compounds are included in it. The primary component of licorice root, glycyrrhizin (also known as glycyrrhizic acid or glycyrrhizinic acid), is a triterpenoid saponin molecule that is 50–170 times sweeter than sucrose [71]. The anti-inflammatory, hepatoprotective, neuroprotective, anxiolytic, estrogenic, antiretroviral, antitumor, antibacterial, and antioxidant actions of these various compounds contribute to their many therapeutic qualities. They also have positive effects on the skin [69]. This herb's extracts are well recognized for improving brain function, stimulating the central nervous system (CNS) by boosting blood flow, and moderating blood sugar levels [72].

According to some studies, *G. glabra* exhibits anti-inflammatory properties similar to those of steroid hormone-like hydrocortisone by lowering the activity of the phospholipase A2 enzyme, which is essential for several inflammatory processes. Additionally, an *in vitro* experiment showed that glycyrrhizic acid inhibits prostaglandin E2 production and cyclooxygenase activity, thus decreasing platelet aggregation [73]. Licorice extracts showed benefits against several neurodegenerative illnesses, such as AD, according to research on the therapeutic efficacy of distinct *Glycyrrhiza* species as neurological defenders against disorders like dementia and AD [74]. In addition to inhibiting mitochondrial oxidative phosphorylation, the neurotoxin 1-methyl-4-phenylpyridinium also inhibits glutathione (GSH), an essential component of the brain's antioxidative system, leading to the production of ROS and cytotoxicity. These effects are countered by glycyrrhizin [74, 75]. Its roots are potential sources of antioxidants and urease inhibitors [76]. In mice, *G. glabra* has demonstrated potential as a memory-improving substance [77]. Moreover, in older male Wistar albino rats, its aqueous root extract has been demonstrated to improve cognitive function [78]. When combined with aerobic exercise, *G. glabra* extract can prevent or stop the onset of moderate cognitive decline in the elderly by enhancing their cognitive states, likely through reducing inflammatory variables [79]. Both exteroceptive and interoceptive memory models demonstrated the potential of *G. glabra* as a memory enhancer [80]. *Glycyrrhiza* works by lowering brain cell damage, increasing nerve cell activity, and suppressing memory deterioration to reduce oxidative stress connected to various types of dementia. The effect of isoliquiritigenin on mitochondrial function may be related to the oxidative stress action of *Glycyrrhiza* [81]. When compared to the corresponding vehicle-treated control groups, the aqueous extract of *G. glabra* (150 mg/kg administered orally for 7 consecutive days) substantially reduced acetylcholinesterase activity [82]. Glabridin reduces the body weight and hyperglycemia of diabetic rats by combining its antioxidant, neuroprotective, and anticholinesterase properties. The results show that glabridin shielded rats from the detrimental effects of diabetes on memory and learning [83]. A natural substance termed 2,2′,4′-trihydroxy chalcone (TDC) from *Glycyrrhiza* worked as a potent non-competitive inhibitor against the BACE1 enzyme in human embryonic kidney cells known as APPswe cells [84].

7.7.3.1 CLINICAL DATA

In the three groups, *Yashtimadhu* tablets were administered with milk. In Group A, seven students received one tablet BID (two times per day), in Group B, two tablets BID, and Group C, two tablets TID for seven days. It is found to be useful in the enhancement of neuropharmacological activity (medha: intelligence, memory) in adolescents. According to the study, consuming *Yashtimadhu* enhances overall intellect rather than short-term memory [83]. Figure 7.3 represents the major properties namely *Rasa*, *Guna*, *Virya*, and *Vipaka* of the four mentioned drugs used as *Medhya Rasayanas*.

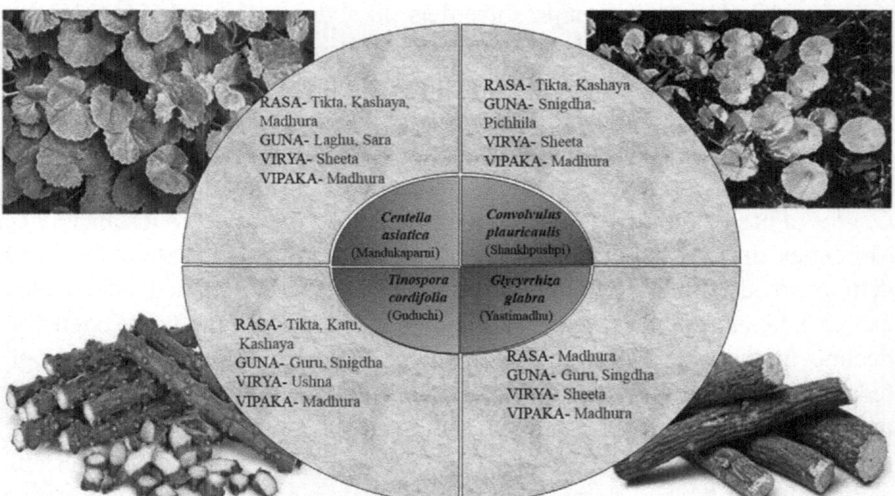

FIGURE 7.3 Four major herbal drugs are mentioned as Medhya Rasayana in Ayurveda.

7.7.4 GUDUCHI (TINOSPORA CORDIFOLIA)

Tinospora cordifolia (*Guduchi*) is a glabrous, large, and deciduous climbing shrub in the Menispermaceae family. It is widespread in the tropical Indian subcontinent and China, and it can reach heights of 300 m. In Hindi, the plant is frequently referred to as 'Giloe' [84]. Because *T. cordifolia* has no detrimental effects on DNA integrity, blood lymphocytes, or bone marrow, it is regarded as a safe feed additive. *T. cordifolia* contains a variety of phenolics, steroids, alkaloids like berberine, palmatine, tembetarine, choline, glycosides, diterpenoid lactones, aliphatic compounds, Tinosporide, and polysaccharides. The major constituents namely Tinocordiofoloside, Tinocordiside, and Cordioside are responsible for the neuroprotective activity of this plant. The therapeutic usage of entire plant juice is known as medhya. Additionally, it's used as a powder, decoction, and Satwa (starch extract of the stem). Their trace element and antioxidant composition help to explain their neuroprotective and therapeutic effects. It improves the blood profile and has lead-scavenging properties. *T. cordifolia* has been reported to have anti-stress, antioxidant, and learning and memory-enhancing properties [31]. The therapeutic potential of the plant in humans includes hepatoprotective, antioxidant, antihyperglycemic, antimicrobial, hypolipidemic, and antipyretic, anti-inflammatory, heart protective, neuroprotective, osteoprotective, and analgesic, antianxiety, antistress, and antidiarrheal activities. The plant also contains iron, manganese, zinc, calcium, phosphorus, copper, and other elements. Treatment with *T. cordifolia* reduces oxidative stress, activates PPAR-ϒ, CREB, and SREBP-1 through the dopamine D1 receptor-mediated signaling molecules cAMP and protein kinase A, and reduces hyperlipidemia [84–86].

Tinospora cordifolia 50% ethanolic extract may help with the treatment of sleep deprivation-related stress and the improvement of cognitive functioning, either by itself or in combination with other memory-enhancing drugs. In addition to its radio- and chemoprotective properties, *T. cordifolia* has been found to have neuroprotective potential by altering the antioxidant enzymatic activity of brain tissue. *T. cordifolia* has also been demonstrated to alleviate cyclosporine-induced memory impairments and enhance cognition (learning and memory) in normal rats. The Hebb William maze learning scores were decreased, and retention memory was increased by *T. cordifolia* alcoholic and aqueous extracts, indicating improved learning and memory. Neurodegenerative changes were seen in the hippocampus of cyclosporine-treated rats, although *T. cordifolia* protected them from these changes [87].

7.7.4.1 CLINICAL DATA

In a 21-day, double-blind, placebo-controlled research, volunteers were randomly divided into two groups of 15 and administered medication (coded box) containing 500 mg of *T. cordifolia* or a matched placebo for 21 days. With breakfast in the morning, one *T. cordifolia* tablet or placebo was administered orally. When compared to a placebo, *T. cordifolia*, 500 mg per day, enhances verbal learning and memory as well as logical memory (both immediate and short-term) [88]. Another trial involving 30 healthy individuals was conducted. They were divided into three groups at random. One capsule (500 mg) of Ashwagandha, one capsule (Guduchi), and a placebo were given to each group twice daily for six months as treatment. Guduchi and Ashwagandha calm Tridoshas and keep everything in check; by keeping Tridoshas in an equilibrium state, they may be able to keep the oxidation process going. *Guduchi* and *Ashwagandha* were beneficial in reducing oxidative stress and early aging [89]. The major bioactive compounds, which are responsible for acting as *Medha Rasayana* from all four plants, have been described in Figure 7.4.

7.8 VARIOUS FORMULATIONS CONTAINING MEDHYA RASAYANA DRUGS

Anxiety, impaired cognition, and lack of attention are among the mental problems for which Brahma Rasayana is advised as a phytomedicine. *Mandukaparni*, *Shankhpushpi*, and other plant extracts are included. *Rajata Bhasma* and Shankhpushpi taken as a syrup boosted hippocampal protein production while improving learning in test animals [90]. The herb *Shankhpushpi*, a memory enhancer utilized as a brain tonic to stimulate cognition and brain function, is found in Shankhpushpi Kalka. One of the *Medhya Rasayanas*, liquorice (Yastimadhu), is found in Yashtimadhu Taila [91]. *Yashtimadhu churna* is a traditional remedy made from the root extract of *Yashtimadhu (Mulethi)*, which is used to cure throat irritation, gastroesophageal reflux disease, stomach ulcers, and other conditions. *Vata-Pitta dushti* is lessened by *Yashtimadhu Kwath Aschantana*. *Brahmi, Vacha, Kushta, Shankhapushpi*, and Punarnava are all herbs that are included in the Ayurvedic composition known as *Brahmi Ghrita*. The "*Guduchyadi Churna*" is made up of *Apamarga Shirovirechaka*, *Kushtha kaphaVatahara*, and *Vidanga krumighna* in addition to *Shankhpushpi, Vacha, Haritaki, Shatavari, Guduchi,* and *Ghrita*, all of which have Medhya and Rasayana qualities.

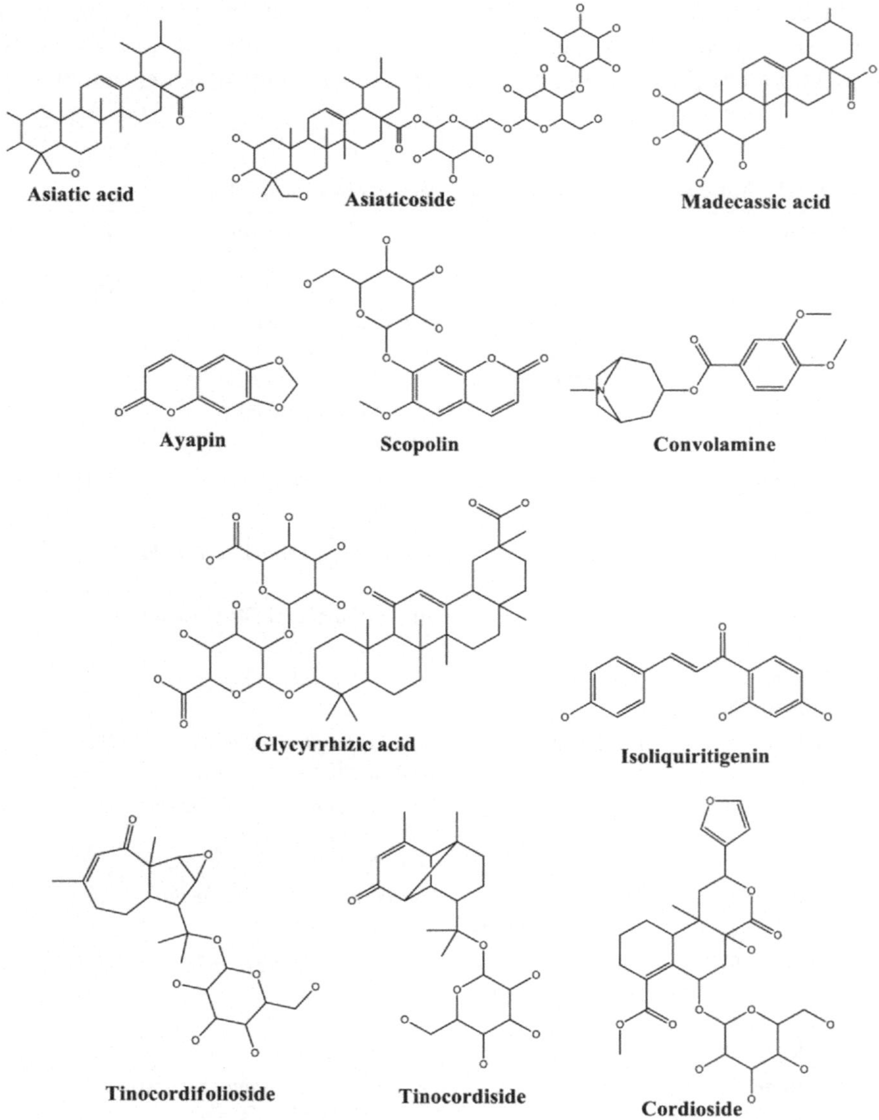

FIGURE 7.4 Major phytocompounds from four major herbal drugs used as Medhya drugs in Alzheimer's disease.

Guduchi Satva, a dried *T. cordifolia* extract, is used to treat various febrile illnesses [92]. *Guduchi Ghritas* is a Ghritas-containing composition. Ghritas are medicinal ghee preparations that include the substances' fat-soluble components [93]. Using Ksheera (milk), fresh Guduchi stem is used to make

Guduchi taila. In India, "Geriforte," a blend of various plant compounds that also includes Mandukaparni and Yastimadhu, is used as a rejuvenating tonic in old age [92, 94]. Table 7.1 describes various formulations containing Medhya Rasayana drugs.

TABLE 7.1 Various Formulations Including Medhya Rasayana Drugs

Sl. No.	Name	Formulation	Medhya Rasayans Included	References
1.	Brahma Rasayana	Phytomedicine includes extracts of different plants in the form of pellets.	*Centella asiatica (Mandukaparni), Convolvulus pluricaulis (Shankhpushpi)*	[90]
2.	Shankhpushpi syrup	Syrup	*Convolvulus pluricaulis (Shankhpushpi)*	
3.	Shankhpushpi Kalka	Kalka (paste)	*Convolvulus pluricaulis (Shankhpushpi)*	[91]
4.	Yastimadhu churna	Churna (a fine powder)	*Glycyrrhiza glabra (Yashtimadhu)*	
5.	Yashtimadhu kwath Aashchontana	Kwath (filtered decoction)	*Glycyrrhiza glabra (Yashtimadhu)*	
6.	Shirodhara with Yashtimadhu Taila	Taila (oil)	*Glycyrrhiza glabra (Yashtimadhu)*	
7.	Brahmi Ghrita	Polyherbal formulation	*Convolvulus pluricaulis (Shankhpushpi)*	[92]
8.	Guduchyadi Churna	Churna	*Tinospora cordifolia (Guduchi), Convolvulus pluricaulis (Shankhpushpi)*	[93]
9.	Guduchi Satva	Satva (Smooth, amorphous powder)	*Tinospora cordifolia (Guduchi)*	
10.	Guduchi ghrita	Guduchi with Ghritas (medicated ghee preparations)	*Tinospora cordifolia (Guduchi)*	
11.	Guduchi taila	*Taila*	*Tinospora cordifolia (Guduchi)*	
12.	Geriforte	Powder	*Centella asiatica (Mandukaparni), Glycyrrhiza glabra (Yashtimadhu)*	[94]

7.9 CONCLUSION

Dementia and ADs are neurological disorders in which the mental ability of an individual is challenged and compromised. The treatment available in modern medicine is not able to manage these conditions. One of the oldest medical systems is Ayurveda, in which herbs, minerals, and other natural ingredients are used to cure mental illness. Hence, there is a ray of hope to provide care and treatment to patients who are suffering from AD, dementia, and related complications. The concept of Medhya Rasayana is reported as an effective way to treat such diseases. Traditional Ayurvedic medicines are useful in treating illnesses, according to scientific literature. Such herbs need to be validated through further specific protocols designed to evaluate their effectiveness against neurological disorders.

7.10 FUTURE PERSPECTIVE

The role of traditional systems in memory and CNS-related diseases is a concern of medical research as it can serve as a discovery lead to design or develop new medicine for AD and related neurological complications. The data published and available so far showing attributes of herbs and Ayurvedic polyherbal, Herbo-mineral formulations are not sufficient enough and also not reported to consider them as a promising candidate for drug discovery. More specific protocols and double-blind clinical trials are needed to support and validate the traditional claims of the healers. The concept of Medhya Rasayana is a technically developed method of treatment mentioned in Ayurvedic texts. Modern science must study the concept and mechanism of treatment utilized for certain diseases of memory loss and behavioral changes.

KEYWORDS

- **Alzheimer's disease**
- **cognitive dysfunction**
- **dementia**
- **herbo-mineral formulations**
- **Medhya Rasayana**
- **medicinal plants**
- **neurological disorders**

REFERENCES

1. Malik, J., Munjal, K., & Deshmukh, R. (2015). Attenuating effect of standardized lyophilized *Cinnamomum zeylanicum* bark extract against streptozotocin-induced experimental dementia of Alzheimer's type. *Journal of Basic and Clinical Physiology and Pharmacology, 26*(3), 275–285. https://doi.org/10.1515/jbcpp-2015-0027.
2. De-Paula, V. J., Radanovic, M., Diniz, B. S., & Forlenza, O. V. (2012). Alzheimer's disease. In J. R. Harris (Ed.), *Protein Aggregation and Fibrillogenesis in Cerebral and Systemic Amyloid Disease* (pp. 329–352). Springer Netherlands. https://doi.org/10.1007/978-94-007-4351-5_14.
3. Schachter, A. S., & Davis, K. L. (2000). Alzheimer's disease. *Dialogues in Clinical Neuroscience, 2*(2), 91–100. https://doi.org/10.31887/DCNS.2000.2.2/aschachter.
4. Dou, K. X., Tan, M. S., Tan, C. C., Cao, X. P., Hou, X. H., Guo, Q. H., Tan, L., Mok, V., & Yu, J. T. (2018). Comparative safety and effectiveness of cholinesterase inhibitors and memantine for Alzheimer's disease: A network meta-analysis of 41 randomized controlled trials. *Alzheimer's Research & Therapy, 10*(1), 126. https://doi.org/10.1186/s13195-018-0428-5.
5. Kobayashi, H., Ohnishi, T., Nakagawa, R., & Yoshizawa, K. (2016). The comparative efficacy and safety of cholinesterase inhibitors in patients with mild-to-moderate Alzheimer's disease: A Bayesian network meta-analysis. *International Journal of Geriatric Psychiatry, 31*(8), 892–904. https://doi.org/10.1002/gps.4435.
6. Haye, A., Ansari, M., Saini, A., Ahmed, Z., Munjal, K., Shamsi, Y., & Sharma, M. (2022). Polyherbal formulation improves glucose-lipid metabolism and prevents hepatotoxicity in streptozotocin-induced diabetic rats: Plausible role of IRS-PI3K-Akt-GLUT2 signaling. *Pharmacognosy Magazine, 18*, 52. https://doi.org/10.4103/pm.pm_522_21.
7. Farooqui, A. A., Farooqui, T., Madan, A., Ong, J. H. J., & Ong, W. Y. (2018). Ayurvedic medicine for the treatment of dementia: Mechanistic aspects. *Evidence-Based Complementary and Alternative Medicine, 2018*, 2481076. https://doi.org/10.1155/2018/2481076.
8. Khare, C. P. (2004). *Indian Herbal Remedies: Rational Western Therapy, Ayurvedic, and Other Traditional Usage, Botany*. Springer Science & Business Media. https://doi.org/10.1007/978-1-4615-1420-3.
9. Satyavert, Gupta, S., Choudhury, H., Jacob, S., Nair, A. B., Dhanawat, M., & Munjal, K. (2021). Pharmacokinetics and tissue distribution of hydrazinocurcumin in rats. *Pharmacological Reports, 73*(6), 1734–1743. https://doi.org/10.1007/s43440-021-00287-5.
10. Singh, R. H., Narsimhamurthy, K., & Singh, G. (2008). Neuronutrient impact of Ayurvedic Rasayana therapy in brain aging. *Biogerontology, 9*(6), 369–374. https://doi.org/10.1007/s10522-008-9168-8.
11. Dubey, T., & Chinnathambi, S. (2019). Brahmi (*Bacopa monnieri*): An Ayurvedic herb against Alzheimer's disease. *Archives of Biochemistry and Biophysics, 676*, 108153. https://doi.org/10.1016/j.abb.2019.108153.
12. Mehla, J., Gupta, P., Pahuja, M., Diwan, D., & Diksha, D. (2020). Indian medicinal herbs and formulations for Alzheimer's disease: From traditional knowledge to scientific assessment. *Brain Sciences, 10*(12), 954. https://doi.org/10.3390/brainsci10120954.
13. Lad, V. (2002). *Textbook of Ayurveda*. Ayurvedic Press New Mexico. Vol. 1.

14. Hankey, A. (2001). Ayurvedic physiology and etiology: Ayurvedo Amritanaam. The doshas and their functioning in terms of contemporary biology and physical chemistry. *The Journal of Alternative & Complementary Medicine, 7*(5), 567–574. https://doi.org/10.1089/107555301317032440.
15. Hankey, A. (2005). The scientific value of Ayurveda. *Journal of Alternative & Complementary Medicine, 11*(2), 221–225. https://doi.org/10.1089/jac.2005.11.221.
16. Priyadarshini, S., & Nagarjun, V. (2019). Alzheimer's disease and Ayurveda: First descriptions in medical literature. *Journal of Clinical and Diagnostic Research, 13*(4), 12–18. https://doi.org/10.7860/JCDR/2019/38766.12890.
17. Mangalasseri, P., & Chandran, S. (2017). A brief insight into the pathogenesis and management of Alzheimer's disease in Ayurvedic parlance. *International Journal of Green Pharmacy, 11*. https://doi.org/10.4103/0973-8258.208670.
18. Amarprakash, D. (2021). Alzheimer's disease management: An integrated overview. *Journal of Interdisciplinary Cycle Research, 13*, 360–373. https://doi.org/10.37380/jicr.v13i3.400.
19. Ponnusankar, S., Pandit, S., Babu, R., Bandyopadhyay, A., & Mukherjee, P. K. (2011). Cytochrome P450 inhibitory potential of Triphala—A Rasayana from Ayurveda. *Journal of Ethnopharmacology, 133*(1), 120–125. https://doi.org/10.1016/j.jep.2010.10.020.
20. Munjal, K., Sharma, S., Sharma, S., Kumar, D., Choudhary, A., Berwal, R., & Kumar, A. (2021). Comparison of serum 25-hydroxyvitamin D levels after a single oral dose of vitamin D3 formulations in mild vitamin D3 deficiency. *Indian Journal of Clinical Biochemistry, 12*(4), 163–167. https://doi.org/10.1007/s12291-021-01092-7.
21. Balasubramani, S. P., Venkatasubramanian, P., Kukkupuni, S. K., & Patwardhan, B. (2011). Plant-based Rasayana drugs from Ayurveda. *Chinese Journal of Integrative Medicine, 17*(2), 88–94. https://doi.org/10.1007/s11655-011-0650-4.
22. Barathe, R. (2021). A conceptual study on Rajonivritti with special reference to the menopausal syndrome in Ayurveda. *Journal of Ayurveda and Integrated Medical Sciences, 6*(3), 154–159. https://doi.org/10.21760/jaims.6.3.22.
23. Kciuk, M., Mujwar, S., Rani, I., Munjal, K., Gielecińska, A., Kontek, R., & Shah, K. (2022). Computational bioprospecting guggulsterone against ADP ribose phosphatase of SARS-CoV-2. *Molecules, 27*, 8287. https://doi.org/10.3390/molecules27238287.
24. Singh, H. (2015). Identity and attributes of Ayurvedic medicinal plant Brahmi/Aindri from antiquity to the modern age. *Indian Journal of History of Science, 50*, 15–20. https://doi.org/10.16943/ijhs/2015/v50i1/48148.
25. Gauttam, V., Munjal, K., Mujwar, S., Sawale, J., Rohilla, M., & Gupta, S. (2022). Comparative study of developed formulation and market formulation for antidiabetic potential in alloxan-induced diabetic Wistar rats. *Journal of Young Pharmacists, 14*, 387–393. https://doi.org/10.5530/jyp.2022.14.53.
26. Joshi, H., Charan, C., & Alkanad, M. (2018). Neuroprotective potentials of Ayurvedic Rasayana *Desmodium triquetrum* on brain aging and chemically induced amnesia in animal models relevant to dementia. *Journal of Traditional Medicine & Clinical Naturopathy, 7*(272), 1–2. https://doi.org/10.4172/2573-4555.1000272.
27. Kumar, Y., Jatav, R., Singh, R., Singh, C., & Kumar, A. (2022). Rasayana: A boon of Ayurveda. *Journal of Ayurveda and Integrative Medicine, 10*, 130–139. https://doi.org/10.4103/0975-9476.110012.

28. Mishra, Y., Vijay, N., Krunal, T., Nagaraj, B., & Shubhasri, B. (2016). Role of Rasayana in geriatric care: A review. *Journal of Ayurveda and Integrated Medical Sciences, 1*(1), 52–55. https://doi.org/10.21760/jaims.1.1.11.
29. Ray, S. (2015). Medhya Rasayanas in brain function and disease. *Medicinal Chemistry, 5*, 1–10. https://doi.org/10.4172/2161-0444.1000221.
30. Munjal, K., Ahmad, S., Gupta, A., Haye, A., Amin, S., & Mir, S. (2020). Polyphenol-enriched fractions and the compounds isolated from *Garcinia indica* fruits ameliorate obesity through the suppression of digestive enzymes and oxidative stress. *Journal of Ethnopharmacology, 16*(70), 236–245. https://doi.org/10.1016/j.jep.2020.112999.
31. Kulkarni, R., Girish, K. J., & Kumar, A. (2012). Nootropic herbs (Medhya Rasayana) in Ayurveda: An update. *Pharmacognosy Reviews, 6*(12), 147–153. https://doi.org/10.4103/0973-7847.99940.
32. Rathee, P., Tanwar, V., Kumar, V., Dewan, S., & Kumari, S. (2018). Role of Medhya Rasayana (nootropic herbs) in present scenario: An Ayurvedic overview. *International Journal of Research in AYUSH and Pharmaceutical Sciences, 1*(5), 172–176. https://doi.org/10.4103/0974-8520.110272.
33. Rawat, N., & Roushan, R. (2018). Medhya Rasayana: A potential anxiolytic drug in Ayurveda. *Journal of Ayurveda and Integrative Medicine, 9*, 263–271. https://doi.org/10.4103/0974-8520.168868.
34. Munjal, K., Uniyal, R., Kumar, A., Arora, A., Gupta, A., & Haye, A. (2020). Development of validated HPTLC method for quantification of luteolin in *Eclipta alba* and its formulation. *Journal of Chromatographic Science, 2685–2695*, 1–11. https://doi.org/10.1093/chromsci/bmaa063.
35. Munjal, K., Amin, S., Mir, S. R., Gauttam, V., & Gupta, S. (2022). Furanocoumarins and lectins as food toxins. In *Food Safety and Toxins* (pp. 67–80). Springer. https://doi.org/10.1007/978-3-030-92812-5_7.
36. Kulkarni, R., Kumar, A., & Kn, S. K. (2013). Formulation and standardization of Medhya Rasayana: A novel Ayurvedic compound nootropic drug. *Pharmacognosy Journal, 5*, 72–76. https://doi.org/10.1016/j.jsps.2013.01.005.
37. Upadhyay, S. D., Lodha, S., Ahmad, Y., Kohli, S., & Sharma, R. (2021). A review on Medhya Rasayanas: A brain bracer. *Pharmacognosy Communications, 11*(4), 172–180. https://doi.org/10.4103/2230-9142.120508.
38. Gourishetti, K., Ghetia, S., Jacob, L., Mallik, S. B., Nayak, P. G., Kishore, A., Nandakumar, K., Alnaseer, S. M., & Hussain, S. M. (2019). Medhya Rasayana restores memory function against doxorubicin-induced cognitive decline: Possibly by its neuroprotective effect. *Indian Journal of Pharmaceutical Education and Research, 53*(s104–s111). https://doi.org/10.5530/ijper.53.2s.55.
39. Tiwari, S. K., & Pandey, Y. K. (2012). Ayurvedic drugs in prevention and management of age-related cognitive decline: A review. *International Journal of Pharmaceutical Sciences and Drug Research, 4*(3), 183–190. https://doi.org/10.4103/0974-6943.99951.
40. Sun, B., Wu, L., Wu, Y., Zhang, C., Qin, L., Hayashi, M., Kudo, M., Gao, M., & Liu, T. (2020). Therapeutic potential of *Centella asiatica* and its triterpenes: A review. *Frontiers in Pharmacology, 11*, 568032. https://doi.org/10.3389/fphar.2020.568032.
41. James, J. T., & Dubery, I. A. (2009). Pentacyclic triterpenoids from the medicinal herb, Centella asiatica (L.) Urban. *Molecules, 14*(10), 3922–3941. https://doi.org/10.3390/molecules14103922.

42. Jantwal, A., Durgapal, S., Upadhyay, J., Rana, M., Tariq, M., Dhariwal, A., & Joshi, T. (2021). *Centella asiatica*. In *Medicinal Plants of South Asia* (pp. 257–269). Elsevier. https://doi.org/10.1016/B978-0-12-819986-1.00010-6.
43. Orhan, I. E. (2012). *Centella asiatica* (L.) Urban: From traditional medicine to modern medicine with neuroprotective potential. *Evidence-Based Complementary and Alternative Medicine, 2012*, 946259. https://doi.org/10.1155/2012/946259.
44. Puttarak, P., Dilokthornsakul, P., Saokaew, S., Dhippayom, T., Kongkaew, C., Sruamsiri, R., Chuthaputti, A., & Chaiyakunapruk, N. (2017). Effects of Centella asiatica (L.) Urb. on cognitive function and mood-related outcomes: A systematic review and meta-analysis. *Scientific Reports, 7*(1), 10646. https://doi.org/10.1038/s41598-017-10963-5.
45. Vaidya, A. D. B., & Devasagayam, T. P. A. (2007). Current status of herbal drugs in India: An overview. *Journal of Clinical Biochemistry and Nutrition, 41*(1), 1–11. https://doi.org/10.3164/jcbn.2007001.
46. Katz, M., Adar Levine, A., Kol-Degani, H., & Kav-Venaki, L. (2010). A compound herbal preparation (CHP) in the treatment of children with ADHD: A randomized controlled trial. *Journal of Attention Disorders, 14*(3), 281–291. https://doi.org/10.1177/1087054709356173.
47. Abbas, S., Latif, M., Shafie, N., Ghazali, M., Abidin, N., Mustafa, M., & Kormin, F. (2021). A review of antioxidant and anti-acetylcholinesterase activities of Centella asiatica (L.) Urb. for the treatment of Alzheimer's disease. *Food Research, 5*(2), 1–17. https://doi.org/10.26656/fr.2017.5(2).201.
48. Hafiz, Z. Z., Amin, M. A. M., Johari James, R. M., Teh, L. K., Salleh, M. Z., & Adenan, M. I. (2020). Inhibitory effects of raw-extract Centella asiatica (RECA) on acetylcholinesterase, inflammations, and oxidative stress activities via in vitro and in vivo. *Molecules, 25*(4), 892. https://doi.org/10.3390/molecules25040892.
49. Gray, N. E., Alcazar Magana, A., Lak, P., Wright, K. M., Quinn, J., Stevens, J. F., Maier, C. S., & Soumyanath, A. (2018). Centella asiatica: Phytochemistry and mechanisms of neuroprotection and cognitive enhancement. *Phytochemistry Reviews, 17*(1), 161–194. https://doi.org/10.1007/s11101-017-9528-0.
50. Fujimori, H., Ohba, T., Mikami, M., Nakamura, S., Ito, K., Kojima, H., Takahashi, T., Iddamalgoda, A., Shimazawa, M., & Hara, H. (2022). The protective effect of Centella asiatica and its constituent, araliadiol, on neuronal cell damage and cognitive impairment. *Journal of Pharmacological Sciences, 148*(1), 162–171. https://doi.org/10.1016/j.jphs.2021.12.004.
51. Dev, R. D. O., Mohamed, S., Hambali, Z., & Samah, B. A. (2009). Comparison of cognitive effects of Centella asiatica in healthy middle-aged female and male volunteers. *European Journal of Scientific Research, 31*(4), 553–565.
52. Sonali, V., Sumeet, G., Rina, D., Kavita, M., Meenakshi, D., Dinesh Kumar, M., Gurudev, G., & Anshu, G. (2023). Unraveling the approaches to treat osteoarthritis: A focus on the potential of medicinal plants. *Pharmacognosy Research, 15*(1), 13–25.
53. Tiwari, S., Singh, S., Patwardhan, K., Gehlot, S., & Gambhir, I. (2008). Effect of Centella asiatica on mild cognitive impairment (MCI) and other common age-related clinical problems. *Digest Journal of Nanomaterials and Biostructures, 3*(4), 215–220.
54. Agarwa, P., Sharma, B., Fatima, A., & Jain, S. K. (2014). An update on Ayurvedic herb Convolvulus pluricaulis Choisy. *Asian Pacific Journal of Tropical Biomedicine, 4*(3), 245–252. https://doi.org/10.1016/S2221-1691(14)60240-0.

55. Mishra, S. H., & Sethiya, N. K. (2010). Review on ethnomedicinal uses and phytopharmacology of memory-boosting herb "Convolvulus pluricaulis" Choisy. *Australian Journal of Medical Herbalism, 22*(1), 19–25.
56. Sethiya, N. K., Nahata, A., Mishra, S. H., & Dixit, V. K. (2009). An update on Shankhpushpi, a cognition-boosting Ayurvedic medicine. *Journal of Chinese Integrative Medicine, 7*(11), 1001–1022. https://doi.org/10.3736/jcim20091102.
57. Dubey, N., Kumar, R., & Tripathi, P. (2004). Global promotion of herbal medicine: India's opportunity. *Current Science, 86*(1), 37–41.
58. Bhowmik, D., Kumar, K. S., Paswan, S., Srivatava, S., Yadav, A., & Dutta, A. (2012). Traditional Indian herbs Convolvulus pluricaulis and its medicinal importance. *Journal of Pharmacognosy and Phytochemistry, 1*(1), 44–51.
59. Gregory, J., Vengalasetti, Y. V., Bredesen, D. E., & Rao, R. V. (2021). Neuroprotective herbs for the management of Alzheimer's disease. *Biomolecules, 11*(4), 543. https://doi.org/10.3390/biom11040543.
60. Olakkaran, S., & Antony, A. (2019). *Convolvulus pluricaulis* (Shankhapushpi) ameliorates human microtubule-associated protein tau (hMAPτ) induced neurotoxicity in Alzheimer's disease Drosophila model. *Journal of Chemical Neuroanatomy, 95*, 115–122. https://doi.org/10.1016/j.jchemneu.2018.10.005.
61. Bihaqi, S. W., Sharma, M., Singh, A. P., & Tiwari, M. (2009). Neuroprotective role of Convolvulus pluricaulis on aluminum-induced neurotoxicity in rat brain. *Journal of Ethnopharmacology, 124*(3), 409–415. https://doi.org/10.1016/j.jep.2009.05.046.
62. Bihaqi, S. W., Singh, A. P., & Tiwari, M. (2012). Supplementation of Convolvulus pluricaulis attenuates scopolamine-induced increased tau and amyloid precursor protein (AβPP) expression in rat brains. *Indian Journal of Pharmacology, 44*(5), 593–598. https://doi.org/10.4103/0253-7613.100390.
63. Rachitha, P., Krupashree, K., Jayashree, G. V., Kandikattu, H. K., Amruta, N., Gopalan, N., Rao, M. K., & Khanum, F. (2018). Chemical composition, antioxidant potential, macromolecule damage, and neuroprotective activity of Convolvulus pluricaulis. *Journal of Traditional and Complementary Medicine, 8*(4), 483–496. https://doi.org/10.1016/j.jtcme.2018.03.002.
64. Malik, J., Karan, M., & Vasisht, K. (2016). Attenuating effect of bioactive coumarins from Convolvulus pluricaulis on scopolamine-induced amnesia in mice. *Natural Product Research, 30*(5), 578–582. https://doi.org/10.1080/14786419.2015.1043645.
65. Sharma, K., Bhatnagar, M., & Kulkarni, S. (2010). Effect of Convolvulus pluricaulis Choisy and Asparagus racemosus Willd on learning and memory in young and old mice: A comparative evaluation. *Pharmaceutical Biology, 48*(10), 1023–1029. https://doi.org/10.3109/13880200903232162.
66. Amin, H., Sharma, R., Vyas, H., Vyas, M., Prajapati, P. K., & Dwivedi, R. (2014). Nootropic (medhya) effect of Bhāvita Śaṇkhapuṣpī tablets: A clinical appraisal. *Ancient Science of Life, 34*(2), 109–112. https://doi.org/10.4103/0257-7941.150768.
67. Amin, H., & Sharma, R. (2015). Nootropic efficacy of Satvavajaya Chikitsa and Ayurvedic drug therapy: A comparative clinical exposition. *International Journal of Yoga, 8*(2), 109–116. https://doi.org/10.4103/0973-6131.158480.
68. Sarokte, A. S., & Rao, M. V. (2013). Effects of Medhya Rasayana and Yogic practices in improvement of short-term memory among school-going children. *Ayu, 34*(4), 383–389. https://doi.org/10.4103/0974-8520.127731.

69. Pastorino, G., Cornara, L., Soares, S., Rodrigues, F., & Oliveira, M. B. P. (2018). Liquorice (*Glycyrrhiza glabra*): A phytochemical and pharmacological review. *Phytotherapy Research, 32*(12), 2323–2339. https://doi.org/10.1002/ptr.6178.
70. Hayashi, H., & Sudo, H. (2009). Economic importance of licorice. *Plant Biotechnology, 26*(1), 101–104. https://doi.org/10.5511/plantbiotechnology.26.101.
71. Badr, S. E. A., Sakr, D. M., Mahfouz, S. A., & Abdelfattah, M. (2013). Licorice (*Glycyrrhiza glabra* L.): Chemical composition and biological impacts. *Research Journal of Pharmaceutical, Biological and Chemical Sciences, 4*(3), 606–621.
72. Rathee, P., Chaudhary, H., Rathee, S., & Rathee, D. (2008). Natural memory boosters. *Pharmacognosy Reviews, 2*(4), 249–256. https://doi.org/10.4103/0973-7847.47335.
73. Harwansh, R., & Patra, K. (2011). Pharmacological studies on *Glycyrrhiza glabra*. *Journal of Medicinal Plant Research, 5*(7), 1286–1290. https://doi.org/10.5897/JMPR.9000071.
74. Chang, K. H., Chen, I. C., Lin, H. Y., Chen, H. C., Lin, C. H., Lin, T. H., Weng, Y. T., Chao, C. Y., Wu, Y. R., & Lin, J. Y. (2016). The aqueous extract of *Glycyrrhiza inflata* can upregulate unfolded protein response-mediated chaperones to reduce tau misfolding in cell models of Alzheimer's disease. *Drug Design, Development, and Therapy, 10*, 885–895. https://doi.org/10.2147/DDDT.S98153.
75. Dringen, R. (2000). Metabolism and functions of glutathione in brain. *Progress in Neurobiology, 62*(6), 649–671. https://doi.org/10.1016/S0301-0082(99)00060-X.
76. Lateef, M., Iqbal, L., Fatima, N., Siddiqui, K., Afza, N., Zia-ul-Haq, M., & Ahmad, M. (2012). Evaluation of antioxidant and urease inhibition activities of roots of *Glycyrrhiza glabra*. *Pakistan Journal of Pharmaceutical Sciences, 25*(1), 99–102.
77. Dhingra, D., Parle, M., & Kulkarni, S. K. (2004). Memory enhancing activity of *Glycyrrhiza glabra* in mice. *Journal of Ethnopharmacology, 91*(2), 361–365. https://doi.org/10.1016/j.jep.2004.01.011.
78. Chakravarthi, K. K., Avadhani, R., & Narayan, R. S. (2012). Effect of *Glycyrrhiza glabra* root extract on learning and memory in Wistar albino rats. *Drug Invention Today, 4*(7), 387–390.
79. Kohanpour, M. A., Peeri, M., & Azarbayjani, M. A. (2017). The effects of *Glycyrrhiza glabra* L. extract use with aerobic training on inflammatory factors and cognitive state in elderly with mild cognitive impairment. *Journal of HerbMed Pharmacology, 6*(4), 178–184. https://doi.org/10.15171/jhp.2017.31.
80. Parle, M., Dhingra, D., & Kulkarni, S. K. (2004). Memory-strengthening activity of *Glycyrrhiza glabra* in exteroceptive and interoceptive behavioral models. *Journal of Medicinal Food, 7*(4), 462–466. https://doi.org/10.1089/jmf.2004.7.462.
81. El-Saber Batiha, G., Magdy Beshbishy, A., El-Mleeh, A., Abdel-Daim, M. M., & Prasad Devkota, H. (2020). Traditional uses, bioactive chemical constituents, and pharmacological and toxicological activities of *Glycyrrhiza glabra* L. (Fabaceae). *Biomolecules, 10*(3), 352. https://doi.org/10.3390/biom10030352.
82. Dhingra, D., Parle, M., & Kulkarni, S. K. (2006). Comparative brain cholinesterase-inhibiting activity of *Glycyrrhiza glabra*, *Myristica fragrans*, ascorbic acid, and metrifonate in mice. *Journal of Medicinal Food, 9*(2), 281–283. https://doi.org/10.1089/jmf.2006.9.281.
83. Teltumbde, A., Wahurwagh, A. K., Lonare, M. K., & Nesari, T. M. (2013). Effect of Yashtimadhu (*Glycyrrhiza glabra*) on intelligence and memory function in male

adolescents. *Journal of Ayurveda and Integrative Medicine, 4*(4), 244–249. https://doi.org/10.4103/0975-9476.123746.
84. Tyagi, S., Raghvendra, Singh, U., Kalra, T., & Munjal, K. (2010). Practical applications of proteomics: A technique for large-scale study of proteins: An overview. *Proteomics, 10*(10), 188–193. https://doi.org/10.1002/pmic.200900223.
85. Tyagi, S., Singh, U., Kalra, T., & Munjal, K. (2010). Applications of metabolomics: A systematic study of the unique chemical fingerprints: An overview. *Journal of Biotechnology and Biomaterials, 20*(5), 107–112. https://doi.org/10.1002/pmic.200900223.
86. Shirolkar, A., Sharma, B., Lata, S., & Dabur, R. (2016). Guduchi Sawras (*Tinospora cordifolia*): An Ayurvedic drug treatment modulates the impaired lipid metabolism in alcoholics through dopaminergic neurotransmission and an antioxidant defense system. *Biomedicine & Pharmacotherapy, 83*, 1265–1277. https://doi.org/10.1016/j.biopha.2016.08.055.
87. Mishra, R., Manchanda, S., Gupta, M., Kaur, T., Saini, V., Sharma, A., & Kaur, G. (2016). *Tinospora cordifolia* ameliorates anxiety-like behavior and improves cognitive functions in acute sleep-deprived rats. *Scientific Reports, 6*, 25564. https://doi.org/10.1038/srep25564.
88. Bairy, K. L., Rao, Y., Kumar Das, S., & Kumar, K. B. (2004). Efficacy of Tinospora cordifolia on learning and memory in healthy volunteers: A double-blind, randomized, placebo-controlled study. *Iranian Journal of Pharmacology and Therapeutics, 3*(2), 57–0.
89. Kuchewar, V. V., Borkar, M. A., & Nisargandha, M. A. (2014). Evaluation of the antioxidant potential of Rasayana drugs in healthy human volunteers. *Ayu, 35*(1), 46–49. https://doi.org/10.4103/0974-8520.141939.
90. Guruprasad, K. P., Mascarenhas, R., Gopinath, P. M., & Satyamoorthy, K. (2010). Studies on Brahma rasayana in male Swiss albino mice: Chromosomal aberrations and sperm abnormalities. *Journal of Ayurveda and Integrative Medicine, 1*(1), 40–44. https://doi.org/10.4103/0975-9476.59827.
91. Kumar, S., Patel, D., Tiwari, A., Dwivedi, A., Prajapati, B. L., & Verma, M. (2019). A review of the role of Shankhpushpi Kalka and Yashtimadhu Taila Shirodhara towards the management of Anidra. Journal of Drug Delivery and Therapeutics, 9(4–A), 884–886. https://doi.org/10.22270/jddt.v9i4-A.3565.
92. Yadav, K. D., Reddy, K. R., & Agarwal, A. (2013). Preliminary physico-chemical profile of Brahmi Ghrita. *AYU (An International Quarterly Journal of Research in Ayurveda), 34*(3), 294. https://doi.org/10.4103/0974-8520.123130.
93. Ashok, B. K., Ravishankar, B., Prajapati, P. K., & Bhat, S. D. (2010). Antipyretic activity of Guduchi Ghrita formulations in albino rats. *Ayu, 31*(3), 367–370. https://doi.org/10.4103/0974-8520.77157.
94. Singh, N., Nath, R., & Mishra, N. K. (1978). An experimental evaluation of anti-stress effects of 'Geriforte' (an Ayurvedic drug). *The Indian Journal of Medical Research, 10*(6), 423–427.

CHAPTER 8

Management of Alzheimer's Disease in the Light of Ayurveda

SUNAYNA CHOUDHARY,[1] KAVITA MUNJAL,[2*] and VINOD KUMAR GAUTTAM[3]

[1]*Department of Pharmacognosy, M.M. College of Pharmacy, Maharishi Markandeshwar (Deemed to be University), Mullana, Ambala, Haryana, India*

[2]*Amity Institute of Pharmacy, Amity University, Noida, Uttar Pradesh, India*

[3]*Department of Pharmacognosy, Shiva Institute of Pharmacy, Bilaspur, Himachal Pradesh, India*

*Corresponding author.

ABSTRACT

Alzheimer's disease (AD) is an age-linked neurodegenerative disorder associated with dementia (*Smritibuddhihrass*) and impaired cognitive functions. It is the fifth leading cause of mortality worldwide. Currently, no reliable treatment is available in conventional medicine to halt the progression of the disease. Ayurveda categorizes AD and dementia as a *Manas* vyadhi that can be associated with Jara janya Smrutibhramsh. Moreover, the three bioenergies (Dosha), seven bodily tissues (*Dhatu*), and three wastes (*Mala*) are vital to the maintenance of the human body. Abnormality in *Dosha* and *Vata* influences *Majja Dhatu*, which manifests neurological problems in the cerebral cortex and hippocampus. *Rasayana* and *Panchkarma* therapies play a crucial role in the treatment of dementia. These therapeutic techniques can potentially halt the disease's progression and improve patients' cognitive deficits. The holistic approach, including a healthy lifestyle, cleansing via Panchkarma, and

Neuro-Nutraceuticals and Drug Discovery and Delivery in Alzheimer's Disease, Volume 1: Targeting Key Pathological Pathways. Varinder Singh, Amit Kumar, Parul Sood (Eds.)

integrated palliative care, would undoubtedly help treat *Manas* vyadhi, particularly concerning dementia associated with AD. Various Ayurvedic medicinal herbs have shown promising benefits to AD pathology. However, the blood-brain barrier (BBB) restricts the availability of phytoconstituents to the central nervous system (CNS), posing the most significant obstacle to medication delivery. Ayurveda offers many unique ways like NASYA administration (intranasal administration of dry herbal powders or medicinal oils) and the MEND program (metabolic enhancement for neurodegeneration) to reverse cognitive decline. This chapter discusses the possible pathogenesis of dementia in terms of Ayurvedic concepts and suggests treatment from Ayurvedic perspectives that can be utilized advantageously for managing the disease.

8.1 INTRODUCTION

Alzheimer's disease (AD) is a neurodegenerative brain disorder that causes behavior and personality changes in addition to a gradual decline in cognitive and memory function, often known as dementia. The hallmarks of the disease include atrophy, tau hyperphosphorylation, and amyloid plaque accumulation. Once an uncommon illness, AD has become a burden on society, medicine, and the economy [1, 2]. The only approved drugs for treating AD are acetylcholinesterase (AChE) and butyrylcholinesterase (BChE) inhibitors, which delay the advancement of symptoms for a limited time [3]. Organizations like the World Health Organization are coming around to the idea that indigenous traditional knowledge systems may play a significant role in preventing and treating a broad range of clinical problems [4]. It has been proposed that communities consider integrating old knowledge systems with other everyday activities to maintain a healthy population. Among the many ancient medical practices still in use today, Ayurveda is most prevalent in South Asian countries like India, Sri Lanka, Nepal, and surrounding neighborhoods. The first written evidence of Ayurveda goes back to the fourth century BC. The Ayurvedic scripture outlines eight sub-disciplines known as '*Samhitas*' in Sanskrit, where the system was applied. The three most popular Ayurvedic texts, or *Samhitas*, are the *Charaka Samhita, Sushruta Samhita,* and *Ashtanga Hridaya* [5].

Ayurveda emphasizes using a customized style of living, proper nutrition, and other treatments to prevent and control disease. Traditional herbal remedies from the *Rasayana* (formulations with revitalizing effects) category have the most promising results in treating cognitive impairment. The Rasayana treatment has the ability to monitor the aging *Dhatu Vaigunya* (defect) and

Kshaya (degeneration). Studies of various plants and plant-based compounds under this category have exhibited neuroprotective and antioxidant activities in different clinical and preclinical investigations [6]. Many plants, including *Convolvulus pluricaulis* (Chois.), *Withania somnifera* (Linn.), *Centella asiatica* (Linn.), and *Nardostachys jatamansi* (DC), have been investigated for their possible nootropic effects [7]. Various pharmaceutical preparations such as *Svarasa* (fresh juices), *Kwatha* (decoctions), *Churna* (dried powders), *Kalka* (pastes), *Vati* (pills), *Asava-arista* (fermented medicinal liquids), *Taila* (therapeutic oils), *Ghrita* (medicinal ghee), and *Avalehas* (semisolid formulations) are used in Ayurveda for the treatment of diseases [4].

8.2 ETIOPATHOGENESIS OF DEMENTIA ASSOCIATED WITH AD (WITH REFERENCE TO AYURVEDA)

The primary symptom of Alzheimer's disease is the degeneration of brain cells leading to causes of dementia [8]. According to Ayurveda, the human body is comprised of five elements: Earth (*Bhumi/Prithvi*) for the skeleton and internal organs; Water (*Varuna/Jal*) for the circulatory system; Fire (*Agni*) for the metabolism; Air (*Vayu*) and Space (*Dyaus/Akash*). The three elemental energies—*Vata* (air and ether, or wind), *Pitta* (fire and water, or bile), and *Kapha* (earth and water, or phlegm) must be kept in harmony. If these three forces are in balance, Ayurveda claims that the body will remain well; otherwise, it will become ill in different ways [9]. Moreover, the human framework is made up of *Sharir* (body), *Satva* (mind), and *Aatma* (soul) components. In addition, *Satva* is comprised of three elements: *Dhee* (innate intelligence), *Dhriti/Dhairya* (courage), and *Smruti* (memory). The three aims of *Manas Vishaya* (mind region) are *Chintya* (thinking), *Vichar* (analyzing), and *Uhya* (inference). Mann also commands the *Jnyanendriya* (sense organs) and the *Karmendriya* (physical organs) [10].

Ayurveda identifies three vital bio-energies (*Dosha*), seven tissues (*Dhatu*), and three wastes (*Mala*) that are essential to human health. Different neurological diseases develop when *Dosha* impacts *Majja Dhatu* (nervous system) [11]. An imbalance of *Vata* (the physiological air spirit or power that passes through the brain and the nerves) was believed to cause nervous system illnesses, known as *'Vata Vyadhi'* in Sanskrit. This means that *Vata* dysregulations often result in fragility, instability, or hypersensitivity of the neurological system [12]. Since *Vata* is arid and chilly in character, an overload of *Vata* flowing in *Majja* Dhatu causes atrophy of the cortex and hippocampus, producing a void in the brain, eventually resulting in AD [11]. Furthermore, the *Dhatus* (tissues) become depleted; and *satva guna* (the quality of mind that speaks to sanctity and consciousness) becomes weak due to the dominance of *rajas* (the trait of the brain that typically speaks to strength and liveliness) and *tamas* (the characteristic of the subconscious that generally talks to the absence of participation and oblivion). When *Vata dosha* aggravates the *Manovaha srotas* (channels transporting rhythmic energies primarily responsible for memory), the person is affected and mentally deteriorates [3].

8.2.1 PROCESS OF THINKING

1. *Manas* (mind) bestows *Arthas* (objects) onto *Indriya* (sense organs). For this kind of insight to be possible, there must be a connection between Artha, Indriya, *Manas*, and Atma. This thinking is termed *Uha* [13].
2. Then *Manas* begins the actual analytical process, which includes *Chintan* (thinking), *Vichara* (reasoning), *Uhya* (judgment), and *Samkalpa* (imagination). In this way, perception becomes decisive. Therefore, the first half of the physiology of *Manas* is comprised of the process of going from vision to decision, also known as *Adhyavasaya* or *Nischayatmaka Buddhi* [14].
3. *Manas's* second half of physiology is linked to the *Karmendriyas*. *Manas* is considered *Ubhayatmaka Indriya* (controls sensory and motor functions) and ensures that *Jnanendriya* and *Karmendriya* work together. *Manas*, with the assistance of the decided knowledge, i.e., *Nischayatmaka Buddhi*, is responsible for coordinating the performance of the necessary desired reflex action after the information received by the *Jnanendriyas.* The command is taken further by the *Karmendriyas* to perform an action [15].

Moreover, the brain is home to *Indriyas*, *Manas*, and *Prana* (inspiration or life force), and *Buddhi* (knowledge or *Prajnya*) is the greatest accomplishment of these three. When there is a structural or physiological change in the brain, it has an immediate effect on *Prajnya* (wisdom). Premature aging and memory loss are caused by brain tissue degenerating at an unnaturally rapid rate and are influenced by food, lifestyle, and mental health [16]. Thus, they are responsible for *Srotovarodh* (blockage of bodily pathways), *Dhatukshaya* (tissue degradation), *Ojokshaya* (reduction of vigor), *Manas Dushti* (disruption of cognitive states and sensory abilities), *Smritibuddhihrass* (dementia), and *Vatic* ailments (neurodegenerative disorders). *Smritivibhransha* is called when pure knowledge cannot be retained because the mind is confused by emotion and illusion. This condition is referred to as a "disorder of memory," as it affects a person's ability to recall specific details [13].

8.3 CLASSIFICATION OF AD (ACCORDING TO AYURVEDA)

1. *Vata*-**Type Alzheimer's Disease (VTAD):** It occurs during the *Vata* stage of life and is consistent with the biochemical parameters in type II AD, which is defined by the removal of neurotrophic assistance and loss in hormone assistance [17]. VTAD is caused by a *Vata*-provoking lifestyle combined with irregular habits, tension, and consuming a dry, chilly, and light diet. *Prana Vayu* (inhalation; uptake of perceptions), *Samana Vayu* (impulses traveling from sensory organs to CNS; movement of thinking), *Vyana Vayu* (impulses traveling from CNS to sensory organs; handling of opinions), *Udana Vayu* (cognition and recollection), and *Apana Vayu* (absorption and distribution of perceptions) may all be out of balance, indicating a problem with collecting and assimilating information from the five senses. In the long run, it affects the way of thinking and behavior in individuals experiencing behavioral and personal problems [18]. Patients may experience memory loss, confusion, emotional instability, and difficulty sleeping. They may struggle to learn new things and have trouble expressing themselves. These individuals may also face significant issues with constipation. Insulin resistance, known as *Madhumeha* (diabetes), a subtype of *Vataja Prameha* (body excretes more urine than usual), and premature loss of female hormones (*Artava Kshaya*, disorders related to menstruation), are two other *Vata*-type disorders associated with this syndrome [19, 20]. VTAD patients are typically a bit older, often in their 80s [21, 22]. Fluorodeoxyglucose-positron emission tomography (FDG-PET) has revealed that decreases in glucose consumption are mainly linked to shrinkage or degradation caused by *Vata*, particularly in the temporoparietal areas [23, 24].
2. ***Pitta*-Type Alzheimer's Disease (PTAD):** The molecular characteristics of type 1 AD are consistent with PTAD (inflammatory AD). Despite Alzheimer's disease mostly being a *Vata* ailment, it may manifest in individuals of *Pitta* nature who exhibit surplus heat due to a *Pitta*-vitiating way of living, leading to the degradation of the hippocampus and cortical cells [17]. The expression of proinflammatory cytokines, inflammatory microglia, stimulated astroglia,

chemokines, and other indicators of inflammation in AD brains is a crucial symptom demonstrating the involvement of *Pitta*. Regular consumption of spicy, sour, salty, highly acidic, and fermented foods is one factor that might aggravate *Pitta*. Drinking, anger, violence, and prolonged heat stress are all potential contributors to PTAD [24, 25].

3. ***Krimi*-Type Alzheimer's Disease (KTAD):** In Ayurveda, the term '*Krimi*' refers to parasite infection and toxin poisoning. Individuals with AD who do not fit into the *Vata* or *Pitta* categories are classified as having *Krimi*-type AD because they share two extrinsic factors: (i) risk to toxins, aflatoxins, and infections; and/or (ii) exposure to hazardous substances. Patients with *Krimi*-AD have a somewhat different profile than those with the first two subtypes of AD, with an earlier age of onset and a more common 3/3 ApoE genotype [17, 26, 27]. Insomnia, sadness, and extreme stress often precede the onset. Patients in this category can form new memories, but they have trouble remembering the past. FDG-PET scans show extensive fronto-temporoparietal abnormalities and brain shrinkage. Patients with these symptoms may have been exposed to toxins such as molds found in water-damaged houses, bacterial infections, aflatoxins like those that induce Lyme disease, or high amounts of heavy metals. These individuals also reported low blood zinc levels, and zinc deficiency is linked to impairments in various processes important for cognitive function and AD [24, 26, 28, 29]. The herbs used to treat various AD types according to Ayurveda are listed in Table 8.1.

TABLE 8.1 Common Drugs Used in *Manas Vyadhi* as per Dosha

Role of Herbs	Ratio	Vata	Pitta	Krimi
Main	8	*Withania somnifera*	*Centella asiatica*	*Commiphora mukul*
Aid-1	2	*Bacopa monnieri*	*Curcuma long)*	Shilajit
Aid-2	2	*Convolvulus pluricaulis*	*Commiphora mukul*	Triphala (*Emblica officinalis, Terminalia bellirica, Terminalia chebula*)
Aid-3	2	*Centella asiatica*	*Convolvulus pluricaulis*	*Centella asiatica*
Assistance-1	1	Shilajit	*Bacopa monnieri*	*Bacopa monnieri*
Assistance-2	1	*Tinospora cordifolia*	*Withania somnifera*	*Withania somnifera*
Assistance-3	1	Triphala	Triphala	*Curcuma longa*

8.4 COMMON DRUGS USED IN *MANAS* VYADHI/SMRUTI BRAMSH

8.4.1 CELASTRUS PANICULATUS (MALKANGANI, FAMILY: CELASTRACEAE)

C. paniculatus (CPa), also called "Jyotishmati" or "Tree of Life," is a highly coveted medicinal plant used in Ayurveda to enhance cognitive function, namely memory and focus [30]. Oil extracted from the plant's seeds has been shown to enhance memory and vigilance [31, 32]. The CPa plant has several traditional medicinal uses, including antimalarial, anti-TB, diuretic, antiflatulence, and antidysentery [33]. The plant contains compounds such as Malkanguniol, Paniculatadiol, and Malkangunin; alkaloids like Celapanin, Celapagin, Celapanigin, and Celastrine; and triterpenoids such as Pristimerin [34, 35]. Some of the fatty acids found in the seed oil are palmitic, stearic, linoleic, benzoic, and linolenic acids [36, 37] (Table 8.2).

As a result of their free radical scavenging property and their capacity to modulate glutamate receptor activity, CPa extracts protected neuronal cells against H_2O_2 and glutamate-induced damage [38, 39]. Memory performance was also enhanced by a dose-dependent cholinergic activity in the aqueous extract of CPa seeds [40]. In another investigation, extracts of CPa seeds were shown to have antioxidant and acetylcholinesterase inhibitory activity [41, 42]. Myelination and phospholipid concentration in the brain have both been improved by CPa seed extract [43, 44]. Current efforts to treat AD have centered on improving cholinergic function, most often by employing acetylcholinesterase (AChE) inhibitors (AChEIs) or cholinergic receptor agonists. In AD treatment, AChEIs should increase endogenous AChE levels in the brain, thereby improving cholinergic neurotransmission and memory. *Celastrus paniculatus* (CPa) seeds were shown to have antioxidant and acetylcholinesterase inhibitory activity. This results in improved memory affected by AD [45]. Moreover, myelination and phospholipid concentration in the brain have both been improved by CPa seed extract, which increases impulse conduction.

8.4.2 CENTELLA ASIATICA LINN (JAL BRAHMI, FAMILY: APIACEAE)

Centella asiatica L. (CA) is also known as Gotu kola, Mandukparni, Jal-Brahmi, and Indian pennywort [47]. As a result of its beneficial effects on memory and its potential to prevent age-related brain problems, Ayurveda classifies it as Medhya Rasayana. So far, CA has been shown to have a number of interesting neuropharmacological effects, including antiepileptic, anxiolytic [47], memory boosting, neurite elongation, and nerve regenerative properties [48, 49]. It contains triterpenoid saponins such as Asiatic acid, madecassic acid, madasiatic acid, asiaticoside, madecassoside, brahmoside, and brahminoside [50].

CA exhibited a neuroprotective effect against colchicine and streptozotocin-induced cognitive defects and oxidative damage in the brains of rats [51, 52]. It has been shown to induce CREB phosphorylation in both neuroblastoma cell lines expressing amyloid beta 1–42 (Aβ) and rat embryonic cortex primary cell culture [53]. *Centella asiatica* triterpene, Asiatic acid, has been shown to protect neurons from oxidative damage after exposure to excess glutamate [54] and aluminum chloride-induced amyloid load [55] in scientific studies. The CA ethanol extract inhibits acetylcholinesterase, butyrylcholinesterase, and tyrosinase activity [56]. Moreover, CA extract enhances memory by improving neuronal morphology by promoting dendritic arborization in CA3 neurons in the hippocampus [57]. In addition, CA extract decreases the number of β-amyloid plaques in the hippocampus of PSAPP mice [58] and protects neuroblastoma cells from amyloid β-induced oxidative stress and mitochondrial dysfunction in MC65 and SH-SY5Y cultures [59]. Triterpene components and the aqueous extract of CA have been demonstrated to reduce amyloid β-induced spine loss, suggesting a potential therapeutic role other than AD [44, 60].

8.4.3 GLYCYRRHIZA GLABRA L. (MULHATTI, FAMILY: FABACEAE)

Glycyrrhiza glabra Linn. (GG), also known as Yashtimadhuha, Mulhatti, and Liquorice, is used as a demulcent, expectorant, anti-tussive, laxative, and sweetener in the ancient Siddha medical system [61]. The main chemical constituent of the plant is Glycyrrhizic acid (a saponin) found in the roots [62]. Memory and learning abilities were greatly enhanced by GG aqueous extract in diazepam and scopolamine-induced amnesia [63]. Licorice root treatment also boosted succinate dehydrogenase levels in brain regions [64]. However, *Glycyrrhiza uralensis*, more commonly known as Chinese licorice, showed a protective effect against cognitive impairment produced by $A\beta_{(25-35)}$ peptide in mice via antioxidant action [65].

Glycyrrhizin has shown promising results in a number of trials, suggesting that it may be a useful agent for treating memory-related illnesses by reducing neuroinflammation and restoring cognitive function [66, 67]. It also reduced acetylcholinesterase (AChE) activity in the hippocampus of obese rats [68].

High-mobility group box 1 (HMGB1) acts as a signal molecule in many neurodegenerative illnesses and is also connected with tau phosphorylation in Alzheimer's disease (AD) pathogenesis; pre-treatment with glycyrrhizin (orally) reduces HMGB1-induced neuroinflammation [69]. Therefore, glycyrrhizin might be useful in treating neuroinflammation associated with AD. Isoliquiritigenin blocked NMDA receptors and inhibited caspase-3 in rats with cerebral ischemia-reperfusion damage [70, 71]. Diabetic rats treated with glabridin have markedly enhanced learning and memory. These findings were linked to glabridin's antioxidant, neuroprotective, and anticholinesterase characteristics, which raise the possibility of using this compound in treating dementia [44, 72].

8.4.4 CONVOLVULUS PLURICAULIS CHOIS. (SHANKHPUSHPI, FAMILY: CONVOLVULACEAE)

In Ayurveda, *Convolvulus pluricaulis* (CP) is referred to as a *Medhya Rasayana* and is primarily recommended in neurostimulation and rejuvenation therapies [73]. Scopoletin, scopolin, kaempferol, β-sitosterol; primary alcohols like n-triacontanol, and n-hexaconasol; fatty acids including myristic and linoleic acid have been isolated from the plant [74]. More than 40 Ayurvedic and herbal preparations available in the Indian market contain CP as a principal element to treat memory and other neurodegenerative disorders. Various plants, including Evolvulus alsinoides, *Clitoria ternatea*, and Canscora decussata, were being sold and consumed as shankpushpi throughout the nation. It was observed that memory-improving potential was highest in CP, with *C. ternatea* coming in the second [75]. Because of its acetylcholinesterase inhibitory and antioxidant effects, CP has been shown to aid memory enhancement against scopolamine-induced amnesia [76, 77].

Furthermore, 70% hydroalcoholic extract of CP inhibited Aβ production in mouse neuroblastoma cells expressing the Swedish APP (N2a-SweAPP). It increases the activity of amyloid-degrading enzymes (such as insulin-degrading enzymes or neprilysin) [78]. The plant extract inhibited the growth and survival of Aβ fibrils *in vitro*, demonstrating anti-amyloidogenic action [79]. CP extract (150 mg/kg) given orally reduces Aβ levels in scopolamine-induced neurotoxicity in male Wistar rats via lowering tau, APP protein, and mRNA levels [80]. It also reduced the accumulation of Aβ and tau protein in rat brains [81]. Scopoletin and scopolin isolated from the plant exhibited acetylcholinesterase inhibitory activity against scopolamine-induced memory impairment [82].

Clinical research using healthy volunteers aged 16 to 25 confirms the nootropic effects of Shankhpushpi. Information was gathered using Wechsler's Memory Scale both before and after the two-month intervention. Improvements in auditory and visual recognition, as well as delayed auditory and visual constructs, were seen in those given Shankhpushpi tablets (made from the powder and juice of CP) compared to those given a placebo [83, 84]. Neuroprotective effects of CP were also seen in aluminum, hydrogen peroxide, and 2,2′-Azobis-(2-methylpropionamidine) dihydrochloride (AAPH)-generated neuronal damage [85, 86]. AChE activity is suppressed, Na^+/K^+ ATPase activity is maintained, lipid and protein damage are prevented, mRNA levels for muscarinic receptor 1, choline acetyltransferase, and nerve growth factor-tyrosine kinase A receptor are maintained, and cyclin-dependent kinase 5 (CDK5) expressions are enhanced when CP is given on a regular basis. Moreover, it reduced lactate dehydrogenase leakage, blocked reactive oxygen species formation and mitochondrial membrane depolarization, and controlled expression of apoptosis indicators (superoxide dismutase, catalase, tumor suppressor gene p53, and caspase-3) [85, 86]. Shankhpushpi had a soothing impact on the body because it inhibited the synthesis of adrenaline and cortisol, two stress chemicals [44, 87].

8.5 TREATMENT (CHIKITSA) FOR DEMENTIA

8.5.1 DAIVAVYAPASHRAYA CHIKITSA (DIVINE THERAPY)

Daivavyapashrayam is based on the concept of *Adrushtam* (which cannot be observed with the naked eye). It includes *Mangalakarma* (auspicious rites), *Bali* (religious sacrifice), *Upahara* (offerings to God), *Homa* (offering ghee to fire), *Niyama* (promise or vow), *Prayashcitta* (redemption), *Upavasa* (fasting), *Swastyayana* (auspicious religious songs), *Pranipata* (paying homage), *Gamanam* (journey to sacred places), and other procedures based on *Adrushtaphala* (karma or deeds) [88].

8.5.2 SATTVAVJAYA CHIKITSA (ASSURANCE THERAPY)

It is a nonpharmacological method for restricting the mind from harmful *Artha* (things) or stresses. *Sattvavajaya Chikitsa*, also known as "therapy through self-control," involves removing one's focus from negative circumstances and shifting to positive thinking for a purposeful life [89]. All of *Astanga Yoga's* (yogic techniques) and *Manonigraha's* practices (mind-controlling techniques) are included in the therapy [90].

TABLE 8.2 Common Drugs Used in *Manas Vyadhi/Smruti Bramsh*

Name	Major Constituent	Functions
Celastrus paniculatus (Jyotishmati) 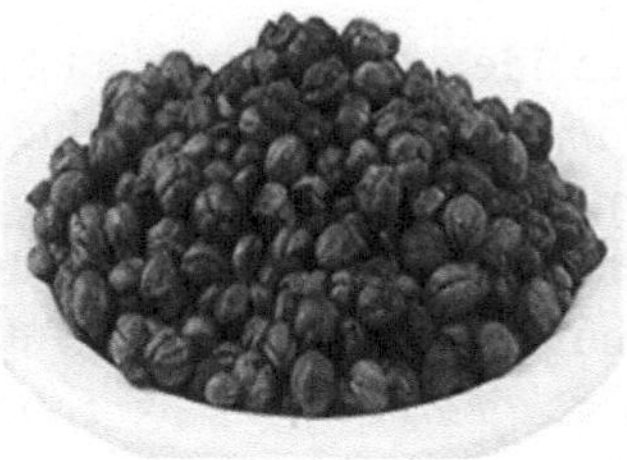	Malkangunial, paniculatadiol, malkangunin, celapanin, celapanigin, palmitic acid	Enhance memory and vigilance.
Centella asiatica (Gotu kola mandukparni) 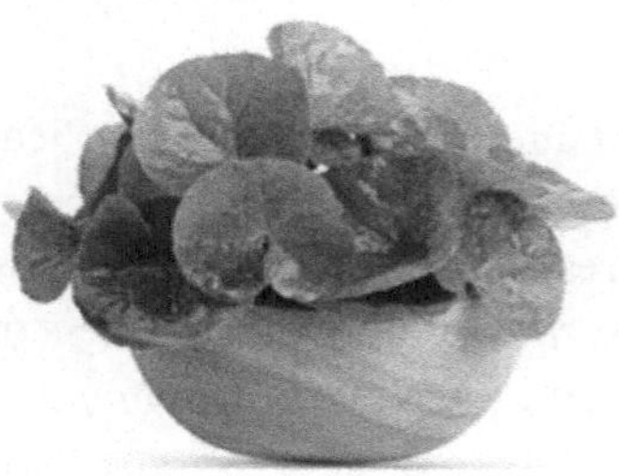	Asiatic acid, madecassic acid, madasiatic acid, asiaticoside, madecassoside.	Treats age-related neuro problems.
Glycyrrhiza glabra (Yashtimadhuha) 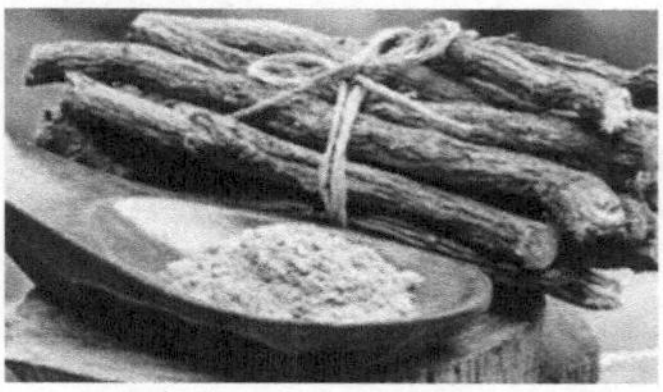	Glycyrrhizic acid	Treats amnesia, neuroinflammation, and Alzheimer's disease.
Convolvulus pluricaulis (Shankhpuspi) 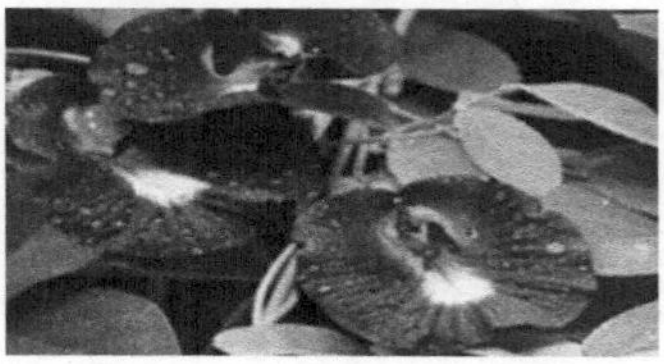	Scopoletin, scopolin, kaempferol, n-triacontanol, linoleic acid	Improves auditory and visual recognition.

8.5.3 YUKTIVYAPASHRAYA CHIKITSA (RATIONAL THERAPY)

It is based on the concepts of Ayurveda and the principle that the body's systems should be restored to their proper order via the use of pharmacological treatments and foods that promote health [91, 92]. It includes:

1. ***Antah parimarjana* (to Cleanse from Inside):** It is further subcategorized into *Samshodhana* and *Samshana. Samshodhana* includes the use of techniques like *Vamana* (vomiting), *Virechana* (purging), *Vasti* (enema), and *Nasya* (nasal administration of drugs) to cure impaired *Dosha*. It has been discovered that *Manorogas* (mental disorders) can be cured with this *Panchakarma* therapy (body cleansing treatment). On the other hand, *Samshamana* prescribes several medications like *Medhya Rasayanas* (e.g., Haridra, Mandukaparni, Brahmi, Shankhpushpi), a healthy diet, and daily exercise to treat the afflicted *Doshas* [91–93].
2. ***Bahir parimarjana* (to Cleanse from Outside):** It includes the application of therapeutic oils externally (at the site of pathology) as a part of the *Purvakarmas* (preparatory measures) of *Panchakarma* therapy (purification technique). It also contains *Snehana* (producing oiliness or softness in the body), *Swedana* (application of heat), and *Dhumapana* (inhalation of medicated smoke) procedures to cure *Manovikara* (mental disorders) [91, 92]. Figure 8.1 defines *chikitsa* or dementia.

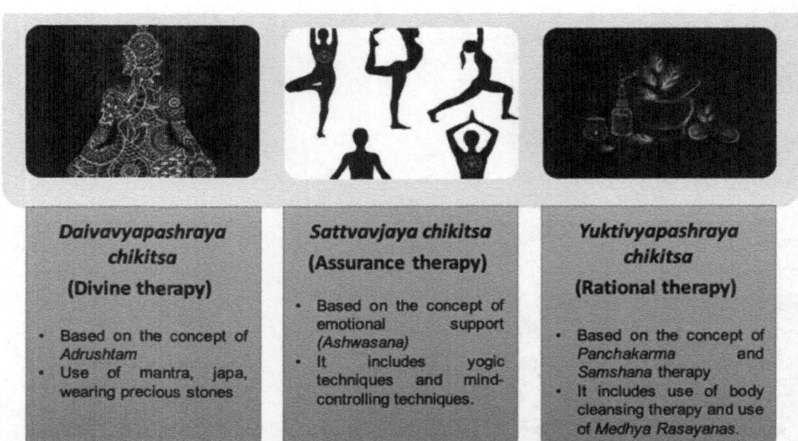

FIGURE 8.1 *Chikitsa* for dementia.

Source: Reprinted/Adapted from Ref.[92]. https://creativecommons.org/licenses/by/4.0/

8.6 DRUG ADMINISTRATION TECHNIQUES USED IN AYURVEDA

The Ayurveda system of medicine follows its principles, some of which are similar to the modern allopathy system. Like the modern system, in Ayurveda, drug formulations are categorized into four different dosage forms: Solid, Powder, Semisolid, and Liquid [94].

According to Ayurveda, drug absorption in the body depends on two criteria:

1. **Properties of the Drug:** Such as solubility in lipid/water, molecular/particle size, physical form, chemical nature, dosage form, concentration, etc.
2. **Site of Administration:** pH of the fluid, vascularity, presence of other substances, disease condition, etc.

   Various routes, as explained in Figure 8.2, are used to administer the dosage forms in the body cavity, known as *Aushadha sevana Margas.*

   There are mainly eight routes (*Srotas*) prescribed in Ayurveda for drug administration.

   - Oral route (*Mukha*);
   - Nasal route (*Netra*) (Nose);
   - Ear route (*Karna*);
   - Dermal route (*Twak*);
   - Eye route (*Akshi*)
   - Rectum route (*Guda*);
   - Urethral route (*Mutra marga*); and
   - Vaginal route (*Yoni marga*).

Ayurveda believes that there are three major causes of CNS-related disorders: neural hyperfunctioning (*Vata vriddhi*), neural hypofunction (*Vata ksaya*), and masked functioning (*avarana).* Ayurveda considers the majority of CNS disorders as non-curable with the help of medicine-based therapy alone. Therefore, several therapy regimens, such as "panchakarma" (five actions), yoga, massage, and combinations of herbs and minerals, have been described in Ayurvedic writings [95]. These can improve the quality of life and lengthen lifespan. Yoga and "Satvavajaya," or mind-control-based Ayurveda psychotherapy, were used to help a patient regain their strength, intelligence, and memory [96, 97].

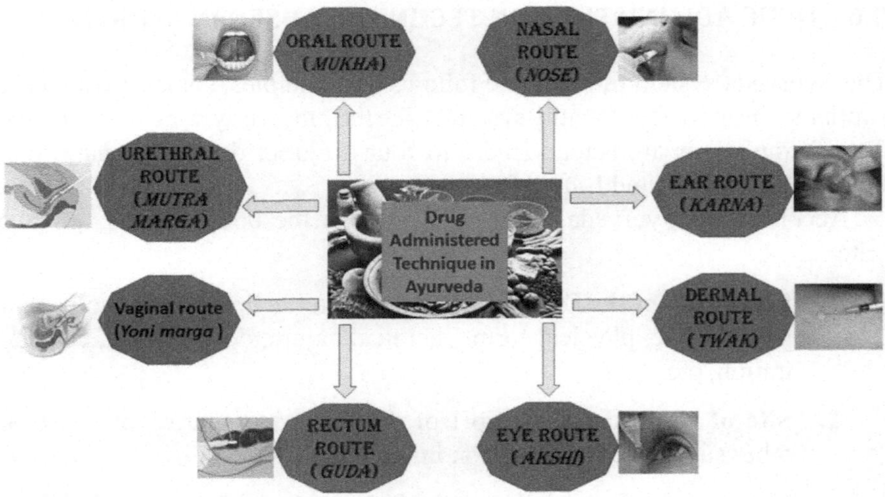

FIGURE 8.2 Routes (*Srotas*) are prescribed in Ayurveda for the drug administration.

We discuss drug administration for the treatment of AD and related illnesses in the current chapter. It includes "Nasya" (one of the commonly used processes in "panchkarma"), massage, and metabolic enhancement for neurodegeneration (MEND), the most effective way of treatment of AD and related disorders in Ayurveda [98].

The treatment of AD needs the entry of medicine into the CNS for which the chemical has to cross the blood-brain barrier (BBB). Therefore, Ayurvedic practitioners started opting for novel drug delivery-based methods to deliver the desirable parts of the brain. "Nasya" is one of the popular techniques used in Ayurveda for the administration of herbs or their constituents directly to the site of action. In this method, dry herbal powders and medicated oil can be administered directly to the CNS. This method is rapid, simple, and non-invasive to deliver the medicine into the CNS. The dried herbs are powdered in such a manner that their particle size is reduced to the nano-level; hence they can be inhaled directly and reach the CNS while crossing the BBB [20, 99].

The drugs or herbs that cannot be administered directly in a powdered form are cooked over a low flame with a 1:4 ratio of oil and water. The heating should continue until all the water has evaporated. The end product, oil, allows the transportation of lipid-soluble molecules across the BBB barrier by solubilizing/dissolving all the lipid-soluble compounds from the herbs [100]. *Nasya* has gained popularity as a non-invasive drug delivery method since it has many advantages for the CNS [101, 102]. Moreover, this method guarantees quick delivery, avoids the BBB, aids in targeting the CNS, lowers systemic exposure, and minimizes side effects [103–106].

Another easy way to administer medication is through massage, which involves applying medicinal oil to specific body parts or regions with light or firm hand strokes. Regarding this method's ability to facilitate the passage of phytochemicals via the BBB, there is no concrete data. Yet, indirect data from a recent study supports this intriguing notion. Massage is reported to increase cerebral blood flow and significantly activate brain functions. It aids in lowering serum cortisol and arginine vasopressin levels while simultaneously raising circulatory lymphocytes and local cerebral blood flow [107–110]. Therefore, it can be further useful in the management of AD-related consequences up to certain limits. In Ayurveda, medicated oil is also administered through a non-systemic and non-invasive technique called transcranial oleation therapy.

In this technique, four procedures are mainly applied including:

- The medicinal oil is gently dripped onto the forehead (*Shirodhara*).
- A patient's shaved head is covered with a special leather cap, and therapeutic oil is poured over it and left on for 30 to 45 minutes (*Shirobasti*).
- A little massage is given after applying medicinal oil to the head (*Shiroabhyanga*).
- A steady stream of medicated oil is poured over the head (*Shiroseka*).

Similar to how Ayurveda massages impact hormonal and cerebral blood flow levels, so does this technique. The possibility that endothelial cells facilitate the entry of the solutes through the frontal lobe and prefrontal cortex is once more raised by recent work, despite the fact that scientific studies regarding the penetration of the herbal components into the CNS through this therapy are still being conducted [111–113]. In Ayurveda, aromatherapy is one of the popular methods, which involves the use of essential oils for healing, mood elevation, and cognitive functions. In this technique, the essential oils are either directly applied to the face and arms or assimilated by steam inhalation. It has been found to have some promise for enhancing cognitive performance, especially in patients with AD, and it may also assist in calming agitated dementia patients [114–116].

Recently, a new concept of therapy has been introduced to treat AD based on the principles of Ayurveda. In this concept, clinical symptoms alone are not considered sufficient to create effective treatment, but diet and lifestyle also play a vital role in the treatment of the disease. In Ayurveda, in addition to herbal-based medications, diet, and lifestyle balancing are considered equally significant factors. Therefore, it recommends a diet plan and herbs to balance *Vata*, *Pitta*, and *Kapha*. In this regard, some studies have been carried out by researchers to understand the concept of diet in the progression and treatment of AD in patients [17]. This extensive approach, known as metabolic enhancement for neurodegeneration (MEND), has been created and applied to achieve the reversal of AD-associated cognitive deterioration. Following the approach exactly has led to a consistent reversal of cognitive decline in hundreds of individuals, along with long-lasting improvements [117–119].

In this method, metabolic profiling of patients is created, and the personal response is recorded. Several people with early-stage Alzheimer's disease or pre-AD symptoms, mild cognitive impairment, or subjective cognitive impairment found that optimizing these metabolic parameters was helpful. In the study, three main subtypes of AD, including inflammatory, non-inflammatory, and cortical AD, were classified as a result of the involvement of several metabolic factors in the AD process [29, 120, 121]. The clinical details and metabolic profiles of AD patients also contributed to the classification of AD patients into the three Ayurveda subtypes of *Vata*, *Pitta*, and *Krimi*. From the perspective of specific subtype-based therapies, this classification is found to be helpful in individuals with cognitive decline and those at risk for such decline. In order to effectively treat the patients against AD, several diet regimens and herb combinations were given to the patients according to their subtypes [122].

8.7 CONCLUSION

The most prevalent type of dementia affecting elderly people in both developed and developing countries is AD. Alzheimer's disease (AD) is an untreatable, progressive neurological condition that causes memory loss, deterioration in cognitive function, and abnormal patient behavior. The disease makes life miserable; patients with AD face stress and require comprehensive care. Modern medicines available for treatment are not up to the expectations and are capable of treating only symptoms but fail to cure them completely. Traditional systems of medicine like Ayurveda offer several options to modify the progress and symptoms of AD. Ayurveda not only provides the incorporation of traditional herbs but also follows novel practices to support safe and possible care for AD patients. Some of the pre-clinical and clinical studies are evidence of the efficacy of Ayurveda as a medicine system to support the clinical manifestations of AD. Around a hundred new products are currently in the clinical development stage, and the use of medicinal herbs backed by literature found in the texts of Ayurveda or other traditional systems of medicine has been a successful source of leads for the development of new pharmaceuticals.

However, scientific studies are available confirming the use of various Ayurvedic herbs or preparations for the treatment of AD, but their mechanisms are still unclear. The phytochemical screening of such plants indicates the presence of therapeutic compounds, such as lignans, polyphenols, flavonoids, tannins, terpenoids, sterols, alkaloids, etc., that show a wide spectrum of pharmacological activities. These ingredients can contribute towards the management and cure of AD and also serve as a lead in drug discovery for AD [46]. Bioavailability of the phytochemicals is the great challenge faced during the treatment of AD with medicinal herbs by practitioners. To address this, medicated oil and the treatment process are modified by progressive healers. The results of Nasya, massage, aromatherapy, MEND, and other therapies are impressive and optimistic. Therefore, the scientific evaluation and validation of Ayurvedic formulations and approaches to drug administration procedures can play a crucial and significant role in the treatment of AD. Furthermore, the recently introduced therapy regimen in Ayurveda, MEND, opens a new area of research in the field of managing AD. Diet management can contribute significantly to treating AD; this individualized protocol can help in curing the condition. The concept of balancing *"tridosha"* through diet and certain herbs has shown significant hope and promise in managing certain other CNS-related disorders.

8.8 FUTURE PERSPECTIVES

The treatment of AD is the biggest challenge for modern medical science. The importance of medicinal herbs and traditional systems to cure different diseases and ailments is time-tested. In the context of AD, Ayurveda offers a complete treatment regimen including medicinal herbs, routes of administration, and procedures to deliver the medicament to the site of action. To utilize the knowledge and practices of Ayurveda to treat AD needs to be validated scientifically. However, scientific literature to support the success of medicinal herbs and Ayurveda principles in the treatment of AD is available. The studies reported are generally carried out as primary ones to collect evidence of the efficacy of the herbs in the treatment of AD. However isolated compounds have failed to reproduce the results and are not supported by the establishment of the mechanism of action and ADME. The potential of the herbs, procedures, and therapy styles used by Ayurveda needs more specific clinical trials to generate more evidence and also to develop newer approaches by modern medical sciences.

In the future, Ayurveda therapy needs to be validated through proper scientific rationale, information on uptake, dosage, and contraindications. This can surely help in the expansion of new horizons for finding keys to cure complex CNS disorders, including AD. Besides the study of the pharmacological effect of the single herb or combination of active constituents present in the herbs, in order to examine the lifestyles, regimens, and yoga recommended as part of the treatment regimen, Ayurvedic therapy needs to move beyond the current paradigm of diagnosis, prognosis, cure, and post-treatment follow-up. The deep knowledge of Ayurvedic principles coupled with combinatorial sciences and high-throughput screening techniques of treatment and medicinal plants can serve the medical sciences in the form of newer leads and treatment regimens, which can help society by reducing the medical burden and also provide a better life expectancy for patients suffering from CNS-related disorders. Moreover, the role of MEND needs to be studied more for its probable mechanism, and coupling this with a modern scientific approach can further lead medical science closer to an effective treatment regimen for patients suffering from AD and other cognitive deficit diseases.

KEYWORDS

- **Alzheimer's disease**
- **ayurveda**
- **CNS disorders**
- **majja dhatu**
- **Panchakarma**
- **Rasayana**
- **therapeutic compounds**
- **traditional systems**

REFERENCES

1. Polis, B., & Samson, A. O. (2019). A new perspective on Alzheimer's disease as a brain expression of a complex metabolic disorder. *Alzheimer's Disease [Internet]*.
2. Malik, J., Munjal, K., & Deshmukh, R. (2015). Attenuating effect of standardized lyophilized Cinnamomum zeylanicum bark extract against streptozotocin-induced experimental dementia of Alzheimer's type. *J Basic Clin Physiol Pharmacol, 26*(3), 275–285. https://doi.org/10.1515/jbcpp-2014-0131.
3. Bhattacharjee, A. (2019). Scientific basis of ayurvedic medicine: In the hunt for a cure to Alzheimer's disease. In S. Paul (Ed.), *Application of Biomedical Engineering in Neuroscience* (pp. 63–83). Springer Singapore. https://doi.org/10.1007/978-981-13-0611-0_4.
4. Sharma, S., Singh, G., & Patwardhan, K. (2023). Effects of two Ayurvedic formulations, Dhanwantaram Kashaya and Saraswatarishta on life history parameters and toxic aggregates in Drosophila models of Huntington's and Alzheimer's disease. *Journal of Ethnopharmacology, 305*, 116080. https://doi.org/10.1016/j.jep.2023.116080.
5. Patwardhan, K., et al. (2011). The Ayurveda education in India: How well are the graduates exposed to basic clinical skills? *Evidence-Based Complementary and Alternative Medicine, 2011*, 197391. https://doi.org/10.1093/ecam/nen073.
6. Farooqui, A. A., et al. (2018). Ayurvedic medicine for the treatment of dementia: Mechanistic aspects. *Evidence-Based Complementary and Alternative Medicine, 2018*. https://doi.org/10.1155/2018/2481076.
7. Balasubramani, S. P., et al. (2011). Plant-based Rasayana drugs from Ayurveda. *Chinese Journal of Integrative Medicine, 17*(2), 88–94. https://doi.org/10.1007/s11655-011-0638-x.
8. Albert, M. S., et al. (2011). The diagnosis of mild cognitive impairment due to Alzheimer's disease: Recommendations from the National Institute on Aging-Alzheimer's Association workgroups on diagnostic guidelines for Alzheimer's disease. *Alzheimer's & Dementia, 7*(3), 270–279. https://doi.org/10.1016/j.jalz.2011.03.008.
9. Sharma, D., et al. (2021). Indigenous therapeutics of Alzheimer: A review of Ayurvedic herbs from its ethnobotany to phytotherapy. *Journal of Ethnopharmacology, 11*(4), 4178–4191.
10. Amarprakash, D. (2021). Alzheimer's disease management: An integrated overview. *Journal of Interdisciplinary Cycle Research, 13*, 360–373.
11. Majhi, V., Choudhury, B., & Paul, S. (2020). Prevention and treatment of Alzheimer's disease in the light of Ayurveda. In *Phytomedicine and Alzheimer's Disease* (pp. 85–96). CRC Press. https://doi.org/10.1201/9780429460141-7.
12. Manyam, B. V. (1999). Dementia in Ayurveda. *The Journal of Alternative and Complementary Medicine, 5*(1), 81–88. https://doi.org/10.1089/acm.1999.5.81.
13. Shastri, K., & Chaturvedi, G. N. (1984). Charak Samhita with Vidyotini Hindi Commentary. *Sharira sthana, 8*(48), 951.
14. Samhita, C., Shastri, K., & Varanasi, C. G. (2004). *Chaukhamba Bharti Academy*. Google Scholar, 917.
15. Tiwari, R. S., & Tripathi, J. S. (2013). A critical appraisal of dementia with special reference to Smritibuddhihrass. *Ayu, 34*(3), 235–242. https://doi.org/10.4103/0974-8520.123121.
16. Narayana Reddy, G., Ramu, M., & Venkataram, B. (1987). Concept of manas (psyche) in Ayurveda. *NIMHANS Journal, 21*(2).

17. Bredesen, D. E. (2015). Metabolic profiling distinguishes three subtypes of Alzheimer's disease. *Aging (Albany NY), 7*(8), 595–600. https://doi.org/10.18632/aging.100801.
18. Rao, R. V., et al. (2012). Ayurvedic medicinal plants for Alzheimer's disease: A review. *Alzheimer's Research & Therapy, 4*(3), 22. https://doi.org/10.1186/alzrt132.
19. Gauttam, V., et al. (2022). Comparative study of developed formulation and market formulation for antidiabetic potential in alloxan-induced diabetic Wistar rats. *Journal of Young Pharmacists, 14*, 387–393. https://doi.org/10.5530/jyp.2022.14.70.
20. Sonali, V., et al. (2023). Unravelling the approaches to treat osteoarthritis: A focus on the potential of medicinal plants. *Pharmacognosy Research, 15*(1), 13–25.
21. Sharma, A., et al. (2021). Combination effect of Spirulina fusiformis with rutin or chlorogenic acid in lipopolysaccharide-induced septic cardiac inflammation in experimental diabetic rat model. *Pharmacognosy Magazine, 17*, 257.
22. Haye, A., et al. (2022). Polyherbal formulation improves glucose-lipid metabolism and prevents hepatotoxicity in streptozotocin-induced diabetic rats: Plausible role of IRS-PI3K-Akt-GLUT2 signaling. *Pharmacognosy Magazine, 18*, 52.
23. Manyam, B. V., & Kumar, A. (2013). Ayurvedic constitution (prakruti) identifies risk factor of developing Parkinson's disease. *Journal of Alternative and Complementary Medicine, 19*(7), 644–649. https://doi.org/10.1089/acm.2012.0412.
24. Bredesen, D. E., & Rao, R. V. (2017). Ayurvedic profiling of Alzheimer's disease. *Alternative Therapies in Health and Medicine, 23*, 46–50.
25. Ninivaggi, F. J. (2010). *Ayurveda: A Comprehensive Guide to Traditional Indian Medicine for the West*. Rowman & Littlefield.
26. Bredesen, D. E. (2016). Inhalational Alzheimer's disease: An unrecognized—and treatable—Epidemic. *Aging (Albany NY), 8*(2), 304–313. https://doi.org/10.18632/aging.100896.
27. Lad, V. (2002). *Textbook of Ayurveda: A Complete Guide to Clinical Assessment.* Ayurvedic Press.
28. Kciuk, M., et al. (2022). Computational Bioprospecting Guggulsterone against ADP Ribose Phosphatase of SARS-CoV-2. *Molecules, 27*, 8287. https://doi.org/10.3390/molecules27238287.
29. Munjal, K., et al. (2022). Furanocoumarins and Lectins as Food Toxins. In *Proceedings of the International Conference on Food Safety and Food Security* (pp. 67–80).
30. Bhanumathy, M., et al. (2010). Nootropic activity of *Celastrus paniculatus* seed. *Pharmaceutical Biology, 48*(3), 324–327. https://doi.org/10.3109/13880200903186967.
31. Lekha, G., et al. (2010). Cognitive enhancement and neuroprotective effect of *Celastrus paniculatus* Willd. seed oil (Jyothismati oil) on male Wistar rats. *Journal of Pharmaceutical Science and Technology, 2*(2), 130–138.
32. Munjal, K., et al. (2022). Scope and limitations of digital learning's in developing countries: A real-time survey. *Annals of Phytomedicine: An International Journal, COVID-19 Special, 11(3), S58–S63.*
33. Shen, Y., et al. (2019). Traditional uses, secondary metabolites, and pharmacology of Celastrus species – a review. *Journal of Ethnopharmacology, 241*, 112024. https://doi.org/10.1016/j.jep.2019.111944.
34. Shashank, D., Rajendra, S. V., & Mistry, A. (2017). An overview of phytoconstituents and pharmacological activities of *Celastrus paniculatus* Willd. *Journal of Pharmaceutical Research, 16*(4), 307–313.

35. Munjal, K., et al. (2020). Development of validated HPTLC method for quantification of luteolin in Eclipta alba and its formulation. In *Proceedings of the International Conference on Chromatographic Analysis* (pp. 2685–2695).
36. Sengupta, A., & Bhargava, H. N. (1970). Chemical investigation of the seed fat of *Celastrus paniculatus*. *Journal of the Science of Food and Agriculture, 21*(12), 628–631. https://doi.org/10.1002/jsfa.2740211203.
37. Satyavert, et al. (2021). Pharmacokinetics and tissue distribution of hydrazinocurcumin in rats. *Pharmacological Reports, 73*(6), 1734–1743. https://doi.org/10.1007/s43440-021-00237-8.
38. Kumar, M. H., & Gupta, Y. K. (2002). Antioxidant property of *Celastrus paniculatus* Willd.: A possible mechanism in enhancing cognition. *Phytomedicine, 9*(4), 302–311. https://doi.org/10.1078/0944-7113-00121.
39. Godkar, P. B., et al. (2006). *Celastrus paniculatus* seed oil and organic extracts attenuate hydrogen peroxide- and glutamate-induced injury in embryonic rat forebrain neuronal cells. *Phytomedicine, 13*(1–2), 29–36. https://doi.org/10.1016/j.phymed.2004.06.004.
40. da Rocha, M. D., et al. (2011). The role of natural products in the discovery of new drug candidates for the treatment of neurodegenerative disorders II: Alzheimer's disease. *CNS & Neurological Disorders Drug Targets, 10*(2), 251–270. https://doi.org/10.2174/187152711794480340.
41. Alama, B., & Haque, E. (2011). Anti-Alzheimer and antioxidant activity of *Celastrus paniculatus* seed. *Iranian Journal of Pharmaceutical Sciences, 7*(1), 49–56.
42. Vinutha, B., et al. (2007). Screening of selected Indian medicinal plants for acetylcholinesterase inhibitory activity. *Journal of Ethnopharmacology, 109*(2), 359–363. https://doi.org/10.1016/j.jep.2006.07.024.
43. Bidwai, P. P., Wangoo, D., & Bhullar, N. K. (1987). Effect of *Celastrus paniculatus* seed extract on the brain of albino rats. *Journal of Ethnopharmacology, 21*(3), 307–314. https://doi.org/10.1016/0378-8741(87)90031-0.
44. Malik, J., & Choudhary, S. (2021). Indian traditional herbs and Alzheimer's disease: Integrating ethnobotany and phytotherapy. In *Evidence Based Validation of Traditional Medicines: A Comprehensive Approach* (pp. 1129–1151).
45. Talesa, V. N. (2001). Acetylcholinesterase in Alzheimer's disease. *Mechanisms of Ageing and Development, 122*(16), 1961–1969. https://doi.org/10.1016/S0047-6374(01)00303-4.
46. Munjal, K., et al. (2020). Polyphenol-enriched fraction and the compounds isolated from *Garcinia indica* fruits ameliorate obesity through suppression of digestive enzymes and oxidative stress. *Journal of Food Science and Technology, 16*(70), 236–245. https://doi.org/10.1007/s11483-020-09769-2.
47. Gohil, K. J., Patel, J. A., & Gajjar, A. K. (2010). Pharmacological review on Centella asiatica: A potential herbal cure-all. *Indian Journal of Pharmaceutical Sciences, 72*(5), 546–556. https://doi.org/10.4103/0250-474X.78519.
48. Lokanathan, Y., et al. (2016). Recent updates in neuroprotective and neuroregenerative potential of *Centella asiatica*. *Malaysian Journal of Medical Sciences, 23*(1), 4–14.
49. Soumyanath, A., et al. (2005). *Centella asiatica* accelerates nerve regeneration upon oral administration and contains multiple active fractions increasing neurite elongation in-vitro. *Journal of Pharmacy and Pharmacology, 57*(9), 1221–1229. https://doi.org/10.1211/002235705684794.

50. James, J. T., & Dubery, I. A. (2009). Pentacyclic triterpenoids from the medicinal herb, *Centella asiatica* (L.) Urban. *Molecules, 14*(10), 3922–3941. https://doi.org/10.3390/molecules14103922.
51. Kumar, A., Dogra, S., & Prakash, A. (2009). Neuroprotective effects of *Centella asiatica* against intracerebroventricular colchicine-induced cognitive impairment and oxidative stress. *International Journal of Alzheimer's Disease, 2009, 972178*. https://doi.org/10.4061/2009/972178.
52. Kumar, M. H. V., & Gupta, Y. K. (2003). Effect of *Centella asiatica* on cognition and oxidative stress in an intracerebroventricular streptozotocin model of Alzheimer's disease in rats. *Clinical and Experimental Pharmacology and Physiology, 30*, 336–342. https://doi.org/10.1046/j.1440-1681.2003.03842.x.
53. Xu, Y., et al. (2008). Gotu Kola (*Centella asiatica*) extract enhances phosphorylation of cyclic AMP response element binding protein in neuroblastoma cells expressing amyloid beta peptide. *Journal of Alzheimer's Disease, 13*(3), 341–349. https://doi.org/10.3233/JAD-2008-13306.
54. Lee, M. K., et al. (2000). Asiatic acid derivatives protect cultured cortical neurons from glutamate-induced excitotoxicity. *Research Communications in Molecular Pathology and Pharmacology, 108*(1–2), 75–86.
55. Rather, M. A., et al. (2019). Asiatic acid attenuated aluminum chloride-induced tau pathology, oxidative stress, and apoptosis via AKT/GSK-3β signaling pathway in Wistar rats. *Neurotoxicity Research, 35*(4), 955–968. https://doi.org/10.1007/s12640-019-00020-x.
56. Orhan, I., et al. (2008). Inhibitory effect of Turkish Rosmarinus officinalis L. on acetylcholinesterase and butyrylcholinesterase enzymes. *Food Chemistry, 108*(2), 663–668. https://doi.org/10.1016/j.foodchem.2007.11.037.
57. Rao, S. B., Chetana, M., & Devi, P. U. (2005). *Centella asiatica* treatment during the postnatal period enhances learning and memory in mice. *Physiology and Behavior, 86*(4), 449–457. https://doi.org/10.1016/j.physbeh.2005.08.020.
58. Dhanasekaran, M., et al. (2009). *Centella asiatica* extract selectively decreases amyloid beta levels in the hippocampus of Alzheimer's disease animal model. *Phytotherapy Research, 23*(1), 14–19. https://doi.org/10.1002/ptr.2564.
59. Gray, N. E., et al. (2015). *Centella asiatica* attenuates amyloid-β-induced oxidative stress and mitochondrial dysfunction. *Journal of Alzheimer's Disease, 45*(3), 933–946. https://doi.org/10.3233/JAD-142993.
60. Gray, N. E., et al. (2017). *Centella asiatica*: Phytochemistry and mechanism of neuroprotection and cognitive enhancement. *Phytochemistry Reviews, 17*(1), 161–194. https://doi.org/10.1007/s11101-017-9516-5.
61. Kaur, R., Kaur, H., & Dhindsa, A. S. (2013). *Glycyrrhiza glabra*: A phytopharmacological review. *International Journal of Pharmaceutical Sciences and Research, 4*(7), 2470–2477.
62. Pastorino, G., et al. (2018). Liquorice (*Glycyrrhiza glabra*): A phytochemical and pharmacological review. *Phytotherapy Research, 32*(12), 2323–2339. https://doi.org/10.1002/ptr.6178.
63. Dhingra, D., Parle, M., & Kulkarni, S. K. (2004). Memory enhancing activity of *Glycyrrhiza glabra* in mice. *Journal of Ethnopharmacology, 91*(2–3), 361–365. https://doi.org/10.1016/j.jep.2004.01.018.

64. Oganisyan, A. O., Oganesyan, K. R., & Minasyan, S. M. (2005). Changes in succinate dehydrogenase activity in various parts of the brain during combined exposure to vibration and licorice root. *Neuroscience and Behavioral Physiology, 35*(5), 545–548. https://doi.org/10.1007/s11055-005-0095-1.
65. Ahn, J., et al. (2006). Protective effects of *Glycyrrhiza uralensis* Fisch. on the cognitive deficits caused by beta-amyloid peptide 25–35 in young mice. *Biogerontology, 7*(4), 239–247. https://doi.org/10.1007/s10522-006-9001-7.
66. Wang, W., et al. (2016). Glycyrrhizin attenuates isoflurane-induced cognitive deficits in neonatal rats via its anti-inflammatory activity. *Neuroscience, 316*, 328–336. https://doi.org/10.1016/j.neuroscience.2015.12.065.
67. Song, J. H., et al. (2013). Glycyrrhizin alleviates neuroinflammation and memory deficit induced by systemic lipopolysaccharide treatment in mice. *Neuroscience Letters, 18*(12), 15788–15803. https://doi.org/10.1016/j.neulet.2013.11.011.
68. Madhavadas, S., & Subramanian, S. (2015). Combination of spirulina with glycyrrhizin prevents cognitive dysfunction in aged obese rats. *Indian Journal of Pharmacology, 47*(1), 39–44. https://doi.org/10.4103/0253-7613.150314.
69. Kong, Z. H., et al. (2017). The oral pretreatment of glycyrrhizin prevents surgery-induced cognitive impairment in aged mice by reducing neuroinflammation and Alzheimer's-related pathology via HMGB1 inhibition. *Journal of Molecular Neuroscience, 63*(3), 385–395. https://doi.org/10.1007/s12031-017-0989-5.
70. Zhan, C., & Yang, J. (2006). Protective effects of isoliquiritigenin in transient middle cerebral artery occlusion-induced focal cerebral ischemia in rats. *Pharmacological Research, 53*(3), 303–309. https://doi.org/10.1016/j.phrs.2005.11.009.
71. Tewari, D., et al. (2018). Ethnopharmacological approaches for dementia therapy and significance of natural products and herbal drugs. *Frontiers in Aging Neuroscience, 10*(3), 1–24. https://doi.org/10.3389/fnagi.2018.00003.
72. Hasanein, P. (2011). Glabridin as a major active isoflavan from *Glycyrrhiza glabra* (licorice) reverses learning and memory deficits in diabetic rats. *Acta Physiologica Hungarica, 98*(2), 221–230. https://doi.org/10.1556/APhysiol.98.2011.2.9.
73. Bhowmik, D., et al. (2012). Traditional Indian herbs *Convolvulus pluricaulis* and its medicinal importance. *Journal of Pharmacognosy and Phytochemistry, 1*(1), 44–51.
74. Agarwa, P., et al. (2014). An update on Ayurvedic herb *Convolvulus pluricaulis* Choisy. *Asian Pacific Journal of Tropical Biomedicine, 4*(3), 245–252. https://doi.org/10.1016/S2221-1691(14)60239-0.
75. Malik, J., Karan, M., & Vasisht, K. (2011). Nootropic, anxiolytic and CNS depressant studies on different plant sources of Shankhpushpi. *Pharmaceutical Biology, 49*(12), 1234–1242. https://doi.org/10.3109/13880209.2011.620059.
76. Bihaqi, S. W., Singh, A. P., & Tiwari, M. (2011). In vivo investigation of the neuroprotective property of *Convolvulus pluricaulis* in scopolamine-induced cognitive impairments in Wistar rats. *Indian Journal of Pharmacology, 43*(5), 520–525. https://doi.org/10.4103/0253-7613.84973.
77. Nahata, A., Patil, U. K., & Dixit, V. K. (2008). Effect of *Convolvulus pluricaulis* Chois. on learning behavior and memory enhancement activity in rodents. *Natural Product Research, 22*(15), 1472–1482. https://doi.org/10.1080/14786410802289103.
78. Suh, Y. H., & Checler, F. (2002). Amyloid precursor protein, presenilins, and alpha-synuclein: Molecular pathogenesis and pharmacological applications in Alzheimer's disease. *Pharmacological Reviews, 54*(3), 469–525. https://doi.org/10.1124/pr.54.3.469.

79. Mathew, M., & Subramanian, S. (2012). Evaluation of the anti-amyloidogenic potential of nootropic herbal extracts in vitro. *International Journal of Pharmaceutical Sciences and Research, 3*(11), 4276–4280.
80. Bihaqi, S. W., Singh, A. P., & Tiwari, M. (2012). Supplementation of *Convolvulus pluricaulis* attenuates scopolamine-induced increased tau and amyloid precursor protein (AβPP) expression in rat brain. *Indian Journal of Pharmacology, 44*(5), 593–598. https://doi.org/10.4103/0253-7613.100382.
81. Kizhakke, P. A., et al. (2019). *Convolvulus pluricaulis* (Shankhapushpi) ameliorates human microtubule-associated protein tau (hMAPT) induced neurotoxicity in Alzheimer's disease Drosophila model. *Journal of Chemical Neuroanatomy, 95*, 115–122. https://doi.org/10.1016/j.jchemneu.2018.11.005.
82. Malik, J., Karan, M., & Vasisht, K. (2016). Attenuating effect of bioactive coumarins from *Convolvulus pluricaulis* on scopolamine-induced amnesia in mice. *Natural Product Research, 30*(5), 578–582. https://doi.org/10.1080/14786419.2015.1024162.
83. Amin, H., et al. (2014). Nootropic (medhya) effect of Bhāvita Śaṇkhapuṣpī tablets: A clinical appraisal. *Ancient Science of Life, 34*(2), 109–112. https://doi.org/10.4103/0257-7941.150782.
84. Amin, H., & Sharma, R. (2015). Nootropic efficacy of Satvavajaya Chikitsa and Ayurvedic drug therapy: A comparative clinical exposition. *International Journal of Yoga, 8*(2), 109–116. https://doi.org/10.4103/0973-6131.158476.
85. Bihaqi, S. W., et al. (2009). Neuroprotective role of *Convolvulus pluricaulis* on aluminum induced neurotoxicity in rat brain. *Journal of Ethnopharmacology, 124*, 409–415. https://doi.org/10.1016/j.jep.2009.05.009.
86. Rachitha, P., et al. (2018). Chemical composition, antioxidant potential, macromolecule damage and neuroprotective activity of *Convolvulus pluricaulis*. *Journal of Traditional and Complementary Medicine, 8*(4), 483–496. https://doi.org/10.1016/j.jtcme.2017.08.003.
87. Sethiya, N. K., et al. (2009). An update on Shankhpushpi, a cognition-boosting Ayurvedic medicine. *Zhong Xi Yi Jie He Xue Bao, 7*(11), 1001–1022.
88. Shalini, H. (2020). Daivavyapashraya chikitsa–The mystic & spiritual healing. *International Journal of Ayurveda and Pharma Research*, 66–70.
89. Deepak, K., et al. (2020). Change in bone mineral density in premenopausal women with rheumatoid arthritis managed with or without prednisolone. *Journal of Ayurveda and Integrative Medicine*, 201–210.
90. Amin, H., & Sharma, R. (2015). Nootropic efficacy of Satvavajaya Chikitsa and Ayurvedic drug therapy: A comparative clinical exposition. *International Journal of Yoga, 8*(2), 109–116. https://doi.org/10.4103/0973-6131.158476.
91. Agnivesha. (2000). Charaka samhitha with dipika commentary of chakrapanidatta (Vaidya Yadavji Trikamji Acharya, Ed.). Chaukhambha surbharathi prakashan.
92. Dhanya, T. (2017). Review article on treatment of Manovikara in Ayurveda. *International Journal of Innovative Research in Medical Science, 2*, 1268–1271.
93. Munjal, K., et al. (2022). Traditional uses and phytochemistry of Cinnamomum species: A mini review. *Research Journal of Pharmacy and Technology, 15*, 5363–5367.
94. Chaudhary, P. (2019). Preformulation studies for Ayurveda drugs: A review. *International Research Journal of Pharmacy, 10*, 16–19.

95. Munjal, K., et al. (2021). Comparison of serum 25-hydroxyvitamin D levels after a single oral dose of vitamin D3 formulations in mild vitamin D3 deficiency. *International Journal of Pharmacy and Pharmaceutical Sciences, 12*(4), 163–167.
96. Ashwini, A., & Rajashekhar, C. V. (2019). Role of Satvavajaya Chikitsa in the management of depression in current scenario. *Journal of Ayurveda and Integrated Medical Sciences, 4*(04), 275–278.
97. Bramhankar, R., et al. (2021). Insight into traditional dosage forms in light of Ayurvedic pharmaceutics. *International Journal for Pharmaceutical Research Scholars, 13*, 3925–3933.
98. Behere, P. B., et al. (2013). Ayurvedic concepts related to psychotherapy. *Indian Journal of Psychiatry, 55*(Suppl 2), S310–S314. https://doi.org/10.4103/0019-5545.105545.
99. Sood, S., Jain, K., & Gowthamarajan, K. (2014). Intranasal therapeutic strategies for management of Alzheimer's disease. *Journal of Drug Targeting, 22*(4), 279–294. https://doi.org/10.3109/1061186X.2014.886777.
100. Ling, T. S., et al. (2021). The potential benefits of nanotechnology in treating Alzheimer's disease. *Biomedical Research International, 2021*, 5550938. https://doi.org/10.1155/2021/5550938.
101. Fonseca, L. C., et al. (2021). Intranasal drug delivery for treatment of Alzheimer's disease. *Drug Delivery and Translational Research, 11*(2), 411–425. https://doi.org/10.1007/s13346-020-00828-5.
102. Rani, I., et al. (2023). Artificial Intelligence and Machine Learning-Based New Drug Discovery Process with Molecular Modelling. *Journal of Pharmaceutical Sciences, 19*(1), 19–35.
103. Lobaina Mato, Y. (2019). Nasal route for vaccine and drug delivery: Features and current opportunities. *International Journal of Pharmaceutics, 572*, 118813. https://doi.org/10.1016/j.ijpharm.2019.118813.
104. Pires, A., et al. (2009). Intranasal drug delivery: How, why and what for? *Journal of Pharmacy and Pharmaceutical Sciences, 12*(3), 288–311. https://doi.org/10.18433/J3NC79.
105. Craft, S., et al. (2012). Intranasal insulin therapy for Alzheimer disease and amnestic mild cognitive impairment: A pilot clinical trial. *Archives of Neurology, 69*(1), 29–38. https://doi.org/10.1001/archneurol.2011.233.
106. Dhuria, S. V., Hanson, L. R., & Frey, W. H. (2010). Intranasal delivery to the central nervous system: Mechanisms and experimental considerations. *Journal of Pharmaceutical Sciences, 99*(4), 1654–1673. https://doi.org/10.1002/jps.21924.
107. Margenfeld, F., Klocke, C., & Joos, S. (2019). Manual massage for persons living with dementia: A systematic review and meta-analysis. *International Journal of Nursing Studies, 96*, 132–142. https://doi.org/10.1016/j.ijnurstu.2019.04.008.
108. Kim, Y. J., et al. (2021). Effects of electrical automatic massage on cognition and sleep quality in Alzheimer's disease spectrum patients: A randomized controlled trial. *Yonsei Medical Journal, 62*(8), 717–725. https://doi.org/10.3349/ymj.2021.62.8.717.
109. Keir, S. T. (2011). Effect of massage therapy on stress levels and quality of life in brain tumor patients–observations from a pilot study. *Supportive Care in Cancer, 19*(5), 711–715. https://doi.org/10.1007/s00520-010-0877-7.
110. Ouchi, Y., et al. (2006). Changes in cerebral blood flow under the prone condition with and without massage. *Neuroscience Letters, 407*(2), 131–135. https://doi.org/10.1016/j.neulet.2006.09.034.

111. Pathirana, W., et al. (2009). Transcranial route of brain-targeted delivery of methadone in oil. *Indian Journal of Pharmaceutical Sciences, 71*(3), 264–269. https://doi.org/10.4103/0250-474X.56028.
112. Uebaba, K., et al. (2008). Psychoneuroimmunological effects of Ayurvedic oil-dripping treatment. *Journal of Alternative and Complementary Medicine, 14*(10), 1189–1198. https://doi.org/10.1089/acm.2008.0165.
113. Xu, F., et al. (2008). Pharmaco-physio-psychologic effect of Ayurvedic oil-dripping treatment using an essential oil from Lavandula angustifolia. *Journal of Alternative and Complementary Medicine, 14*(8), 947–956. https://doi.org/10.1089/acm.2008.0095.
114. Lin, L., et al. (2022). Effect of aromatherapy in patients with Alzheimer's disease: A randomized controlled clinical trial. *Research Square, 9(4), 173–179.* https://doi.org/10.1111/j.1479-8301.2009.00299.x.
115. Jimbo, D., et al. (2009). Effect of aromatherapy on patients with Alzheimer's disease. *Psychogeriatrics, 9*(4), 173–179. https://doi.org/10.1111/j.1479-8301.2009.00299.x.
116. Ballard, C. G., et al. (2009). Management of agitation and aggression associated with Alzheimer disease. *Nature Reviews Neurology, 5*(5), 245–255. https://doi.org/10.1038/nrneurol.2009.39.
117. Bredesen, D. E., et al. (2016). Reversal of cognitive decline in Alzheimer's disease. *Aging, 8*(6), 1250–1258. https://doi.org/10.18632/aging.100981.
118. Tyagi, S., et al. (2010). Applications of metabolomics–A systematic study of the unique chemical fingerprints: An overview. *Journal of Applied Pharmaceutical Science, 3(1), 019.*
119. Tyagi, S., et al. (2010). Practical applications of proteomics–A technique for large-scale study of proteins: An overview. *Journal of Applied Pharmaceutical Science, 3(1), 87–90.*
120. Bredesen, D. E. (2016). Inhalational Alzheimer's disease: An unrecognized – and treatable–epidemic. *Aging, 8*(2), 304–313. https://doi.org/10.18632/aging.100896.
121. Alkefai, N., et al. (2022). NMR in analysis of food toxins. In *Advances in Food Toxicology* (pp. 131–139).
122. Bredesen, D. E., & Rao, R. V. (2017). Ayurvedic profiling of Alzheimer's disease. *Alternative Therapies in Health and Medicine, 23*(3), 46–50.

CHAPTER 9

Nootropics: Traditional Medicinal Prospective

PREETI MAAN,* NISHA GUPTA, and SHILPI CHAUHAN

Lloyd Institute of Management and Technology, Greater Noida, Uttar Pradesh, India

*Corresponding author.

ABSTRACT

One of the most important characteristics that distinguish humans from other animals is memory. Ayurveda medicine is an Indian medical system that contains a vast treasure trove of cognition-enhancing medications which are now popular all over the world owing to their proven potency. Nootropic herbs are herbs that act on the brain, and their isolated constituents are known as smart drugs. Dementia has emerged as a major global health concern as the world's population has aged over the last few decades. Alzheimer's disease (AD) is the most prevalent kind of dementia. Irrespective of substantial drug development research, there are only a few FDA-approved drugs for Alzheimer's disease. Alternative approaches to AD therapies must be created immediately because conventional medications only alleviate symptoms and are frequently linked to negative effects. One of the major approaches in this regard is ethnopharmacological screening of medicinal plants. People have been using drugs and herbal treatments to enhance their memories for ages. These plants include *Bacopa monnieri, Celastrus paniculatus, Centella asiatica, Ginkgo biloba, Glycyrrhiza glabra, Rhodiola rosea, Tinospora cordifolia, Withania somnifera*, and others. The active phytoconstituents in such plants are solely responsible for their memory-boosting effects. Herbs that improve memory have the ability to cross the blood-brain barrier and increase blood circulation in the brain. By acting on memory, they enhance

Neuro-Nutraceuticals and Drug Discovery and Delivery in Alzheimer's Disease, Volume 1: Targeting Key Pathological Pathways. Varinder Singh, Amit Kumar, Parul Sood (Eds.)

cognitive function in the brain, causing it to become more attentive and focused. Despite the absence of polyphenol or other phytochemical receptors or transporters in brain areas, compounds with multi-target approaches appear to be a promising therapy for the treatment of disorders with a multifactorial or complex etiology.

9.1 INTRODUCTION

Herbal remedies have long been used around the world to improve memory and treat other ailments [1, 2]. Several medicinal plants and extracts have demonstrated nootropic or memory-enhancing properties due to the appropriate nature of their medicinal components [3]. The growing global demand for herbal remedies is due to the fact that natural compounds have fewer side effects as compared to synthetic compounds. Indian Ayurveda possesses a treasure trove of medicinal herbs to improve memory, intelligence, and knowledge. These Ayurvedic herbs have become more and more popular worldwide [4]. Not just Indian Ayurveda but also American, African, European, Japanese, Korean, and traditional Chinese medicine (TCM) contain plenty of medicinal plants that help to restore memory. Herbs that have a positive impact on brain performance are known as "nootropics" and the isolated phytoconstituents are referred to as "smart drugs." Herbal medicine that promotes intelligence is known as "Rasayana" or "Medhya herbs" in Ayurveda. In Ayurveda, compound formulations are extensively employed, with the notion that such combinations give synergistic medicinal effects with lesser adverse effects. Include 10 herbal drugs: Jatamansi, Ashwagandha, Vacha, Jyotishmati, Shankhapushpi, Amalaki, Yashtimadhu, Kavach Beej, Bramhi, and all of these medicinal herbs increase neurotransmitter levels (particularly acetylcholine) in the brain by inhibiting excess acetylcholinesterase (AChE) activity and also improve blood circulation within the brain, supplying adequate oxygen to brain cells [5]. The most ancient yet current traditions are Ayurveda, traditional Indian medicine (TIM), and TCM. Ayurveda is both a science of life and a system of medicine. This branch of natural science is based on a natural therapeutic approach to treat various human ailments. Aging is a natural process of gradual and continuous change, with the brain being the most affected organ. To prevent this change, the *Rasayana* therapy (rejuvenation branch) was developed. *Rasayana* uses a variety of natural drugs that act as brain tonics, promote brain health, and improve memory impairment. *Rasayana* therapies employ a variety of memory-enhancing and rejuvenating plants; *Bacopa monnieri, Acorus calamus, Clitoria ternatea, Terminalia chebula, Nardostachys jatamansi*, and a variety of others are among them. Some home remedies for memory loss can be found in common food plants, such as oils and vegetables [6]. TCM is based on the idea that a vital life force known as Qi flows through the human body. Any Qi imbalance can lead to disease and illness. The illness is caused by a person's lifestyle, pathogens, and a variety of negative effects. Herbal treatment, on the other hand, can restore the balance. Chinese people have thousands of years of experience in diagnosis, prevention, and treatment of disease, resulting in a comprehensive theoretical system of medicine. TCM also includes medicinal herbs that improve memory. *Camellia sinensis, Ginkgo biloba, Huperzia serrata, Panax ginseng,* and other plants are used in TCM to improve memory. According to the World Health Organization (WHO), 80% of the world's population currently uses herbal remedies to improve their health [7].

The human brain can be called the most complex organ of the body. Memory is the foremost skill required for survival. Memory can be defined in many ways but in an overall view sensory stimuli, events, pieces of information, etc., and retained over short or long periods and recalled the same whenever needed at a later date. When we discuss memory, it is not only pertaining to retaining information but also includes intelligence, cognitive abilities, and concentration.

Neurodegenerative disorders (ND) have emerged as one of the most significant issues facing the 21st century. There is currently no highly effective treatment for Alzheimer's disease, AD-associated dementia, or other neurodegenerative disorders. Neurodegeneration is the progressive loss of neuron structure and function. ND are a group of diseases characterized by progressive neuron malfunction and loss. Proteolytic events are increasingly being misidentified as primary mechanisms in the emergence of major neurodegenerative diseases. There are various types of neurodegenerative diseases, but the most common are Alzheimer's disease (AD), Huntington's disease, and Parkinson's disease (PD). Treatment options that are available only provide symptomatic relief, temporarily improving memory and intellectual problems, and their clinical effect are ambiguous. Over the past decade, drug discovery and development have targeted active substances from plants that can slow the progress of the disease or delay its onset. Here comes the use of several plants from different medicinal systems like Ayurvedic, Chinese, Unani, Sindhi, and Homeopathy. The fundamental law of Ayurveda for the treatment of different ailments is to act in harmony with nature. Among all these diseases, AD and PD are the major ones and cause more than 40% of all ND. Among the available treatments for AD, only provide symptomatic relief to the patient. This disease was earliest recognized by Alois Alzheimer in 1906; It is an incurable, gradual brain disease that progressively worsens memory and cognitive skills. It is estimated that around 47 million people are affected by AD worldwide. Age is the biggest known risk factor for 1 in 10 of those over 65 years. It is anticipated that around 131 million people will be affected by these neurodegenerative diseases. Over the past decade, various medications have been approved for the treatment of AD. These drugs have their limitations regarding efficacy, safety, and various factors.

9.2 CLASSIFICATION

Depending on the source, nootropics are divided into two categories: natural nootropic agents and synthetic nootropics [3].

9.2.1 NATURAL NOOTROPICS

Natural nootropics include herbal drugs that improve cognitive functions due to their antioxidant, anti-apoptotic properties, and neurotransmitter modulating properties.

For example, *Ginkgo biloba*, *Nicotiana rustica*, *Panax quinquefolius*, *Duboisia hopwoodii*, *Panax ginseng*, *Bacopa monnieri*, *Nicotiana tabacum*, *Hericium erinaceus, Asclepias syriaca, Rhodiola rosea, Mucuna pruriens, Centella asiatica, Montmorency cherry, Withania somnifera*, etc.

9.2.2 SYNTHETIC NOOTROPICS

Based on the mechanism, synthetic nootropic agents can be further classified into three subclasses which are discussed in subsections.

9.2.2.1 DOPAMINERGIC NOOTROPICS

They have an effect on the neurotransmitter dopamine levels throughout the brain. They are direct agonists and indirect agonists at the Dopamine (D1) receptor. They may include dopamine reuptake inhibitors, antidepressants, and enzymes. For example, Bromantane, L-Theanine, DL-Phenylalanine (DLPA), L-Dopa, Phenylethylamine (PEA), Mucuna Pruriens, Selegiline, Rasagiline.

9.2.2.2 ADRENERGIC NOOTROPICS

They are adrenergic receptor agonists and direct and indirect agonists of the alpha ($\alpha 2$) adrenoceptor. For example, amphetamines, methylphenidate, caffeine, armodafinil, and modafinil.

9.2.2.3 RACETAMS

Racetams are 2-oxopyrrolidineacetamide derivatives that are structurally similar but differ only in the side chain. Members of this class all have the ability to reverse amnesia caused by scopolamine, electroconvulsive shock, and hypoxia. These nootropic agents are among the pharmacologically safe drugs that act at the acetylcholine-Muscarinic (M1) receptor and AMPA-glutamate receptor and are used in the management of stroke, alcoholism, Parkinsonism, epilepsy, AD, schizophrenia, dyslexia, and dementia. For example, piracetam, pramiracetam, oxiracetam, aniracetam, rolziracetam [10].

One more classification can be given for nootropics which is based on mechanism because some synthetic and natural nootropics may have the same mechanism. A classification is compiled in Table 9.1 according to the mechanism.

9.3 MECHANISM OF ACTION OF NOOTROPICS

It has been stated that nootropics exert a highly complex action on cortical cells. Although nootropics may not work by emitting neurotransmitters directly, they can increase the energy reserve of the brain by stimulating the transformation of adenosine diphosphate (ADP) into adenosine triphosphate (ATP) (antihypoxic effects), as well as promoting physiological information communication between the two hemispheres via the corpus callosum [12]. Depending on the available literature, the mechanism of action can be categorized into four classes: (i) energy metabolism-related effects; (ii) cholinergic effects; (iii) effects on excitatory glutaminergic functions; and (iv) miscellaneous [13].

TABLE 9.1 Classification of Nootropics According to Mechanism [3, 5, 11–18, 20]

SL. No.	Class	Mechanism of Action	Examples
1.	Cholinergic system activators:	Agents that enhance central cholinergic transmission.	Acetylcholine
	Subclasses: a. Acetylcholinesterase inhibitors	These nootropics increase acetylcholine availability in central synapses by inhibiting the catabolic enzyme acetylcholinesterase.	Physostigmine, Tacrine, Galanthamine, Donepezil, Bacopa monnieri, Huperzine A.
	b. Muscarinic receptor agonists	They emit acetylcholine through interactions with postsynaptic M1 receptors.	Sabcomeline, Xanomeline
	c. Nicotinic receptor agonists	They produce acetylcholine by activating intact nicotinic acetylcholine receptors.	Nicotine, N-(3-pyridylmethyl) pyrrolidine (PMP).
	d. Allosteric modifiers	They allosterically potentiate nicotinic and muscarinic responses by causing receptor conformational changes toward open channel conformation.	Gallamine
	e. Acetylcholine release and storage modulators	These nootropics increase acetylcholine release, which increases neuronal activity and restores central cholinergic tone.	Potassium channel blockers: Linopridine, Fampridine; ACE inhibitors: Captopril; Serotonin receptor antagonists: Zacopride, Ondansetron; Benzodiazepine receptor inverse agonists: ZK 93426; Panax quinquefolius, Panax ginseng.
	f. Non-specific cholinergic agents	Their relationship with the cholinergic system is not clearly understood.	Minaprine, Salbutiamine.
	g. Neurotrophic factor stimulants	They increase the synthesis of nerve growth factors.	TMQ, Guanosine, Hericium erinaceus.

TABLE 9.1 *(Continued)*

SL. No.	Class	Mechanism of Action	Examples
2.	GABAergic system modulators	They have an effect on GABA neurotransmission, which is known to reduce arousal and stress levels in the central nervous system.	GABA, Phenibut, Picamilon, Muscimol, (–)-Nipecotic acid.
3.	Dopaminergic system modulators	They influence levels of the neurotransmission dopamine throughout the brain.	Rasagiline, Selegiline, Stablon (Tianeptine), Sulbutiamine, Suntheanine.
4.	Adrenergic (α2) receptor agonist	These agents are direct or indirect agonist of adrenergic (α2) receptor.	Amphetamines, Gingko biloba
5.	Serotonergic system	They work by stimulating the serotonin system in the brain. They also exert a tonic inhibitory control over acetylcholine release.	5 HTP (5-Hydroxytryptophan), Griffonia simplicifolia, tryptophan.
6.	Psychostimulants	They increase physical and mental arousal by stimulating dopamine production in the brain and activating the sympathetic nervous system.	Adderall, Caffeine, Cylert (Pemoline), Dextroamphetamine, Ephedrine, and Guanfacine (Intuniv).
7.	Ampakines	They have an effect on the AMPA receptor, which is responsible for glutamate binding.	3-hydroxy-2,4-dinitro-DL-phenylalanine NMDA antagonists: MK-801, 7-nitro-5-(N-oxyaza) quinoxaline, ketamine, phencyclidine.
8.	Metabolic enhancers	These supplements increase metabolic processes and energy among neurons. These can also provide more energy to brain cells and are thought to improve cognition.	Hydergine, Vinpocetine
9.	Neuroprotective agents	They support healthy brain function by stimulating nerve growth, repairing damage, and preserving neuronal health. Many of them are consumed for their antioxidant properties, which help in the prevention of cognitive decline and maintenance of optimal cognition.	Bacopa monnieri, Kapikacchu (Mucuna pruriens), Co-Enzyme Q10, Idebenone

TABLE 9.1 *(Continued)*

SL. No.	Class	Mechanism of Action	Examples
10.	Miscellaneous:		
	a. Natural products	These are herbal plants and their extract which elicit their cognitive action by different mechanisms.	Bacopa monnieri, Ginkgo biloba, Panax ginseng, Mitragyna speciosa, Hericium erinaceus, Melissa officinalis
	b. Hormones	These are hormone-based nootropics that may boost arousal and brain stimulation or enhance a sense of calm concentration.	Cortisol, desmopressin (DDAVP), DHEA (dehydroepiandrosterone), melatonin, vasopressin (AVP), and pregnenolone (P5).
	c. Nutraceuticals	They enhance concentration, inhibit cognitive decline, and encourage neuroprotection. It is believed that consuming a variety of healthy nutrients improves overall cognitive function.	Iodine, L-glutamine, omega-3 fatty acids, L-lysine, magnesium, fish oil, krill oil.
	d. Vitamins	They elicit their cognitive action by antioxidant action and scavenging of free radicals.	Vitamin B1, Vitamin B6, Vitamin B3, Vitamin B8, Vitamin B5, Vitamin B12.

9.3.1 EFFECTS ON ENERGY METABOLISM

The induction of adenylate kinase activity by piracetam was one of the pieces of evidence in favor of energy metabolism. These facts were further supported by the augmented uptake of ^{32}P into phosphatidyl inositol and phosphatidyl chloride in nerve cells as well as glial cells improved utilization of glucose under hypoxic conditions and improved recovery in the electroencephalogram. However, some observations showed the reversal of low levels of glucose utilization induced by scopolamine rather than an increase in glucose utilization in response to piracetam [13].

9.3.2 EFFECTS ON CHOLINERGIC MECHANISMS

Acetylcholine (ACh) is an essential neurotransmitter associated with the central cholinergic system. These neuronal nicotinic ACh receptors are located on the presynaptic terminal and have an effect on hippocampal synaptic transmission. Cognitive dysfunction in Alzheimer's disease is related to diminished neuronal cholinergic functions in the hippocampal area. Smart drugs increase choline uptake and prevent acetylcholine depletion in the cortex and hippocampus. Nootropics also increase the density of muscarinic cholinergic receptors in the frontal cortex of aged rats, suggesting the involvement of biochemical modifications in the aging brain [14]. Nootropics have shown significant effects on brain function impairment caused by various harmful stimuli, such as hypoxia, aging, and injury [15]. Furthermore, nootropics also decrease ACh esterase activity and subsequently increase ACh levels in the brain [21].

Moreover, some nootropics, such as *Bacopa monnieri*, can reduce norepinephrine (NE) and increase 5-hydroxytryptamine (5-HT) release in the central cortex, hypothalamus, and hippocampus [22]. In AD, cholinergic system abnormality is associated with the intervention of amyloid protein, specifically neurofibrillary tangles and amyloid β-protein. Amyloid precursor protein (APP) is one of the cellular components that affect synaptic plasticity and contribute to memory formation. Natural nootropics cause upregulation of APP expression and increase learning and memory performance [23]. Furthermore, β-amyloid derived from APP is another fragment causative of the mutilation of short-term working memory. Deposition of β-amyloid peptide and oxidative stress are plausible reasons for the onset of Alzheimer's disease. High amyloid β-protein expression in neurons enhances neuronal apoptosis death via induction of caspase-3 pursuits [20, 24]. Nootropics like *Ginkgo biloba, Panax ginseng*, and *Bacopa monnieri* inhibit the production and aggregation of amyloid-β fibrils and downregulate the activity of caspase-3 [25–27].

9.3.3 EFFECTS ON GLUTAMINERGIC RECEPTOR

Glutamate is a neurotransmitter that plays an important role in cognitive processes. Glutamate receptors are classified into two types: metabotropic receptors and ionotropic (AMPA, NMDA, and kainite receptors) that are distributed on the pre-synaptic and postsynaptic nerve cells. These receptors are responsible for the neuronal network, which allows for synaptic transmission, cognitive performance, and classic learning and memory. However, hyperactivity of glutamate receptors can cause oxidative stress, which can be a reason for cognitive dysfunction. The N-methyl-D-aspartate (NMDA) glutaminergic receptor also aids in the movement of Ca^{2+}, K^{+}, and Na^{+} ions in the hippocampus, cortex, and thalamus. Synaptic plasticity and memory formation are aided by increased Ca^{2+} permeability and voltage-dependent Mg^{2+} blockade. Ca^{2+} elevation also influences protein and gene expression for long-term potentiation (LTP), which may lead to toxicity in neurons due to glutamate overexcitation as seen in Alzheimer's disease [28]. Furthermore, Ca^{2+} is demonstrated to activate protein kinase C (PKC) in the dentate gyrus, a molecule involved in memory and learning processes [29]. PKC activators as well as nootropic drugs were found to improve memory performance, implying the participation of a related pathway, the PKC pathway [30]. Nootropics improve cognitive function possibly by decreasing NMDA-dependent CA1 long-term potentiation (LTP) and increasing NMDA-independent CA1 LTP [31, 32]. A lot of studies have shown that insulin receptors are also important for learning and memory, which are highly found in the hippocampus. These receptors can regulate synaptic activity via NMDA, which then affects the α-amino-3-hydroxy-5-methyl-4-isoxazole-propionate (AMPA) and γ-aminobutyric acid type A ($GABA_A$) receptors. The activation of neuronal insulin will stimulate the cognitive function signaling pathway, which includes the activation of phosphatidylinositol-3-kinase (PI3K), PKC, and mitogen-activated protein kinase (MAPK) [33] (Figure 9.1).

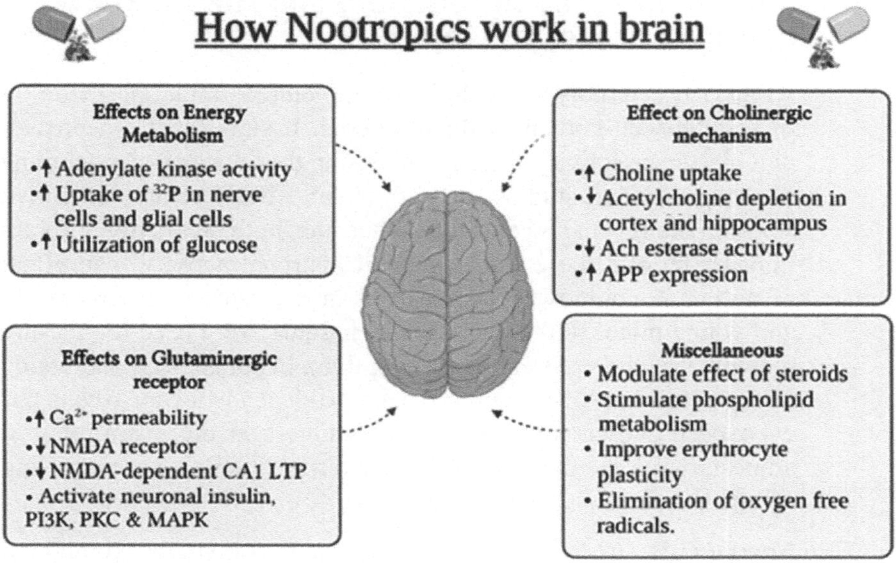

FIGURE 9.1 Mechanism of action of nootropics.

9.3.4 MISCELLANEOUS

Although there is no clear-cut conclusion about the mechanism of piracetam-like nootropics, studies have shown that these nootropics may modulate the effects of corticosterone, cortisol, dexamethasone, and dehydroepiandrosterone-like steroids on memory. Corticosterone can activate both angiotensin I (Ang I) and angiotensin II (Ang II) receptors. Angiotensin II (Ang II) regulates not only blood pressure via vasoconstriction and renal actions but also facilitates cognitive and behavioral processes [34]. In cognitive impairment diseases, Ang II inhibits the release of acetylcholine in the brain, which is a critical neurotransmitter responsible for memory.

In addition to these mechanisms, nootropics also stimulate phospholipid metabolism in neurohormonal membranes and improve neuronal protein and nucleic acid synthesis [35, 36]. Some nootropics have been found to have an anti-aggregation effect, as well as to improve erythrocyte plasticity and the elimination of oxygen-free radicals. This improves blood rheological properties and blood flow to the brain [16].

9.4 EFFECTIVE HERBAL FORMULATIONS FOR THE TREATMENT OF ALZHEIMER'S DISEASE [37–39]

1. **Abana:** It is a polyherbal Indian Ayurvedic formulation made up of sixteen well-known medicinal herbs. It significantly decreases cholinesterase activity, thereby increasing the levels of acetylcholine in the preclinical studies. Its antioxidant effects reduce oxidative stress in brain cells. As a result, Abana aids in the reduction of brain impairment and the enhancement of neuronal activity. The effect of Abana on cognitive processes was investigated in groups of old and young mice. Both behavioral techniques were used to measure memory (exteroceptive and interoceptive). In both elderly and young mice, Abana improves memory in a dose-dependent way. Abana has even been shown to reverse scopolamine and diazepam-induced amnesia. As a result, this polyherbal formulation shows promising results in treating Alzheimer's disease [40].
2. **Mentat (BR-16A):** As *Medhya Rasayana*, the polyherbal compound known as Mentat is used in Ayurvedic medicine to treat memory loss and cognitive impairment brought on by aging and chronic illness. The composition of herbs includes *Triphala, Asparagus racemosus, Evolvulus alsinoides, Withania somnifera, Phyllanthus emblica,* and *Bacopa monnieri*. This has been shown to improve learning retention and acquisition and prevent cognitive deficits caused by increasing age, prenatal malnutrition, postnatal environmental deprivation, aluminum, and electroconvulsive shock-induced amnesia. Clinical studies with Mentat on various age groups showed that the memory quotient of tested subjects improves learning ability in children with minimal brain damage or behavioral problems. Mentat reduces attention fluctuations and increases memory span in healthy adults [41].
3. **Brain-o-Brain:** These capsules are a unique blend of herbs such as Brahmi, Shatavari, and Shankhpushpi that naturally prevent stress and depression. Brain-o-brain is an Ayurvedic memory booster supplement made from potent herbs and natural nutrients that naturally boost brain function, concentration, and mental sharpness. These herbal brain booster tablets are intended to prevent or lessen forgetfulness in people of all ages. Taking Brain-o-brain on a regular basis is effective in increasing grasping power and natural brain ability. This completely natural remedy aids in the treatment of nervous exhaustion and mental fatigue [42].

4. **Brahmi Ghrita (BG):** *Bacopa monnieri* and cow milk ghee are among the four Ayurvedic herbs in *Brahmi ghrita*. The active principle Bacoside A and B are responsible for BG's potential. BG is an Ayurvedic medicinal formulation used to treat memory problems, epilepsy, poor concentration, mental sickness, and impotence. The rise in cerebral glutaminic acid and the transitory increase in gamma-aminobutyric acid caused by BG improved the learning method. In rats, *Brahmi* was evaluated in terms of memory retention. The elevated plus-maze transfer latency was considerably lowered by Brahmi ghrita (30, 50, and 100 mg/kg). It showed a nootropic effect by improving the learning and memory of rats [43].
5. **Chyawanprash:** It is an Ayurvedic tonic made up of more than fifty herbal extracts and medicinal herbs. One of its key constituents is amla, Indian gooseberry (*Emblica officinalis*), very nutritious and one of the richest sources of vitamin C. In Indian households, it is widely consumed. It lowers thiobarbituric acid-reactive substances (TBARS) in the brain while increasing glutathione levels. Pre-clinical studies confirmed Chyawanprash's significant role in protecting against memory impairment. The results reveal free radical reduction and an increase in free radical scavenging properties. As a result, this may be an effective treatment for Alzheimer's disease [42].
6. **Memorin:** It is made up of 21 different herbal extracts. Memorin's experimental studies on rats were conducted in a shuttle box using the passive avoidance learning paradigm. Andrade, 1998 examined the effect of Memorin on memory problems associated with aging and reported positive results in elderly people who exhibited age-related cognitive decline. It was discovered that Memorin (200 mg/kg body weight/day) reduced rats' retrograde and antegrade amnesia. In clinical studies, Memorin has been shown to improve poor memory, mental fatigue, and dementia associated with aging [42].
7. **Optimized-Sopung Sunkiwon (OSS):** It is a multi-herbal formula made up of 6 herbal plants from Sopung Sunkiwon medicinal herbs, commonly used to treat neurodegenerative disorders. OSS improves memory function significantly by inhibiting AChE activity. OSS therapy improves memory function and hippocampus neuron loss caused by AβO. These findings imply that OSS may have an effect on memory impairment by boosting synaptophysin and PSD-95

levels in the brain, implying that OSS might be a possible multitargeted option for AD therapy [42].

8. **Trasina:** It is also a multi-herb formula of potent Indian medicinal plants (*Eclipta alba, Picrorrhiza kurroa, Ocimum sanctum, Tinospora cordifolia, shilajit*, and *Withania somnifera*). Which are classified as *Medhya rasayan* in Ayurveda. It has shown significant memory enhancer effects at doses between 200 and 500 mg/kg. After 14 and 21 days of therapy, in a rat model, it increased both cognition and cholinergic indicators such as acetylcholine levels, choline acetyl transferase, and muscarinic cholinergic receptor binding in the brain. As a result, its nootropic effect might be related to the improvement of cholinergic dysfunction [44].
9. **Shimotsu-To:** It means "four substance decoction." The following four crude herbal extracts are used in this TCM formula: Cnidium rhizome, Rehmannia root, peony root, and Japanese angelica root. In a pre-clinical study, the spatial memory of rats has been improved by Shimotsu-to. Furthermore, the study in rat models suggests that tetramethylpyrazine (Cnidium rhizome) and paeoniflorin (peony root) are important cognitive enhancers [38, 39].
10. **Yukmijihwang-Tang Derivatives (YMJD):** A Chinese polyherbal formulation, is made up of six different herbal medicines that are used to improve cognition and memory. YMJD is mentioned in a Chinese herbal textbook as an anti-aging treatment. Furthermore, it aids in the prevention of memory and learning impairment in mice. YMJD was found to increase neurogenesis in the dentate gyrus (hippocampus) of stressed rats, as well as improve cognitive functions and memory retention [39].

A comprehensive list of plants with their parts used and phytoconstituents is given in Table 9.2.

9.5 PROMISING HERBAL DRUGS AGAINST ALZHEIMER'S DISEASE [37–40]

The development of novel clinical treatments for Alzheimer's disease is at a crossroads. This opens the door to concentrating prospective drug development activities on disease modification, an area where many treatments are

TABLE 9.2 A Comprehensive List of Plants Used as Nootropics [42, 45, 46]

Sl. No.	Common Name	Botanical Name	Family	Parts Used	Phytoconstituents
1.	African egg-plant	*Solanum indicum*	Solanaceae	Fruit	Solasodine and solasonine
2.	Agathi	*Sesbania grandiflora*	Fabaceae	fruits, leaves, and seeds	Betulinic acid
3.	Almond	*Prunus amygdalus*	Rosaceae	Nuts (seeds)	Kaempferol, quercetin, and isorhamnetin
4.	Amla	*Emblica officinalis, Phyllanthus emblica)*	Phyllanthaceae	Fruit (fresh and dried)	Phyllanthin, vitamin C (L-Ascorbic acid), Chebulin, Phyllembin, and Hypophyllanthin
5.	Aparajita	*Clitoria ternatea*	Fabaceae	Roots	Histidine, Threonine, and Tannin
6.	Ashwagandha	*Withania somnifera*	Solanaceae	Roots	Withaferin, Withanolides, and Sitiindosites.
7.	Betal Nut	*Areca catechu*	Arecaceae	nut extract	Tannic acid and arecoline
8.	Bhringaraj	*Eclipta alba*	Astearaceae	Leaves	Alpha-Amyrin, Seclabatin, Urosilic acid, Oleanoic acid & Ecliptasaponin
9.	Bittle leaf	*Piper betle*	Piperaceae	Leaves	Arecoline
10..	Black pepper	*Piper nigrum*	Piperaceae	Fruits	Piperine
11..	Brahmi	*Bacopa monnieri*	Plantaginaceae	Whole plant	Bacosides A and B
12..	Branched sweet-sultan	*Amber boaramosa*	Asteraceae	–	Sesquiterpene lactones: Amberin A, B, C, AND D
13..	Castor oil	*Ricinus communis*	Euphorbiaceae	Beans	Ricinine
14..	Cat's claw	*Uncaria tomentosa*	Rubiaceae	Bark and root	Mitraphylline, Uncarine F, Uncarine C, Rhynchophylline Procyanidin
15..	Chinese skullcap	*Scutellaria baicalensis*	Lamiaceae	Roots	Flavanoid: Oroxylin A
16..	Club moss	*Huperzia serrata*	Lycopodiaceae	Moss	Huperzine A and B
17..	Cocoa	*Theobroma cacao*	Malvaceae	Seeds	Catechin catechol polyphenols glycosides
18..	Common fig	*Ficus carica*	Moraceae	Fruit	Bergapten, psoralen, rutin, and quercetin

TABLE 9.2 *(Continued)*

Sl. No.	Common Name	Botanical Name	Family	Parts Used	Phytoconstituents
19..	Common sage	*Salvia officinalis*	Lamiaceae	Leaves	Monoferpenoid, Camosic acid and Rosemarinic acid
20..	Coriander	*Coriandrum sativum*	Apiaceae	Leaves and Seeds	Linalool, nerylacetate, gamma-terpinene and pinene
21..	Curry leaves	*Murraya koenigii*	Rutaceae	Leaves	Girinimbine and mahanimbin
22..	Daffodil	*Narcissus confuses*	Amaryllidaceae	Crude drug	Galanthamine
23..	Dwarf morning glory	*Evolvulus resinoids*	Convulvulaceae	Leaves	Luteolin and evolvine
24..	Eggplant	*Solanum melongana*	Solanaceae	Fruit	Anthocyanin
25..	Eye wort	*Euphrasia officinalis*	Orobanchaceae	Whole Plant	Iridoid glycosides, Flavonoids, Euphosid, Aucubin, & Tannins
26..	False black pepper	*Embelia ribes*	Primulaceae	Roots	Embelin and quercitol
27..	Fennel	*Foeniculum vulgare*	Apiaceae	Whole Plant	Anethole, Fenechone, and pinene
28..	Five flavor berries	*Schisandra chinensis*	Schisandraceae		Schisandrin A, B & C
29..	Frog orchid	*Coeloglossum viride*	Orchidaceae	Rhizomes	coelovirins A-G
30..	Garlic	*Allium sativum*	Amaryllidaceae	Bulb	(S)-allyl-L-cysteine
31..	Gastrodia tuber	*Gastrodia elata*	Orchidaceae	Root	P-hydroxybenzyl alcohol (HBA) & Gastrodins
32..	Giloy	*Tinospora cordifolia*	Menispermaceae	Whole Plant	Tinosporine and tinosporide
33..	Ginger	*Zingiber officinale*	Zingiberaceae	Rhizome	Gingerin Gingerol Shogaol Zingerone
34..	Ginkgo	*Ginkgo biloba*	Ginkoaceae	Leaves	Terpenoids, flavanoids, Quercetin, Kaempferol, and Terpene lactones (Ginkgolides & Bilobalide)
35..	Ginseng	*Panax ginseng*	Araliaceae	Roots	Ginsenosides (Rg1, Rb2, Rg3), Saponins (Protopanaxatriol and Protopanaxdiol)
36..	Golden root	*Rhodiola rosea*	Crassulaceae	Root and Leaves	Kaempferol, gossypetin, and herbacetin

TABLE 9.2 *(Continued)*

Sl. No.	Common Name	Botanical Name	Family	Parts Used	Phytoconstituents
37..	Goolar	*Ficus racemosa*	Moraceae	Bark	Beta-sitosterol and lupeol
38..	Gorakhmundi	*Sphaeranthus indicus*	Asteraceae	Flowers	Methyl chavicol, eugenol, and alpha terpinene.
39..	Grapes	*Vitis vinifera*	Vitaceae	Seeds	Resveratrol
40..	Green tea	*Camellia sinensis*	Theaceae	Leaves	Flavonoids – Epigalactocatechin-3-gallate (EGCG), Isoflavone daidzein
41..	Gulweed	*Sargassum sagamianum*	Sargassaceae	Whole plant	Sargaquinoic acid, plastoquinone, and sargamchromenol
42..	Haritaki	*Terminalia chebula*	Combretaceae	Rhizomes	Chebulic acid
43..	Hibiscus	*Hibiscus asper*	Malvaceae	Leaves	Gallic acid, catechin rutin and hesperidin
44..	Holy basil	*Ocimum tenuiflorum*	Lamiaceae	Whole Plant	Eugenol, caryophyllene, and rosemarinic acid
45..	Houpu Magnolia	*Magnolia officinalis*	Magnoliaceae	Bark	Magnolol Honokiol
46..	Japanese cornel	*Cornus officinalis*	Cornaceae	Fruits	iridoid glycosides (CIG), polyphenols, Loganin, and saponins
47..	Jatamansi	*Nardostachys jatamansi*	Caprifoliaceae	Whole Plant	Jatamansone and Nardostachone
48..	Java grass	*Cyperus rotundus*	Cyperaceae	Rhizomes	alpha copaene, cyperene, and valerenal
49..	Jyotishmati	*Celastrus paniculatus*	Celastraceae	Seeds	Celapanin, celastrine, Calapagone, Calapanigine, and Paniculatin.
50..	Lemon balm	*Melissa officinalis*	Lamiaceae	Leaves	Rosmarinic acid
51..	Licorice	*Glycyrrhiza glabra*	Fabaceae	Roots	Glycyrrhizin
52..	Marsilea	*Marsilea minuta*	Marsileaceae	Leaves	Marsiline
53..	Mate tea	*Ilex paraguariensis*	Aquifoliaceae	Leaves	Polyphenols, Flavanoid (Quercetin, Kaempferol), Xanthines (Theophylline, Theobromine, caffeine) and Vitamins (B1, B12)

TABLE 9.2 *(Continued)*

Sl. No.	Common Name	Botanical Name	Family	Parts Used	Phytoconstituents
54..	Nakai	*Corydalis ternata*	Papaveraceae	Tuber	Protopine and tetrahydro coptisine
55..	Nutmeg	*Myristica fragrans*	Myristicaceae	Seeds	Myristicin and Elemicin
56..	Paddle weed	*Ecklonia cava*	Lessoniaceae	Whole plant	Bieckol, Dleckol, Eckol, and Phlorofucofukoeckol-A
57..	Palash	*Butea monosperma*	Fabaceae	Leaves	Butin, isobutrin, andbutein
58..	Pomegaranate	*Punica granatum*	Lythraceae	Seeds	Polyphenols (Gallocatechin and Catechin), Tannin
59..	Rosemary	*Rosmarinus officinalis*	Lamiaceae	Leaves	Eucaluptol, Carnosic acid, camphene, and Carnosol
60..	Saffron	*Crocus sativus*	Iridaceae	Whole Plant	Crocin & Crocetin
61..	Sekkoku	*Dendrobium moniliforme*	Orchidaceae	Whole Plant	Dendrocandins F-I
62..	Shankh pushpin	*Convolvulus pluricaulis*	Convolvulaceae	Whole Plant	kaempferol, scopoletin, and convolamine
63..	Shatavari	*Asparagus racemosus*	Liliaceae	Roots	Triterpene saponins: Shatavarin I-IV
64..	Sheng di huang	*Rehmanniaglutinosa*	Orobanchaceae	Roots	Aucubin and catalpol
65..	Solomon's seal	*Polygonatum multiflorum*	Asperagaceae	Roots and Rhizomes	Emodin
66..	Spanish sage	*Salvia lavandulaefolia*	Lamiaceae	Leaves	Essential oils (cineole, Linalool, Luteolin, Carvacrol, and pinene)
67..	St. John's Wort	*Hypericum perforatum*	Hypericaceae	Roots	Prenylated phloroglucinol: Hyperforin, Naphthodianthrone (Hypericin).
68..	Star anise	*Illicium verum*	Schisandraceae	Seed pod, fruit	Sesquiterpenoids: Veranisatins A, B, and C
69..	Sweet flag	*Acorus calamus*	Aracaceae	Rhizomes	a-and b-Asarone, Methyl isougenol
70..	Thankuni	*Centella asiatica*	Apiaceae	Whole Plant	Asiaticoside, Brahmoside, and triterpenic pentacyclic Madicasoside.
71..	Tobacco plant	*Nicotiana tabacum*	Solanaceae	Leaves	Nicotine and Choline

TABLE 9.2 *(Continued)*

Sl. No.	Common Name	Botanical Name	Family	Parts Used	Phytoconstituents
72..	Turmeric	*Curcuma longa*	Zingiberaceae	Rhizomes	Curcuminoids: Curcumin, Bisdemethoxycurcumin-cumin, Desmethoxycurcumin
73..	Vidarikand	*Pueraria tuberose*	Fabaceae	Tubers	Quercetin and genistein
74..	Wedge-leaf T	*Taverniera cuneifolia*	Fabaceae	Roots	Iduronic acid
75..	Yuan zhi	*Polygala tenuifolia*	Polyagalaceae	Roots	Onjisaponins V-Z

already needed. Phytochemicals, or potentially helpful plant substances, are still being researched. Because of their usage in traditional medicine, several plant species have been chosen for testing as nootropic drugs, and research has already identified several intriguing natural compounds that potentially work as cognitive enhancers.

1. ***Brahmi (Bacopa monnieri):*** This drug is traditionally used in the Ayurvedic Medicine system for the treatment of neurodegenerative diseases like AD. Bacosides A, B, betulinic acid, D-mannitol, stigmastanol, β-sitosterol, stigmasterol, and others are active phytoconstituents. Various *in-vivo* and *in-vitro* trials have been carried out to illustrate Brahmi's role in memory and cognition. Around 10 patients were given Sideritis extract, Brahmi extract, and a combination of the two in a clinical trial. Combining Sideritis extract with a low dose of Brahmi extract increased the d2 concentration test score in the studies. In a multicenter clinical trial, 104 patients with mild cognitive impairment (MCI) were given Brahmi, astaxanthin, phosphatidylserine, and tocopherol for sixty days. When compared to the baseline values, the improvement in scores reported after 60 days was found to be statistically significant [47]. Currently, there is a decent amount of literature supporting the claim that Brahmi could be a game-changing alternative therapeutic herb for terminal illnesses like Alzheimer's, but we believe more human-based trials are needed to help make an unassailable case for the use of Brahmi in diseases like Alzheimer's [44].
2. ***Gotu Kola (Centella asiatica):*** Indian pennywort, Asiatic pennywort, and kodavan are all names for this tropical medicinal plant. It is a member of the Apiaceae family. Its major phytoconstituents are asiatic acid and asiaticoside. It suppresses beta-amyloid cell death and toxicity *in vitro*, suggesting that it could play an essential role in the prevention and treatment of Alzheimer's disease. It significantly improves blood circulation all over the body as well as in the brain. Gotu kola has an important place in Indian medicine for millennia in treating and preventing a wide range of ailments and health difficulties, including malignancy, Alzheimer's, wound healing, diabetes, ulcers, skin disorders, nerve and brain cell regeneration, asthma, preventing aging, and more. Human research on the effect of *C. asiatica* on Alzheimer's disease patients is limited. As a result, more attention must be placed on performing human-centered trials

to analyze the benefits and drawbacks of this herb when used to treat Alzheimer's patients. It has the power to alter the brain; in fact, it is utilized in animal models as a nerve tonic and to boost memory and cognitive function [42, 44].

3. ***Shankhpushpi (Convolvulus pluricaulis):*** It is also known as Butterfly pea and is a valued herb in the Ayurvedic system. Active ingredients include convolvine, confoline, convosine, convolidine, kaempferol, and phytosterols. These components are responsible for *C. pluricaulis*' therapeutic properties. *C. pluricaulis* has been shown in several trials to relieve mental stress and fatigue. It has also been shown to be beneficial in patients suffering from anxiety, mental fatigue, and insomnia. An ethanolic extract of *C. pluricaulis* reduces reactive oxygen and improves learning and memory in rats *in vitro*. In another study, neonatal rats were administered shankhpushpi aqueous root extract. Retention and spatial learning performance improved significantly. ACh levels and activity both increased significantly. In a similar study on mice, shankhpushpi administration resulted in a considerable increase in dendritic branching and processes when compared to saline controls. Another investigation on aged and young mice discovered that *C. pluricaulis* caused an improvement in memory retention that was directly proportionate to the amount administered. Memory retention was found to be greater in young mice. Its efficacy as a brain tonic was proven in clinical trials of its polyherbal formulation. The memory and learning behavior improving capabilities of Shankhpushpi have increased in recent years [44].

4. ***Ginkgo (Ginkgo biloba):*** This plant belongs to the Ginkgoaceae family, which is also known as maidenhair tree, Japanese silver apricot, kew tree, and fossil tree. It contains terpenes, trilactones, ginkgolides A, B, C, J, bilobalide, biflavones, alkylphenols, polyphenols, and other substances. It lowers lipid peroxidation by neutralizing free radicals. *Ginkgo biloba* is often used to treat Alzheimer's disease and vascular dementia in its early stages. *In vitro* research has shown that *Ginkgo biloba* medication enhances cognitive capacity in Alzheimer's disease patients in multiple randomized controlled trials. When a nanosized extract of *G. biloba* was used in a study, it was observed that the group of animals given the extract exhibited increased cholinergic

neurotransmitter discharge from many locations of the brain when compared to the control group. Among these, EGb761's bioactive ingredient ginkgolides have neuroprotective and regenerative potential in brain stem cells (NSCs) actions because they interact with the cholinergic system [48]. Ginkgo promotes central nervous system blood circulation and increases nutrition and oxygen distribution in the brain. It also cleanses the body of free radicals, which promotes memory and alertness. Amnesia and Alzheimer's disease are treated using ginkgo extract. Ginkgo is a common element in many herbal nerve tonics. This plant has recently been demonstrated to help with a number of neurological health disorders including depression, psychosis, anxiety, and schizophrenia. *Ginkgo biloba* is a powerful herb that has been shown to improve symptoms in Alzheimer's patients, but its use is limited due to a lack of research data. Because most research to date has used animal models, large-scale clinical studies are needed to understand more about the importance of this herb to aid patients with Alzheimer's disease [40].

5. **Turmeric *(Curcuma longa):*** Turmeric is a well-known medicinal plant obtained from the rhizomes of Curcuma longa, which belongs to the Zingiberaceae family and is commonly grown in Southeast Asian countries. It is widely regarded as a medicine for treating a wide range of diseases in animals, including neuroprotective, hepatoprotective, anti-inflammatory, antibacterial, antineoplastic, antifertility, and immunostimulant properties. The active components of turmeric include the curcumin flavonoid and diferuloylmethane, as well as volatile oils such as atlantone, tumerone, and zingiberone. Additional substances found in turmeric are sugars, resins, and proteins. The primary bioactive phytochemical is curcumin. Curcuma oil has been shown to reduce endothelial cell inflammation following myocardial ischemia/reperfusion. Research has found that curcumin (at doses of 50, 100, or 200 mg/kg) can improve cognitive deficits and mitochondrial malfunction symptoms in mice. Turmeric has also been demonstrated to protect the nervous system, particularly in neurodegenerative diseases. Studies show that curcumin protects the brains of mice from localized ischemia by increasing the expression of the transcription factors nuclear factor erythroid 2-related factor 2 (Nrf2) and heme oxygenase-1 (HO-1) [40, 42].

6. **Withania *(Withania somnifera)*:** It is generally known as ashwagandha belongs to the family Solanaceae. Overall, a dose of 500 mg/kg of *Withania somnifera* was found to have a substantial effect on memory impairment. Because of its ability to increase acetylcholine levels, ashwagandha has been studied for memory enhancement and cognition impairment. Ashwagandha is one of the most well-explored Ayurvedic herbs. Withania roots, just like Ginseng, are one of the most astonishing ingredients in the traditional medicine system. Therefore, it is generally referred to as the Indian Ginseng. In mice, withania root extract improved retention of a passive avoidance test [40].
7. **Tea *(Camellia sinensis):*** This is the world's second most consumed beverage after water, and its medicinal effects are well known. Tea possesses powerful neuroprotective, hepatoprotective, antioxidant, anti-oncogenic, and chemopreventive activities due to its varied chemical contents. Various recent research has revealed that regular and green tea both act as dietary supplements and have a considerable ability to protect cognition and learning impairments, as well as hippocampal oxidative stress, in Alzheimer's disease and ischemia-reperfusion (IR) models. The presence of Epigallocatechin gallate (EGCG) in the brain is responsible for green tea's ability to inhibit neuronal cell degeneration, which implies it has antioxidative properties that can protect the brain from free radicals. According to research, Epigallocatechin gallate present in green tea improved learning and memory ability in Alzheimer's disease in rats. As a result, bioactive teas might be a viable treatment option for neurodegenerative illnesses [40, 44].
8. **Licorice *(Glycyrrhiza glabra):*** It is also known as "Yashti-madhuh or liquorice," and it is a member of the Leguminosae family. Glabridin is the major flavonoid found in licorice and has a variety of pharmacological activities including neuroprotective, anticancer, antidiabetic, antioxidant, immunomodulatory activity, and anticonvulsant effects. Glabridin decreases malondialdehyde (MDA) levels in rats' brains while increasing superoxide dismutase and reducing glutathione levels. In hypoxic rats, dietary *Glycyrrhiza glabra* restored low levels of brain neurotransmitters including glutamate and dopamine while reducing AChE activity. This plant is known as 'Medhya dravya' in Ayurveda and was traditionally used to enhance

memory and intellect. Mouse experiments indicated that a 150 mg/kg dose of aqueous licorice extract significantly improves memory and learning ability. Liquiritigenin (LIQ), a bioactive component found in the root of *Glycyrrhiza glabra*, has been shown to reduce reactive oxygen species (ROS) generation, Ca^{2+} influx, and lipid peroxidation in glutamate-induced hippocampal neuronal cell death. Therefore, LIQ is considered a potent neuroprotective agent with the potential to be a promising treatment for Alzheimer's disease [40, 44].

9. ***Phyllanthus emblica (Emblica officinalis):*** It is also known as *amla*. Parle et al. evaluated amla extract for memory-enhancing activity at three distinct oral doses (50, 100, and 200 mg/kg), and AchE activity was significantly reduced in mice. All of the studies suggested that *Emblica officinalis* could be very beneficial. In scopolamine-induced amnesic mice (150, 300, 450, and 600 mg/kg), cholinergic function and oxidative stress were examined for hydroalcoholic extract.

10. **Ginseng *(Panax ginseng):*** It belongs to the Araliaceae family, which is spread over Northeast Asia. It is one of the plants that is often utilized to increase vitality. The presence of ginsenosides in ginseng root determines its classification. It protects against neuro-degeneration through several methods. Ginsenosides may be able to improve neuroprotection. In animal studies, Ginseng improved the ability to decrease cellular AChE movement and raise its metabolic rate, implying that it may provide neuroprotection. It also reduced beta-amyloid deposition and led to oxidative stress caused by glutamate. It therefore avoids apoptosis and neuronal loss [40, 44].

11. **Blue Pea Flower *(Clitoria ternatea):*** *Shankhpushpi* is another name for it. *Clitoria ternatea* ethanolic root extract was evaluated against stress-induced amnesia in rats orally. In this experiment, a protective effect of shankhpushpi and significant inhibition of nitric oxide were detected. In another study, rats were given dosages of 300 and 500 mg/kg of an alcoholic extract of *Clitoria ternatea* roots and aerial portions to assess their memory and central cholinergic activity. The extract increased memory function in rats by boosting acetylcholinesterase activity and acetylcholine concentration. *Clitoria ternatea* root extract was more effective than aerial parts.

12. **Drumstick *(Moringa oleifera):*** The aqueous extract of *Moringa oleifera* leaves was administered to rats at a dose of 250 mg/kg for Alzheimer's disease. This extract acts on the brain, raising superoxide dismutase (SOD) and catalase levels while lowering lipid peroxidation (LPO) activity in the rat cerebral cortex. The extract was also investigated for Alzheimer's disease and cognitive impairment. Moringa extract was observed to inhibit tau hyperphosphorylation and protect nerve cells in this investigation. In another study, the effects of hydroalcoholic (leaves extract) on cognition impairment and neurodegeneration in age-related dementia animal models at distinct doses in the concentrations of 100, 200, and 400 mg/kg orally [50].
13. **Ginger *(Zingiber officinale):*** *Zingiber officinalis*is a well-known Zingiberaceae plant. It is widely known as ginger. It contains active chemical constituents such as gingerdiol, methoxy gingerol, shogaol, gingerol, shogaol, gingerol, shogaol, gingerol, shogaol, and methoxy gingerol. The anti-Alzheimer activity of the methanolic extract was investigated. All isolated compounds showed strong antioxidant action, as well as improved memory and learning capacities. *Hanumanthacar* et al. studied *Zingiber officinalis*' acetylcholinesterase inhibitor action, which alleviated scopolamine-induced memory impairment. At dosages of 108 and 216 mg/kg, ginger extract was found to be neuroprotective [40, 41].
14. **Saffron *(Crocus sativus):*** It is the dried stigma of *Crocus sativus* flowers. It belongs to the Iridaceae and Crocoideae families. Many countries grow it, including Spain, Afghanistan, Iran, and Turkey. In traditional Iranian medicine, *Crocus sativus* is used to cure mental diseases. Ingredients from saffron have recently been used to treat specific brain diseases and calm smooth muscle. It exhibits anti-Alzheimer and anticonvulsant effects in preclinical and clinical trials. Saffron can treat depression and impact brain neurotransmitter attention and interaction with the opioid system in experimental clinical education. It also reduced neuron loss in the hippocampus of mice [40].
15. ***Jatamansi (Nardostachys jatamansi):*** *Jatamansi* is a well-known Medhya herb that is revered in Ayurvedic medicine. It's most common in Nepal, India's Himalayas, and in China. *Nardostachys jatamansi* roots have anti-ischemic, antioxidant, anticonvulsant,

and neuroprotective effects, according to Ayurvedic medicine [40]. An alcoholic extract of Jatamansi at a concentration of 200 mg/kg considerably increased learning and cognition power in young mice. Moreover, dementia was dramatically reversed. In mice, it also corrected forgetfulness produced by normal aging. Based on these findings, Jatamansi may be an effective treatment for dementia in the elderly [51] (Figure 9.2).

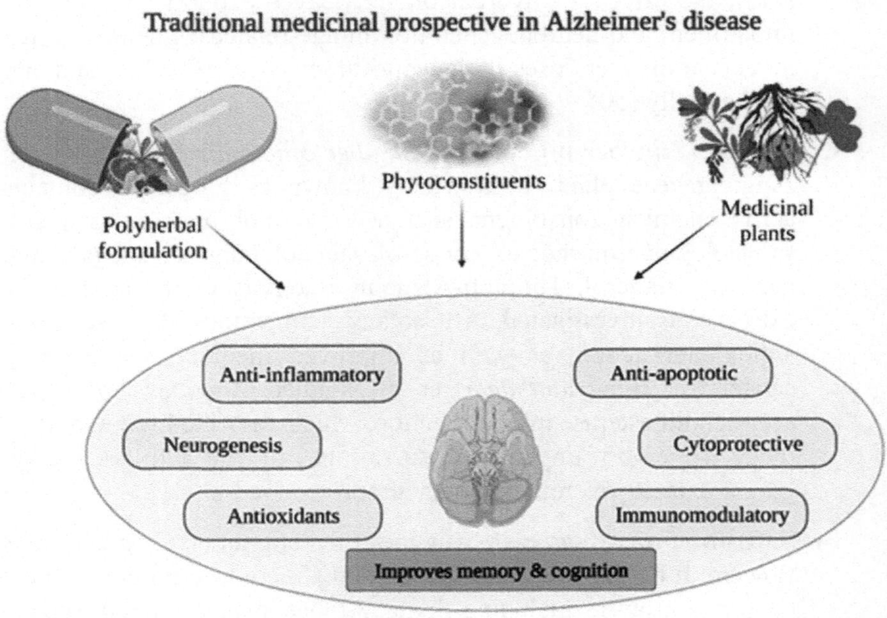

FIGURE 9.2 Traditional medicine approach in Alzheimer's disease.

9.6 EFFICACY, SAFETY CONCERNS, AND CHALLENGES OF HERBAL MEDICINES

1. **Environmental Factor:** The environment has a significant impact on the phytochemical profile of plants. The levels of bioactive constituents in the same species can vary depending on geographical location, weather conditions, soil composition, and other factors. Due to local weather divergence, plant chemical composition differs from year to year, even within the same location. Various factors like altitude, temperature, drought, flood,

etc., greatly affect the biosynthesis process. In general, constituent levels in wild plants are more variable. Standardization of cultivation techniques can help to reduce these negative effects in commercial plants. Plants grown under controlled conditions and derived from a well-characterized and homogeneous genetic source have more stable amounts of bioactive chemicals. The plant processing mechanism determines the concentration of nootropics. The entire plant or its parts (roots, leaves, fruits, and seeds) contain varying levels of secondary metabolites. It is required to use plant parts which have potent and higher concentrations of active metabolites [52].

Adulteration: It is characterized as the partial or complete replacement of an actual herbal medication with another chemical that has a similar appearance but is inferior. Herbs with volatile components are more frequently tampered with. The adulterants could be toxic or have no therapeutic value [53].

2. **Extraction:** These techniques and processing steps can cause variations in active constituent concentration. A combination of chemicals at various concentrations is produced by different extraction techniques. Various factors that affect the final concentration are solvents, temperature, extraction time, and the method used for extraction. The same nootropic can have a variety of biological effects. When compared to synthetic drugs, the main advantage of the natural drug is the presence of multiple potent phytochemicals. Additionally, it's important to find and segregate any potentially dangerous substances. Inadequate separation processes may result in lower amounts of active compounds, resulting in poor bioactivity [52].
3. **Herb-Drug Interaction:** Combining herbal drugs with prescription medications can have serious side effects. Herbal drugs contain a large number of unidentified constituents, making it challenging to determine the type of interactions [54]. Furthermore, while many people believe that herbal medications are safe since they are sourced from nature, several of the plants have lately been proven to have adverse drug interactions [55]. Drug interactions are also complicated by heterogeneity in phytochemicals and dose frequency. CYP450 is involved in the metabolism of drugs used to treat Alzheimer's disease. Therefore, CYP450 inhibition by herbal

medicines should be researched in order to anticipate such herb-drug interactions. Once *Ginkgo biloba* and phenytoin are combined, breakthrough seizures occur owing to CYP2C19 induction. However, when combined with donepezil, it has a significant effect on Alzheimer's disease due to its extra cholinergic activity. Similarly, curcumin and donepezil (a reversible cholinesterase inhibitor) worked synergistically to improve cognition and reduce oxidative stress [56]. To evaluate further, experimental and clinical research is required to assess the herb-drug interaction. Such interactions can be avoided if patients disclose their concurrent use of any other medications and physicians are aware of it. Drug absorption, metabolism, and elimination are already compromised in the elderly population. Concurrent use of herbal medicines may exacerbate the impairment. As a result, in elderly patients, herbal medications should be used with caution [57].

9.7 PHARMACOVIGILANCE FOR HERBAL MEDICINES

Nowadays, modern medicines that have been thoroughly researched must adhere to stringent national and international regulations. However, alternative or traditional medical systems face a lack of or inadequate regulatory guidelines. Because of their natural origins, herbal medicines are widely perceived to be safe. However, as previously discussed, several herbal medications have adverse effects, either by themselves or as a result of unfavorable herb-drug interactions with other medications [58]. In addition to the risks associated with using herbal medicines, unknown composition, inaccurate labeling, inferior quality, lack of standardization, adulteration, contamination, and even quackery can have a negative impact. The inability to communicate with Alzheimer's patients in the later stages of the disease necessitates special consideration in terms of adverse effects and drug-drug interactions.

So, the above-said challenges can be addressed by [9, 19]:

- For higher-quality final products, detailed standardization in plant processing is required.
- Well-labeled formulations can decrease the likelihood of inappropriate use and adverse drug reactions or herb-drug interactions. The label should clearly state the active ingredient composition, the name

of the herbal drug along with the method of administration, storage conditions, shelf life, adverse effects, and any other cautions.

- Natural products are widely assumed to be inherently safe, with no side effects and no risk of overdosing. Although natural products can have negative side effects, herb-herb or herb-drug interactions are possible. As a result, more research is needed to gain a better understanding of nootropic interactions.
- Integrating pharmacovigilance in traditional medicine system.

9.8 FINDINGS AND PROSPECTS FOR THE FUTURE

Plants clearly play an important role in the form of herbal foods and spices, in improving poor memory. Various medicinal plants are used all over the world (e.g., in Ayurveda, African medicine, American medicine, Korean medicine, TCM, and so on), and it has been proven that they improve memory and cognition in animal models. Several phytochemicals present in these medicinal plants have proven to improve cognition, intelligence, concentration, and attention. This is done by controlling the enzyme acetylcholinesterase's (AChE) activity in order to maintain a normal level of the neurotransmitter acetylcholine (ACh) in the brain. Several poly-herbal formulations seem to have a positive effect on the central nervous system. Along with preclinical research, effective clinical studies are being conducted. It's possible that these herbs will soon be used to treat Alzheimer's disease because they have significant effects in animal models of AD-type dementia. Herbal preparations and various plant extracts have been used as an alternative medicine since ancient times. These preparations and extracts have demonstrated their potential for use in Alzheimer's disease. Due to the presence of various phytoconstituents that are active on a wide range of biological targets, medicinal plants are a rich source of potential new drugs. However, there remains plenty of work to be done before this potential can be recognized in the form of actual medicine. Standardization of phytoconstituents is a key necessity in the development of herbal remedies. Potent phytochemicals should be identified, isolated, and thoroughly tested. To confirm the effectiveness of such herbal medicines or herbal formulations for the treatment of Alzheimer's disease, large-scale clinical studies must be conducted.

KEYWORDS

- **acetylcholine**
- **Alzheimer's disease**
- **dementia**
- **ethnopharmacognosy**
- **nootropics**
- **phytochemicals**
- **smart drugs**

REFERENCES

1. Banerjee, S., Anand, U., Ghosh, S., Ray, D., Ray, P., Nandy, S., Deshmukh, G. D., Tripathi, V., & Dey, A. (2021). Bacosides from *Bacopa Monnieri* extract: An overview of the effects on neurological disorders. *Phytotherapy Research, 35*(10), 5668–5679. https://doi.org/10.1002/ptr.7203.
2. Gregory, J., Vengalasetti, Y. V., Bredesen, D. E., & Rao, R. V. (2021). Neuroprotective herbs for the management of Alzheimer's disease. *Biomolecules, 11*(4). https://doi.org/10.3390/biom11040543.
3. Onaolapo, A. Y., Obelawo, A. Y., & Onaolapo, O. J. (2019). Brain aging, cognition and diet: A review of the emerging roles of food-based nootropics in mitigating age-related memory decline. *Current Aging Science, 12*(1), 2–14. https://doi.org/10.2174/1874609812666190311160754.
4. Anand, U., Jacobo-Herrera, N., Altemimi, A., & Lakhssassi, N. (2019). A comprehensive review on medicinal plants as antimicrobial therapeutics: Potential avenues of biocompatible drug discovery. *Metabolites, 9*(11), 258. https://doi.org/10.3390/metabo9110258.
5. Suliman, N. A., Mat Taib, C. N., Mohd Moklas, M. A., Adenan, M. I., Hidayat Baharuldin, M. T., & Basir, R. (2016). Establishing natural nootropics: Recent molecular enhancement influenced by natural nootropic. *Evidence-Based Complementary and Alternative Medicine, 2016*. https://doi.org/10.1155/2016/4391375.
6. Hardman, R. J., Kennedy, G., Macpherson, H., Scholey, A. B., & Pipingas, A. (2016). Adherence to a Mediterranean-style diet and effects on cognition in adults: A qualitative evaluation and systematic review of longitudinal and prospective trials. *Frontiers in Nutrition, 3*. https://doi.org/10.3389/fnut.2016.00022.
7. Srivastava, A., Srivastava, P., Pandey, A., Khanna, V. K., & Pant, A. B. (2019). Phytomedicine: A potential alternative medicine in controlling neurological disorders. In *New Look to Phytomedicine: Advancements in Herbal Products as Novel Drug Leads* (pp. 625–655). https://doi.org/10.1016/B978-0-12-814619-4.00025-2.

8. Zlotnik, G., & Vansintjan, A. (2019). Memory: An extended definition. *Frontiers in Psychology, 10*. https://doi.org/10.3389/fpsyg.2019.02523.
9. *Gazette Notifications*. Retrieved from: https://cdsco.gov.in/opencms/opencms/en/Notifications/Gazette-Notifications/ (accessed on 22 July 2024).
10. Ahmed, A. H., & Oswald, R. E. (2010). Piracetam defines a new binding site for allosteric modulators of alpha-amino-3-hydroxy-5-methyl-4-isoxazole-propionic acid (AMPA) receptors. *Journal of Medicinal Chemistry, 53*(5), 2197–2203. https://doi.org/10.1021/jm901905j.
11. Malik, R., Sangwan, A., Saihgal, R., Paul Jindal, D., & Piplani, P. (2007). Towards better brain management: Nootropics. *Current Medicinal Chemistry, 14*(2), 123–131. https://doi.org/10.2174/092986707779313408.
12. Malík, M., & Tlustoš, P. (2022). Nootropics as cognitive enhancers: Types, dosage, and side effects of smart drugs. *Nutrients, 14*(16), 3367. https://doi.org/10.3390/nu14163367.
13. Mondadori, C. (1994). In search of the mechanism of action of the nootropics: New insights and potential clinical implications. *Life Sciences, 55*(25–26), 2171–2178. https://doi.org/10.1016/0024-3205(94)00398-X.
14. Ghosh, C., Dick, R. M., & Ali, S. F. (1993). Iron/ascorbate-induced lipid peroxidation changes membrane fluidity and muscarinic cholinergic receptor binding in rat frontal cortex. *Neurochemistry International, 23*(5), 479–484. https://doi.org/10.1016/0197-0186(93)90133-P.
15. Müller, W. E., Koch, S., Scheuer, K., Rostock, A., & Bartsch, R. (1997). Effects of piracetam on membrane fluidity in the aged mouse, rat, and human brain. *Biochemical Pharmacology, 53*(2), 135–140. https://doi.org/10.1016/s0006-2952(96)00463-7.
16. Nicholson, C. D. (1990). Pharmacology of nootropics and metabolically active compounds in relation to their use in dementia. *Psychopharmacology, 101*(2), 147–159. https://doi.org/10.1007/bf02244119.
17. Shaji, C., Aleyas, J., & Mathews, S. M. (2016). A review on nootropics. *International Journal of Advanced Research in Biological Sciences, 3*(2), 272–277.
18. Musa Chiroma, S., Mat Taib, C. N., Aris, M., Moklas, M., Taufik, M., Baharuldin, H., Amom, Z., & Jagadeesan, S. (2019). The use of nootropics in Alzheimer's disease: Is there light at the end of the tunnel? *Biomedical Research and Therapy, 6*(1), 2937–2944. https://doi.org/10.15419/bmrat.v6i1.513.
19. *Guidelines Series-I General Guidelines for Drug Development of Ayurvedic Formulations*. Central Council for Research in Ayurvedic Sciences, Ministry of AYUSH, Government of India, New Delhi.
20. Kumar, K. H., Mitta, S., K., Davarika, R., Mounica, G. S., & Sai, M. (2016). Nootropics-memory boosters. *Journal of Pharmaceutical Biology, 6*(1), 14–16.
21. Bhattacharya, S. K., Upadhyay, S. N., &Jaiswal, A. K. (1993). Effect of piracetam on electroshock-induced amnesia and decrease in brain acetylcholine in rats. *PubMed*. Retrieved from: https://pubmed.ncbi.nlm.nih.gov/8276434/.
22. Singh, H., & Dhawan, B. (2023). Neuropsychopharmacology effects of the Ayurvedic nootropic *Bacopa Monniera* Linn. (Brahmi). *Indian Journal of Pharmacology, 29*(5), 359.
23. Huber, G., Bailly, Y., Martin, J. R., Mariani, J., & Brugg, B. (1997). Synaptic β-amyloid precursor proteins increase with learning capacity in rats. *Neuroscience, 80*(2), 313–320. https://doi.org/10.1016/S0306-4522(97)00120-6.

24. Cleary, J., Hittner, J. M., Semotuk, M., Mantyh, P., & O'Hare, E. (1995). Beta-amyloid (1–40) effects on behavior and memory. *Brain Research, 682*(1–2), 69–74. https://doi.org/10.1016/0006-8993(95)00323-I.
25. Luo, Y., Smith, J. V., Paramasivam, V., Burdick, A., Curry, K. J., Buford, J. P., Khan, I., Netzer, W. J., Xu, H., & Butko, P. (2002). Inhibition of amyloid-beta aggregation and caspase-3 activation by the Ginkgo biloba extract EGb761. *Proceedings of the National Academy of Sciences U S A, 99*(19), 12197–12202. https://doi.org/10.1073/pnas.182425199.
26. Heo, J. H., Lee, S. T., Chu, K., Oh, M. J., Park, H. J., Shim, J. Y., & Kim, M. (2008). An open-label trial of Korean red ginseng as an adjuvant treatment for cognitive impairment in patients with Alzheimer's disease. *European Journal of Neurology, 15*(8), 865–868. https://doi.org/10.1111/j.1468-1331.2008.02157.x.
27. Aguiar, S., & Borowski, T. (2013). Neuropharmacological review of the nootropic herb *Bacopa Monnieri*. *Rejuvenation Research, 16*(4), 313. https://doi.org/10.1089/rej.2013.1431.
28. Butterfield, D. A., & Pocernich, C. B. (2003). The glutamatergic system and Alzheimer's disease: Therapeutic implications. *CNS Drugs, 17*(9), 641–652. https://doi.org/10.2165/00023210-200317090-00004.
29. Routtenberg, A. (1986). Synaptic plasticity and protein kinase C. *Progress in Brain Research, 69*(C), 211–234. https://doi.org/10.1016/S0079-6123(08)61061-4.
30. Battaini, F. (2001). Protein kinase C isoforms as therapeutic targets in nervous system disease states. *Pharmacological Research, 44*(5), 353–361. https://doi.org/10.1006/phrs.2001.0893.
31. Lardner, A. L. (2014). Neurobiological effects of the green tea constituent theanine and its potential role in the treatment of psychiatric and neurodegenerative disorders. *Nutritional Neuroscience, 17*(4), 145–155. https://doi.org/10.1179/1476830513Y.0000000079.
32. Takeda, A., Sakamoto, K., Tamano, H., Fukura, K., Inui, N., Suh, S. W., Won, S. J., & Yokogoshi, H. (2011). Facilitated neurogenesis in the developing hippocampus after intake of theanine, an amino acid in tea leaves, and object recognition memory. *Cellular and Molecular Neurobiology, 31*(7), 1079–1088. https://doi.org/10.1007/s10571-011-9707-0.
33. O'Malley, D., Shanley, L. J., & Harvey, J. (2003). Insulin inhibits rat hippocampal neurones via activation of ATP-sensitive K+ and large conductance Ca2+-activated K+ channels. *Neuropharmacology, 44*(7), 855–863. https://doi.org/10.1016/S0028-3908(03)00081-9.
34. Gard, P. R. (2002). The role of angiotensin II in cognition and behavior. *European Journal of Pharmacology, 438*(1–2), 1–14. https://doi.org/10.1016/S0014-2999(02)01283-9.
35. Chekman, I., Belenichev, I. F., Demchenko, A. V., Bobrova, V. I., Kucherenko, L. I., Gorchakova, N. A., & Bukhtiyarova, N. V. (2014). Nootropics in complex therapy of chronic cerebral ischemia. *Scientific Innovations, 10*(4), 56–68. https://doi.org/10.15407/scine10.04.056.
36. McDaniel, M. A., Maier, S. F., & Einstein, G. O. (2002). "Brain-specific" nutrients: A memory cure? *Psychological Science in the Public Interest, 3*(1), 12–38. https://doi.org/10.1111/1529-1006.00007.
37. Mehta, S. P., & Balaraman, R. (2022). A review on herbal remedies for Alzheimer's disease. *Journal of Natural Remedies, 22*(2), 123–135. https://doi.org/10.18311/jnr/2022/29277.

38. Sharma, C., Pal, A., Amar, S., & Singh, P. (2021). Memory potential herb: A review. *World Journal of Current Medical and Pharmaceutical Research, 3*(4), 68–73. https://doi.org/10.37022/wjcmpr.v3i4.180.
39. Abdolmaleki, A., Akram, M., Muddasar Saeed, M., Asadi, A., & Kajkolah, M. (2020). Herbal medicine as a neuroprotective potential agent in human and animal models: A historical overview. *Journal of Pharmaceutical Care, 8*(2). https://doi.org/10.18502/jpc.v8i2.3832.
40. Mehla, J., Gupta, P., Pahuja, M., Diwan, D., & Diksha, D. (2020). Indian medicinal herbs and formulations for Alzheimer's disease, from traditional knowledge to scientific assessment. *Brain Sciences, 10*(12), 1–31. https://doi.org/10.3390/brainsci10120964.
41. Mandal, A., & Prabhavalkar, K. S. (2018). Evaluation of the efficacy of combination therapy of vinpocetine and *Withania somnifera* methanolic extract in cognitive impairment. *World Journal of Pharmacy and Pharmaceutical Sciences, 7*(8), 1295–1322. https://doi.org/10.20959/wjpps20188-12176.
42. Halder, S., Anand, U., Nandy, S., Oleksak, P., Qusti, S., Alshammari, E. M., El-Saber Batiha, G., Koshy, E. P., & Dey, A. (2021). Herbal drugs and natural bioactive products as potential therapeutics: A review on pro-cognitive and brain boosters' perspectives. *Saudi Pharmaceutical Journal, 29*(8), 879–907. https://doi.org/10.1016/j.jsps.2021.07.003.
43. Kumar, S., Namburi, U. R. S., Chiluveri, A. C., Londhe, D., Dora, B. B., Chiluveri, S. K., & Chinchalkar, S. (2021). Scientific review on indication and therapeutic effects of selected nootropic herbs/drugs from *Kashyapa Samhita. Journal of Research in Ayurvedic Sciences, 5*(1), 4. https://doi.org/10.4103/jras.jras_39_21.
44. Bhattacharjee, A., Chakraborty, R., & Sen, S. (2019). Scientific basis for Ayurvedic medicinal plants against Alzheimer's disease. In *Herbal Medicine in India: Indigenous Knowledge, Practice, Innovation and its Value* (pp. 51–67). https://doi.org/10.1007/978-981-13-7248-3_5/cover.
45. Pandey, S. N., Rangra, N. K., Singh, S., Arora, S., & Gupta, V. (2021). The evolving role of natural products from traditional medicinal herbs in the treatment of Alzheimer's disease. *ACS Chemical Neuroscience, 12*(15), 2718–2728. https://doi.org/10.1021/acschemneuro.1c00206.
46. Islam, F., Khadija, J. F., Harun-Or-Rashid, M., Rahaman, M. S., Nafady, M. H., Islam, M. R., Akter, A., Emran, T. B., Wilairatana, P., & Mubarak, M. S. (2022). Bioactive compounds and their derivatives: An insight into prospective phytotherapeutic approach against Alzheimer's disease. *Oxidative Medicine and Cellular Longevity, 2022*, 5100904–5100904. https://doi.org/10.1155/2022/5100904.
47. Zanotta, D., Puricelli, S., & Bonoldi, G. (2014). Cognitive effects of a dietary supplement made from the extract of *Bacopa Monnieri*, astaxanthin, phosphatidylserine, and vitamin E in subjects with mild cognitive impairment: A noncomparative, exploratory clinical study. *Neuropsychiatric Disease and Treatment, 10*, 225–230. https://doi.org/10.2147/ndt.s51092.
48. Luo, Y. (2001). *Ginkgo Biloba* neuroprotection: Therapeutic implications in Alzheimer's disease. *Journal of Alzheimer's Disease, 3*(4), 401–407. https://doi.org/10.3233/jad-2001-3407.
49. Taranalli, A. D., & Cheeramkuzhy, T. C. (2000). Influence of *Clitoria Ternatea* extracts on memory and central cholinergic activity in rats. *Pharmacology Biochemistry and Behavior, 38*(1), 51–56. https://doi.org/10.1076/1388-0209(200001)3811-bft051.

50. Mahaman, Y. A. R., Huang, F., Wu, M., Wang, Y., Wei, Z., Bao, J., Salissou, M. T. M., Ke, D., Wang, Q., Liu, R., Wang, J. Z., Zhang, B., Chen, D., & Wang, X. (2018). *Moringa Oleifera* alleviates homocysteine-induced Alzheimer's disease-like pathology and cognitive impairments. *Journal of Alzheimer's Disease, 63*(3), 1141. https://doi.org/10.3233/jad-180091.
51. Joshi, H., & Parle, M. (2006). *Nardostachys jatamansi* improves learning and memory in mice. *Journal of Medicinal Food, 9*(1), 113–118. https://doi.org/10.1089/jmf.2006.9.113.
52. Parveen, B., Parveen, A., Parveen, R., Ahmad, S., Ahmad, M., & Iqbal, M. (2020). Challenges and opportunities for traditional herbal medicine today with special reference to its status in India. *Advances in Pharmacological Sciences, 9(2), 97–112*. https://doi.org/10.21276/ap.2020.9.2.8.
53. Ahmad Khan, M. S., & Ahmad, I. (2019). Herbal medicine: Current trends and future prospects. In *New Look to Phytomedicine: Advancements in Herbal Products as Novel Drug Leads* (pp. 3–13). https://doi.org/10.1016/b978-0-12-814619-4.00001-x.
54. Choi, Y. H., & Chin, Y. W. (2020). Multifaceted factors causing conflicting outcomes in herb-drug interactions. *Pharmaceutics, 13*(1), 43. https://doi.org/10.3390/pharmaceutics13010043.
55. Wilson, V., & Maulik, S. K. (2018). Herb-drug interactions in neurological disorders: A critical appraisal. *Current Drug Metabolism, 19*(5), 443–453. https://doi.org/10.2174/1389200218666171031123738.
56. Akinyemi, A. J., Oboh, G., Oyeleye, S. I., & Ogunsuyi, O. (2017). Anti-amnestic effect of curcumin in combination with donepezil, an anticholinesterase drug: Involvement of cholinergic system. *Neurotoxicity Research, 31*(4), 560–569. https://doi.org/10.1007/s12640-017-9701-5.
57. Yan, J., Hu, J., Liu, A., He, L., Li, X., & Wei, H. (2017). Design, synthesis, and evaluation of multitarget-directed ligands against Alzheimer's disease based on the fusion of donepezil and curcumin. *Bioorganic & Medicinal Chemistry, 25*(12), 2946–2955. https://doi.org/10.1016/j.bmc.2017.02.048.
58. Barkat, M. A., Goyal, A., Barkat, H. A., Salauddin, M., Pottoo, F. H., & Anwer, E. T. (2020). Herbal medicine: Clinical perspective and regulatory status. *Combustion Chemistry & High Throughput Screening, 24*(10), 1573–1582. https://doi.org/10.2174/1386207323999201110192942.

CHAPTER 10

Ethnopharmacological Approaches for Dementia

KAMICA YADAV,[1*,2] ARUN MITTAL,[2] PARVEEN KUMAR GOYAL,[3]
SATISH SARDANA,[2] and SUMAN KHURANA[2,3]

[1]*Department of Pharmacy, Starex University, Gurugram, Haryana, India*

[2]*Amity Institute of Pharmacy, Amity University Haryana, Amity Education Valley, Manesar, Gurugram, Haryana, India*

[3]*Department of Pharmacy, Panipat Institute of Engineering and Technology (PIET), Samalkha, Panipat, Haryana, India*

*Corresponding author.

ABSTRACT

Dementia is a clinical syndrome wherein a steady decline of an affected person's mental and cognitive capabilities occurs. It has been recognized that symptoms of dementia are gradual, persistent, and progressive. Because of cognitive decline, 90% of patients with dementia are more prone to show behavioral and psychological symptoms, such as psychosis, aggression, agitation, and depression. The pathophysiology of dementia is multifactorial. There are many risk factors associated with dementia and conditions such as improper cerebral blood supply, increased oxidative stress, exposure to toxins, mitochondrial injury, and frequently coexisting with some cerebrovascular and neurodegenerative disorders such as Alzheimer's disease (AD), Huntington's disease (HD), and Parkinson's disease (PD). Other risk factors for dementia are hypertension, stroke, diabetes mellitus, some heart diseases, smoking, consumption of alcohol, and lack of exercise. Currently, several synthetic and semi-synthetic approaches are available for the treatment like reversible acetylcholinesterase (AChE) inhibitor donepezil, the non-selective

Neuro-Nutraceuticals and Drug Discovery and Delivery in Alzheimer's Disease, Volume 1: Targeting Key Pathological Pathways. Varinder Singh, Amit Kumar, Parul Sood (Eds.)

butyrylcholinesterase (BuChE), and AChE inhibitor rivastigmine, but these have several side effects. So, there is a need to shift to traditional medicines. Medicines from various plants (*Ginkgo biloba* L., *Panax ginseng* C.A. Meyer (Ginseng), Curcuminoids from genus *Curcuma, Glycyrrhiza genus*, *Camellia sinensis* Kuntze) derived lead molecules were introduced from time to time which may be beneficial for further medical research. Ethnopharmacology plays a very important role in the development of conventional medicines.

10.1 INTRODUCTION

Dementia is a clinical syndrome and Major Neurocognitive Disorder wherein the steady decline of the mental and cognitive capabilities of an affected person takes place. It has been recognized that symptoms of dementia are gradual, persistent, and progressive. Because of cognitive decline, 90% of patients with dementia are more prone to show behavioral and psychological symptoms, such as psychosis, aggression, agitation, and depression [1]. It has been noticed for some years that young-onset cases are progressively recognized. Dementia is usually a condition that affects older people, and it is a leading contributor to disability and dependence among the older population. Predominantly rapid increases in the number and percentage of older people are forecast for countries like China, India, and Latin America. It has been estimated that by 2050, the number of people aged $\geq$60 years will increase by 1.25 billion which accounts for 22% of the world's population, with 79% living in the world's less developed regions [2].

The causes of dementia can be categorized into reversible and irreversible. The reversible causes of dementia include Dural Arteriovenous Fistula [3], Normal pressure hydrocephalus [4], bioaccumulation of various chemical pollutants [5], Neurosyphilis, Whipple disease, Lyme neuroborreliosis, Collagen-vascular, Systemic lupus erythematosus, Temporal arteritis, Rheumatoid vasculitis, Sarcoidosis, Thrombotic thrombocytopenic purpura, Granulomatous angiitis, Idiopathic hyper-eosinophilic syndrome, endocrine disorders, nutritional deficiencies, Chronic alcoholism, Psychiatric pseudodementia, Obstructive sleep apnea syndrome, Chronic obstructive pulmonary disease, Congestive heart failure, Limbic encephalitis, Radiation-induced dementia, Dialysis encephalopathy, etc. [6]. The irreversible causes of dementia include neurodegenerative diseases such as Alzheimer's disease, PD, and Huntington's disease [7].

The most common type of dementia is caused by a neurodegenerative disorder such as AD, PD, HD, or Amyotrophic Lateral Sclerosis (ALS), and Vascular Cognitive Impairments (VCI) are another type of dementia. These diseases frequently coexist with neurodegenerative dementias [8]. All forms of cognitive disorder associated with cerebrovascular disease are referred to as vascular cognitive impairment resulting in structural and functional connectivity loss, compromising functional networks within the brain. Vascular dementia has overtaken AD as the second most common type of dementia [9]. Numerous gene polymorphisms and other mutations are also connected with the occurrence of dementia. A family with ALS and frontotemporal dementia was found to have a heterozygous R1101K mutation in the p150 subunit of dynactin (DCTN1) (FTD) [10]. The cytoskeletal protein dysfunction in tau is on the pathway that leads to neurodegeneration and dementia. Tau is generated either indirectly, by Aβ42, or directly, in some forms of frontotemporal dementia by mutations in tau itself [11]. Several genetic mutations cause high penetrance, early-onset dementia, also known as familial Alzheimer's disease. These mutations occur in AβPP, the gene for amyloid-β protein precursor (AβPP); or in PSEN1 or PSEN2, genes for proteins that regulate the enzyme secretase, which is important in the cleavage of AβPP to produce the peptide amyloid-β (Aβ) [12].

APOEε4 is involved in the pathogenesis of AD through independent mechanisms involving neurovascular functions, synaptic plasticity, cholesterol homeostasis, and neuroinflammation. The presence of the APOE ε4 allele is thought to be one of the risk factors for AD; more specifically, it is linked to an increased risk of cerebral amyloid angiopathy and age-related cognitive decline during aging [13]. Mutations in the presenilin 1 (*PS1*) and *PS2* genes, as well as the amyloid precursor protein, are autosomal dominantly inherited (APP). An inheritable form of AD (familial Alzheimer's disease) is associated with disease onset before the age of 65 [14].

10.2 PATHOGENESIS OF DEMENTIA

The extracellular accumulation of senile plaques composed of Aβ peptide and intra-neuronal accumulation of neurofibrillary tangles (NFTs) composed of hyperphosphorylated microtubule-binding protein tau (p-tau) are the neuropathological hallmarks of AD. These pathologic indicators are strongly correlated with cognitive decline, neuronal degeneration, neuroinflammation, microglial activation, and malfunction of the Blood-Brain

Barrier (BBB) [15]. It has been observed that there is an alteration of cleavage of Amyloid Precursor Protein (APP), an integral protein on the plasma membrane, by β-secretases (BACE1) and γ-secretases to produce insoluble Aβ fibrils. After that, Aβ oligomerizes, diffuses into synaptic clefts, and disrupts synaptic signaling, leading to polymerization into insoluble amyloid fibrils resulting in aggregation into plaques. The clumps of plaques and tangles are followed by microglial recruitment surrounding plaques. This accelerates the microglial activation and local inflammatory reaction, contributing to neurotoxicity [16].

Dementia in PD is significantly more accurately predicted by the presence of both Lewy bodies and AD pathology than by the degree of either pathology alone. When cerebrospinal fluid biomarker patterns for individuals with dementia with Lewy bodies and Parkinson's disease dementia (PDD) were compared, it was discovered that lower levels of A1–42 (coupled with higher tau levels) are related to dementia with Lewy bodies rather than PDD and that this association is especially noticeable in patients with more quickly progressing dementia [17]. The regulation of α-synuclein aggregation, Lewy bodies production, and neuronal degeneration may be significantly influenced by posttranslational modification. Before the development of Lewy bodies pathology, higher levels of phosphorylated α-synuclein are present in the early stages of Parkinson's disease dementia/dementia with Lewy bodies (PDD/DLB). The severity of the disease is correlated with the level of phosphorylated α-synuclein. The existence of this "alpha-synucleinopathy" was identified as a typical pathological hallmark of Parkinson's disease, whether "sporadic" or "hereditary." The phrase "Hereditary PD" refers to the Mendelian variants of PD. However, the clinical presentations of these genetic illnesses differ from those of "typical" Parkinsonism, and in some cases are suggestive of atypical Parkinsonism [18].

It has been revealed that cerebrovascular disease may be related to dementia, including cerebral embolism caused by thrombotic or burst carotid plaques, targeting distal vessels, persistent cerebral hypoperfusion caused by major artery thrombosis, blood pressure issues that affect the Blood-Brain Barrier (BBB), elevated parenchymal oxidative stress, and inflammation. The distribution of nutrients and oxygen within the brain requires cerebral blood flow with a local metabolic rate. Because normal cerebral blood flow is essential for neuronal activity, disruption of Cerebral Blood Flow (CBF) can cause mortality and brain malfunction. The ability of cerebral blood vessels to maintain steady CBF throughout a wide range of blood pressures is a built-in feature of the blood vessels. This hemodynamic process, known as cerebral autoregulation, protects the brain from unwelcome variations in artery pressure brought on by activities of everyday living and maintains a constant CBF baseline. Studies have shown a significant connection between the development of VCI, CBF lowering, and cerebral endothelial dysfunction [19].

It has been proposed that an imbalance between Aβ production and Aβ clearance causes cerebral amyloid angiopathy. It is believed that this would cause a series of harmful alterations to the vessel walls, such as the loss of smooth muscle cells, which will result in microaneurysms, and fibroid necrosis of the vessel wall, which will cause poor blood flow and vessel fragility [20]. Damage to the limbic system, cortical regions, and signs of neuritis in the brainstem are all characteristics of PDD. Dopaminergic neurotransmission associated with motor circuits slows down as a result of dopaminergic neurons degenerating, which causes a reduction in dopamine in the synaptic cleft. Dopaminergic neurons present in the substantia nigra pars compacta deteriorate due to the enzyme monoamine oxidase, which causes abnormal metabolism of dopamine and the accumulation of toxic hydrogen peroxide [21].

It was revealed by some common findings that Apo-lipoprotein E (ApoE) was a common component of both neurofibrillary plaques and tangles. Apolipoprotein E primarily binds to β-amyloids and thus prevents the oxidative damage of neuronal-glial cells, preserving the integrity of the synaptic junctions. Meanwhile, ApoE, E3 form has been determined to have the highest affinity for tau cells; it inhibits the toxicity caused by amyloids and APP. However, an increased number of E4 were found in Alzheimer's disease. Because of this, it might not be able to stop the aberrant phosphorylation of tau [22].

While increasing mitochondrial Reactive Oxygen Species (ROS) production in the aging substantia nigra pars compacta (SNc) results from deterioration of physiological redox regulation, excessive ROS generation by mitochondria in the PD SNc is associated with severe Electron Transport Chain (ETC) impairment and oxidative damage caused by additional environmental toxins and pesticides, as well as genetic mutations. Many contributors to heightened oxidative stress in the PD SNc have been identified as drivers of nigral oxidative stress in healthy aging, implying that the etiology of PD may include aggravation of molecular mechanisms implicated in healthy aging [21].

Currently available pharmaceutical dementia treatments (Approved Synthetic and Semi-Synthetic Drugs) and recent interventions.

Worldwide, several (semi-)synthetic medications are accessible for the treatment of Alzheimer's disease and some kinds of dementia (Table 10.1). Currently, dementia has no cure. Pharmaceutical therapies aim to slow its progression and ease symptoms. Some of the most widely used therapeutics for Alzheimer's disease-associated dementia are selective, reversible acetylcholinesterase (AChE) inhibitor donepezil, the non-selective butyrylcholinesterase (BuChE) and AChE inhibitor rivastigmine, as well as the N-Methyl-D-aspartate (NMDA) receptor antagonist memantine. A few of these medications, such as semi-synthetic medication rivastigmine, are also approved to treat other kinds of dementia, such as PD-related dementia [23].

Pharmacologic dementia treatments with FDA approval for the use of allopathic drugs in the cognitive, global function, behavior/mood, and quality of life/daily living activities domains. The most popular medications accepted for therapeutic use in Alzheimer's disease and various types of dementia are listed in Table 10.1 [24].

Currently, some neuroleptic/antipsychotic medications, including haloperidol, risperidone, and olanzapine, are used to treat the behavioral and mental symptoms of dementia (BPSD); however, their use is controversial. Numerous research initiatives are focused on the prevention of pathogenesis, such as by directly reducing the Aβ aggregation, improving Aβ clearance, or preventing Aβ formation. Although preventing Aβ aggregation has proven to be difficult, numerous teams are still working to create tiny molecule inhibitors of this mechanism [24].

During the initial phases of the inflammatory response, the myeloid-specific enzyme myeloperoxidase (MPO), which is created and secreted by innate immune system cells, produces free radical species that encourage oxidative damage and result in lipid peroxidation. In the pathogenesis and progression of AD, oxidative damage to neurons and peroxidation of the highly polyunsaturated lipids in the post-mitotic stage of neurons also appear to be an early and crucial occurrence [25]. Potential targets for lowering inflammation include MPO and the oxidants and free radicals it produces. Doing so may also lower the likelihood of developing AD and slow the course of the illness. The current pharmacological option for treating AD involves cholinesterase inhibitors (ChEIs), which improve cholinergic transmission. APP, the protein precursor of amyloid, can be released more easily with the help of ChEIs [26].

A combination of disease-modifying and symptomatic treatments may be successful in the future for those who already have mild Alzheimer's disease symptoms. New symptomatic medications are still being developed. According to an analysis of the 2018 drug development pipeline for Alzheimer's disease,

TABLE 10.1 Recommended (Semi-)Synthetic Drugs Used for the Treatment of Dementia [24]

Drug	Indication	Mechanism of Action	Side-Effects	Half-Life	Recommended Dose per Day
Memantine	Moderate to severe AD, AD-related dementia. Dose adjustment is necessary for patients with moderate to severe renal impairment.	Memantine may reduce the quantity of calcium that enters nerve cells by binding to NMDA receptor sites.	Confusion, dizziness, constipation, and headache.	60–100 Hrs.	Once daily dosing.
Rivastigmine	Mild-to-moderate AD, AD-related dementia.	Slowly reversible, non-selective AChE and BuChE inhibitor.	Nausea, vomiting, loss of appetite. Increased bowl movement frequency.	2 Hrs. (BD dose)	20 mg
Galantamine	Mild-to-moderate AD, AD-related dementia.	Slowly reversible, non-selective AChE and BuChE inhibitor.	Renal and hepatic side effects.	3.5–4 hrs.	18 mg
Donepezil	Mild to moderate dementia.	Reversible, selective AChE inhibitor.	Nausea, vomiting, Anorexia.	70 hrs.	10 mg

the majority of substances now being evaluated in clinical trials have disease-modifying capabilities (63% spanning Phases 1 to 3), followed by cognitive enhancers (23%), and medications intended to treat BPSD (12%) [27]. Aripiprazole is one of the drugs that is used for controlling BPSD. In patients with advanced illness and frailty, it has demonstrated a good safety profile of aripiprazole when compared to other antipsychotics. As a result, aripiprazole has become more significant in current therapy strategies for dementia patients because of its effectiveness in reducing agitation and aggressiveness quickly [28].

The FDA-approved treatments for AD, which are only for AD as of 2021, focus on the neurochemical communication channels involved in learning and memory but not the actual disease. For mild to moderate stages of Alzheimer's dementia, the FDA has approved AChEIs, galantamine hydrobromide, and rivastigmine, while donepezil HCL is approved for mild to severe stages. AChEIs work by inhibiting the enzyme that breaks down acetylcholine, making up for the loss of cholinergic neurons that control memory [29].

Memantine prevents excess glutamate from activating the NMDA receptor and the associated excitotoxicity by inhibiting the NMDA (N-methyl-d-aspartate) receptor. Alzheimer's dementia in its intermediate to advanced stages may be treated with the donepezil and memantine combination [30]. Aducanumab, an amyloid beta-directed monoclonal antibody, was given accelerated clearance by the FDA in June 2021 for the treatment of early Alzheimer's disease. It is believed to stop beta-amyloid from forming plaques and to make it easier for it to be removed from the brain. The most frequent adverse effects included headache, falls, diarrhea, changed mental status, Amyloid-Associated Imaging Abnormalities (ARIA), linked transient swelling in certain brain regions, and headache. For the medicine to be approved more quickly, additional research must be done to demonstrate that it can stop the development of MCI symptoms. According to FDA guidelines, aducanumab must be taken intravenously to cross the blood-brain barrier, where it binds to amyloid and eliminates it with the aid of microglia from the immune system. The FDA advises a gradual (6-week) titration to a therapeutic dosage of 10 mg/kg given over roughly an hour every 4 weeks. Before receiving the seventh and twelfth infusions, a patient must undergo Magnetic Resonance Imaging (MRI) if they exhibit symptoms that point to cerebral enlargement such as ARIA [31]. The efficacy and tolerability of various potential monoclonal antibodies against amyloid, such as donanemab, gantenerumab, solanezumab, and crenezumab, are now being investigated in phase III trials [32].

Floral ozone reduces neuronal cell death, increases synaptic structural plasticity, and has therapeutic promise for VaD. It might be related to transient receptor potential melastatin-related 2 (TRPM2)/N-Methyl-D-aspartate receptor (NMDAR) pathways in the hippocampus. It has been found that Floral ozone (50, 100, 150 mg/kg) dose-dependently alleviated the pathological changes, and decreased oxidative stress injury, which eventually reduced cognitive impairment in BCCAO rats [33].

Mevidalen is a selective positive allosteric modulator (PAM) that acts on dopamine receptor D1. Mevidalen uses a new mode of action that simultaneously improves or stabilizes non-motor symptoms related to conventional dopaminergic therapy while alleviating or stabilizing motor symptoms related to LBD [34].

Vascular Cognitive Disorder (VCD) risk is doubled with diabetes. The common pathology between diabetes and VCI is cerebrovascular dysfunction. It has been hypothesized that improvement of endothelial function in diabetes prevents micro-emboli-mediated white matter injury. By enhancing endothelial integrity, pharmacological treatment with Isosorbide Mononitrate/Cilostazol (ISMN/CZL) before micro-embolic injection protected the diabetic rats from the latter's potentially harmful effects, making it a workable preventative and maybe curative strategy for VCD [35].

Brexpiprazole is an atypical antipsychotic that was authorized by the US FDA in July 2015 and the EU in July 2018 for the treatment of schizophrenia. It is now being investigated for Alzheimer's disease-related agitation. Brexpiprazole is frequently referred to as a third-generation antipsychotic due to its partial D2 agonist action, however when compared to other third-generation antipsychotics, it has less intrinsic activity at the D2 receptor and a stronger binding affinity to 5-HT2A, 5-HT1A, and alpha-1B receptors (aripiprazole, cariprazine). Brexpiprazole, as compared to a placebo, delayed the time to relapse in individuals with schizophrenia, according to the findings of three long-term clinical trials (EQUATOR, ZENITH, and a Japanese extension study), and was linked to ongoing improvement in symptoms and general functioning. Two 12-week, randomized, double-blind, placebo-controlled trials on the efficacy and safety of brexpiprazole for the treatment of agitation in Alzheimer's dementia were carried out. In this trial, on the basis of evidence, it was concluded that brexpiprazole 2 mg/day has the potential to be efficacious, safe, and well-tolerated in the treatment of agitation in Alzheimer's dementia [36].

The use of specialized nutritional supplements in the daily diet, dietary behavior adjustments (such as consuming more of or avoiding certain food categories or beverages), and adherence to complete dietary patterns are all examples of nutritional preventative interventions. Animal models, observational research, and clinical trials all provide proof that nutrition is a crucial, changeable component that affects cognitive performance throughout the course of a person's lifetime [37]. Folate has been tested as a solo intervention, and after 6 months, MCI patients have reported cognitive improvements in general intelligence, attention span, and visuospatial measures [38]. Before dietary components may be included in suggested therapeutic guidelines, bigger, well-designed trials are required to confirm the preliminary positive benefits of folate, vitamin E, omega-3 fatty acids, and several multi-nutrient formulations [37].

Ferroptosis inhibition may help to improve neuronal discrimination and cognitive decline, as ferrostatin-1 also markedly improved cognitive impairment in Vascular Dementia (VaD) rats. Therefore, by suppressing neuronal ferroptosis, GAS can be utilized as an addition to prevent and treat cognitive impairment and can also serve as the foundational component of *G. elata* functional foods [38].

Atomoxetine (2 mg kg^{-1}/4 mg kg^{-1}) and N-acetylcysteine (250 mg kg^{-1}/500 mg kg^{-1}) were used alone as well as in combination were reported to attenuate the memory impairment and behavioral changes in diabetic rats (induced by streptozotocin). It has also been observed that co-treatment of Atomoxetine and N-acetylcysteine was better in comparison to the doses when given alone. As a precursor to glutathione, N-acetylcysteine, an acetylated derivative of cysteine, exhibits antioxidant and anti-inflammatory properties. N-acetylcysteine penetrates the BBB, by which glutathione (GSH) concentration in the brain increases, thereby preventing neuronal damage, degeneration, impaired memory, and cognition that occurs as a result of excitotoxic damage and oxidative stress [39].

MCC950 has been found to ameliorate dementia symptoms at an early age in line M83 mice and reduce hippocampal α-synuclein accumulation. MCC950 was found to inhibit inflammation by directly targeting the NLRP3 ATP-hydrolysis motif. Furthermore, in mice treated with MPTP, 6-OHDA, or α-synuclein PFF, MCC950 protects nigrostriatal dopaminergic neurodegeneration and behavioral impairments [40].

Tacrine works against monoamines and ion channels in addition to being a centrally acting cholinesterase inhibitor. Adrian Albert at the University of Sydney synthesized it for the first time in 1945, and it is now used to treat Alzheimer's disease. It is marketed under the brand name Cognex. Another mechanism of action acts as an inhibitor of histamine N-methyltransferase. Tacrine, according to the PASS, demonstrates better antiviral activity (74.1%) or can be used as a respiratory analeptic (68.4%), but it has poor cholinesterase activity (48.2%) and low activity for treating Alzheimer's disease (41.2%). Velnacrine is a derivative of tacrine and was also used to treat Alzheimer's disease; however, due to the drug's toxicity, the FDA

Advisory Council on Peripheral Drugs and CNS Drugs suggested discontinuing all research regarding this drug in 1994. However, this drug has only minimal efficacy for treating Alzheimer's disease (50.1%), the same efficacy as an acetylcholinesterase inhibitor [41].

The Food and Drug Administration (FDA) recently approved the selective 5-hydroxytryptophan (5-HT) 2A receptor inverse agonist pimavanserin for the treatment of psychosis in PD. It doesn't have significant effects on dopamine or histamine receptors; thus it doesn't have the motor or sedative side effects that are frequently linked to other antipsychotic drugs. Pimavanserin increases the risk of death in older individuals with dementia, similar to other groups of antipsychotic medications. Pimavanserin is now the subject of a phase 3 clinical investigation sponsored by the National Institute on Aging for the recurrence of dementia-related psychosis. Patients with dementia with Lewy bodies, PDD, or other dementias may qualify for the trial if they have been experiencing psychotic symptoms for at least two months and are taking memantine or a cholinesterase inhibitor at a stable dose [42].

Zonisamide is an anticonvulsant drug that inhibits the release of glutamate and carbonic anhydrase as well as sodium and T-type calcium channels. It has received approval in Japan to treat PD [43]. A Phase II clinical trial was conducted on zonisamide as an adjuvant to levodopa in treating the parkinsonism associated with dementia with Lewy bodies for its efficacy and safety. For patients with young-onset PD, dopamine agonist drugs like pramipexole and ropinirole are frequently administered since they are thought to have a lower risk of developing drug-induced motor fluctuations than levodopa. Levodopa, however, is preferred over dopamine agonist drugs in dementia with Lewy bodies due to the agonists' higher tendency to result in hallucinations and sleepiness [44].

CZ-7, a new derivative of *Claulansine F* was found to significantly improve the cognitive deficits induced by chronic cerebral hypoperfusion in rats. The proposed mechanism demonstrated that the neuroprotective effect of CZ-7 (20 mg/kg) significantly improved the surviving pyramid cells of the CA1–CA3 area of the hippocampus of 2VO rats, improved brain white matter injury, diminished the cellular levels of 8-OHdG and ROS, and boosted the antioxidant capacity by upregulating HO-1 and NQO1 through Nrf2 activation. These kinds of pathologies were observed in vascular dementia [45].

It was revealed that ladostigil has a beneficial effect on dementia by blocking the brain's acetylcholinesterase (AChE), butyrylcholinesterase (BuChE), monoamine oxidase (MAO) A and B, and monoamine oxidase (MAO) A and B. Furthermore, it can restore memory deficits, by which this drug can increase cholinergic activity in the brain. Furthermore, it has been noted that ladostigil boosts the expression of neurotrophic factors such as brain-derived neurotrophic factor (BDNF) and glial cell line-derived neurotrophic factor (GDNF). In addition, ladostigil might have the power to reverse the harm that neurogenesis-induced problems do to neurons [46].

10.3 NON-PHARMACOLOGICAL APPROACHES FOR DEMENTIA

A non-pharmacological or behavioral intervention (Figure 10.1) aims to maintain or improve a person's cognitive performance, allow them to carry out their regular daily activities, and/or treat behavioral symptoms that frequently accompany memory loss (e.g., depression, wandering, sleep, agitation, or aggression) [47].

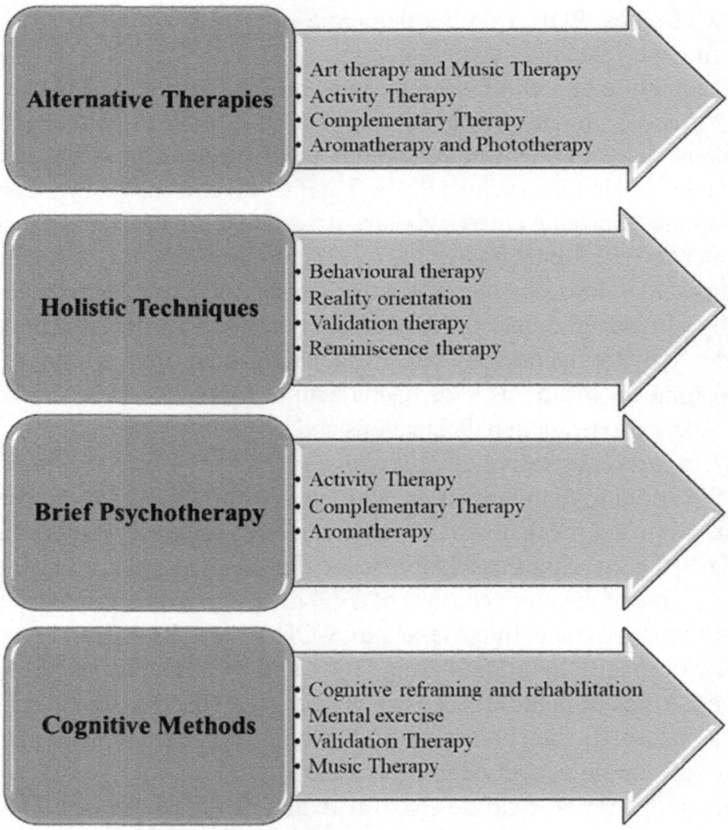

FIGURE 10.1 Non-pharmacological approaches for dementia.

Source: Adapted from Ref. [48]

Since there is no effective long-term pharmacologic treatment for cognitive impairment, experts, people who have been diagnosed, their families, and caregivers are looking for assistance and support in coping with the illness. Professionals and caretakers are particularly looking for methods to deal with BPSD. About 80% of people with cognitive impairment will suffer from BPSD at some point during their chronic illness. Non-pharmacologic therapies are therefore starting to become a viable alternative method for not only treating BPSD but also improving the quality of life for the dementia patient and their care partners [48].

It is becoming more widely accepted that non-pharmacological methods should always be sought first and that pharmacological therapies for dementia should only be used as a last resort. Medicines used in treating dementia do not stop the progression of dementia but, in some cases, can slow it down. The National Institute for Health and Care Excellence (NICE) examined the clinical guidelines of dementia that support people with dementia and their caregivers in health and social care. Some non-pharmacological approaches are listed in Figure 10.1.

10.4 NON-PHARMACOLOGICAL APPROACH FOR COGNITIVE TREATMENT

Non-pharmacological Cognitive Enhancement (NPCE) is recommended following techniques for cognitive treatment (Figure 10.2) [50].

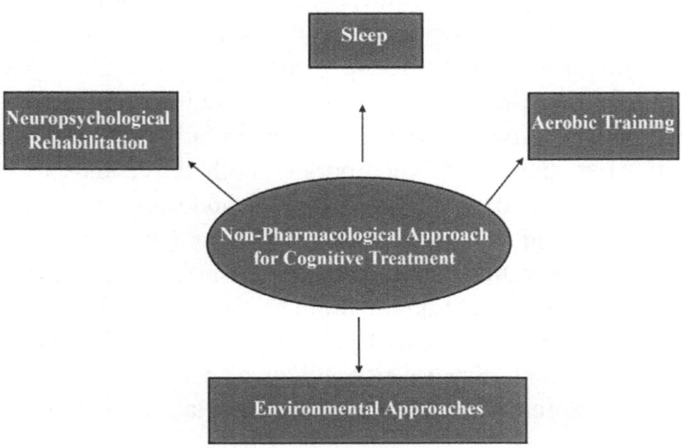

FIGURE 10.2 Techniques for cognitive treatment.

Source: Adapted from Ref. [50]

10.4.1 COMPLEMENTARY AND ALTERNATIVE MEDICINE FOR BPSD

Over the last decade, complementary and alternative medicine (CAM) has grown in popularity and has been utilized to treat a variety of illnesses, including dementia. The main types of CAM are:

- Aromatherapy;
- Music therapy;
- Art therapy;
- Massage;
- Touch.

These NPTs fall within the broad category of sensorial stimulation techniques, or treatments intended to arouse patients' senses [51]. Among CAM, aromatherapy is more familiar to consumers. Pure essential oils from aromatic plants are used in aromatherapy, a branch of phytotherapy, to treat health issues and enhance the quality of life. Essential oils have a wide range of possible effects, including the facilitation of sleep and relaxation and the reduction of pain and depressive symptoms [52]. People with cognitive disorders, those who are confused, or those who have trouble communicating verbally may find aromatherapy to be a helpful remedy, especially if current conventional medication is only partially helpful. Indeed, BPSD, disturbances in sleep, and stimulation of motivational behavior have been treated using aromatherapy [53]. Using music or sound as a nonverbal communication tool, music therapy (MT) can have educational, rehabilitative, or therapeutic impacts on a variety of diseases, including dementia. The majority of music-based therapies involve singing, listening, improvising, or playing musical instruments along with the group or individual patients [54]. MT can be classified into active and passive intervention. Which style of intervention can be more beneficial in dementia is still unknown because the majority of studies on MT incorporated both active and passive strategies [55]. The value and advantages of music and music therapy programs for older persons, and more specifically for those with dementia, are well established in the literature. It has been shown by some studies that sound can have a significant impact on the brain by triggering a variety of cortical and subcortical regions, especially the limbic and paralimbic areas involved in processing emotions. From a psychological perspective, music encourages emotional expression, communication in relationships, and relational processes [53].

According to the American Art Therapy Association (AATA), art therapy is a mental health profession where clients work with a therapist to explore their emotions, resolve emotional conflicts, foster self-awareness, manage behavior and addictions, develop social skills, enhance reality orientation, lessen anxiety, and boost self-esteem through the creation of artwork. According to some experts, patients with right cerebral hemisphere impairment may exhibit abnormal emotional behavior, and engaging in creative activities can control mood by having an impact on this hemisphere [55]. It was observed that using coloring crayons or inks in small groups of patients with mild dementia who were asked to color realistic images of cats, birds, and fruits rather than abstract ones. They were also encouraged to recall and paint happy memories from the past. The control group was asked to perform calculations as much as possible within an acceptable range. The strategy considerably improved mental health and the symptoms of indifference, but it did not affect depression or cognitive function, which was probably related to the intervention's brief duration (just 12 weeks) and small sample size [56].

A relaxation response is elicited by massage/touch therapy, a potential non-pharmacological therapeutic. This reaction lessens the agitation brought on by elevated worry and stress, which have a negative impact on the autonomic nervous system. The C-tactile afferent stimulation that occurs during affective tactile encounters mediates the release of oxytocin. According to research, oxytocin helps dementia patients with their behavioral and social cognitive symptoms [57]. The results of a meta-analysis of 11 RCTs indicated that touch and massage interventions may have a significant impact on verbally aggressive, physically aggressive, and non-aggressive behavior; however, the small sample size and poor quality of the included studies prevent us from drawing any firm conclusions about the impact on BPSD or offering any practical advice for clinical practice [58].

Patients with dementia frequently experience interrupted or disturbed sleep. Sleep disruption is closely linked to feelings of well-being, health, emotion control, productivity and performance, memory and cognitive abilities, and social interaction. Elderly people with dementia may experience sleep disturbances for a variety of reasons, including physical and psychological ones like loneliness, anxiety, discomfort, incontinence, hunger, and constipation, as well as environmental ones like noise, light, and temperature. It has been revealed by the clinical findings that inhalation aromatherapy containing any of piperonal, santol, linalool, or cedrol may improve difficulties in maintaining sleep in elderly persons with dementia [59].

Acupuncture has been used for numerous disorders in Asian countries for hundreds of years and is a common kind of traditional Chinese medicine with few adverse effects on stroke recovery. Usually, 15–30% of stroke survivors experience vascular dementia within three months, and 20–25% experience delayed dementia over time as a result of recurrent stroke. It was indicated in clinical findings that acupuncture could defend neurons in animal models of vascular dementia through enhanced oxygen and glucose metabolism, as well as antioxidant and anti-apoptosis effects [60].

Yoga is a mind-body activity that has its roots in ancient India and is recognized by the National Center for Complementary and Integrative Health as a complementary health strategy. Yoga has advantages for both physical and mental health, as well as for cognitive performance. According to a recent meta-analysis, yoga has a significant impact on memory, executive function, attention, and processing speed, among other areas of cognitive performance in healthy individuals. Around 87 older individuals without dementia participated in a randomized yoga trial at senior housing. They discovered that practicing yoga for six months (including physical postures, breathing exercises, and meditation) significantly enhanced one's short- and long-term verbal memory, short- and long-term visual memory, attention, and processing speed [61]. It was revealed in one study that yoga-plus improved cognitive, affective, ADL, and physical functions in a local elderly population, particularly among below-baseline individuals, indicating the benefits of dementia prevention among elderly individuals [62].

10.4.2 NEW TECHNOLOGIES OF NPI FOR DEMENTIA

An increasing number of studies investigating new technologies' effects on dementia have been conducted as a result of the accessibility of new technologies, their widespread use, and, for some of them, their relatively low cost. Based on the evidence, it can be as follows:

- Application of information and communication technologies (ICT);
- Assistive device;
- Domotics;
- Virtual reality;
- Telemedicine to monitor people with dementia.

ICT, including computational devices, robotics, machine learning algorithms, the miniaturization of sensors and technologies, as well as the decreased costs of these devices, has increased the availability of intelligent devices and technology-embedded environments to support dementia patients and their caregivers in their daily lives and to assess the severity and progression of the disease [63]. A key focus of research is the development of tools that allow individuals with dementia to safely and securely remain outdoors. One of the most advanced areas of ICT research in dementia is tracking systems that utilize the global positioning system (GPS) to track the patient's location and locate them if they become lost [64].

Inertial measurement units (IMUs), a type of wearable sensor technology, have introduced a new method for identifying and monitoring the "quantity" and "quality" of movement and physical activity in individuals with various neurological conditions, including dementia. IMUs worn by patients have been utilized to capture their movement patterns and measure their walking and turning movements using acceleration and angular velocity signals [65]. Agitation is one of the most challenging symptoms for caregivers to address, and ICT can be utilized to evaluate it. ICT applications are rapidly expanding to support clinical and assistive activities in dementia patients, but obstacles to successful implementation include a lack of complete clinical validation and insufficient attention to patient needs. To facilitate the translation of medical engineering research into clinical practice, clinicians, and stakeholders involved in the implementation and management of dementia care through ICT applications should collaborate [66].

Virtual reality (VR) is a combination of technologies that are used to examine the nature of interactions with various environments and virtual environments, as well as to increase memory capacity. VR provides an efficient, secure, and engaging technique for treating people with impairments by combining traditional therapies that call for repetitive training to enhance cognitive and motor skills with computer simulation VR-based procedures. VR can provide perceivable data for human senses, such as visual and auditory stimuli, and maintain well-known features of the real world, such as space and time. VR holds great promise for psychological intervention in general and, more specifically, for the treatment of dementia, which can enhance the quality of life for those who have the disease [67].

Domotics, house automation, and smart homes are phrases that are frequently used interchangeably to refer to the integration of technology and appliances to enhance comfort and functionality in the home. Although domotics was first developed to automate jobs, the diversity of potential applications, coupled with internet access, could significantly improve understanding and management of Parkinson's dementia, resulting in improved clinical decision-making [68].

Telemedicine is a term used to describe a method of delivering healthcare remotely using telecommunications technologies. New options for interventions to raise the caliber and accessibility of healthcare are made possible by technology. Since dementia is a chronic illness with problems requiring ongoing long-term care and having restricted access to medical care, telemedicine may be an effective way to examine and treat dementia patients at home. Follow-up treatment using telemedicine can assist persons with dementia to keep their independence, stay in their own homes, increase their safety, and improve clinical results and access to medical services [69].

10.5 STRATEGIES FOR PREVENTION OF DEMENTIA

On the basis of randomized controlled trials, systematic reviews, meta-analyses, observational studies in humans, and relevant work in model organisms, the relationship between prevention strategies and the progression of diseases is depicted in Figure 10.3 [70].

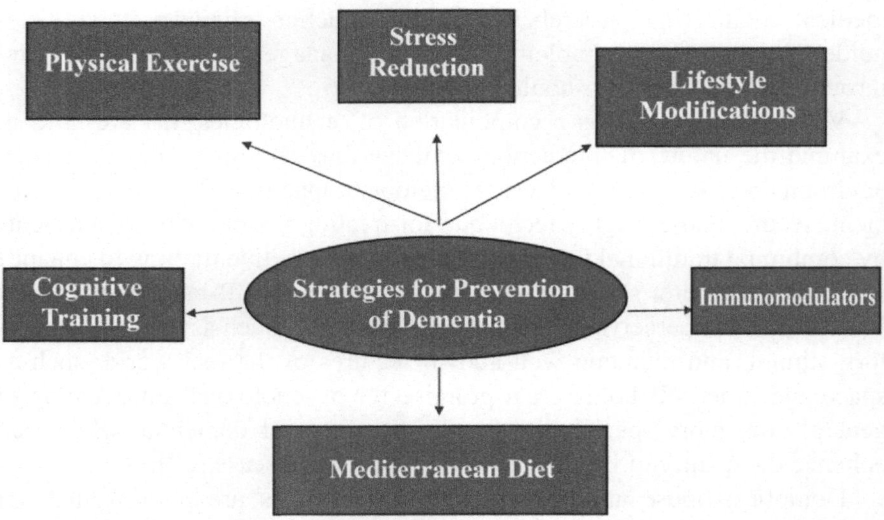

FIGURE 10.3 Strategies for the prevention of dementia.

10.6 MEDICINAL PLANTS AND NATURAL DRUGS USED FOR THE TREATMENT OF DEMENTIA

Modern research on dementia shows that dementia is a complicated disease with various molecular processes implicated in its etiology, which makes it particularly difficult to treat. This insight led to the development of a new paradigm for treating various pathologies: treatments for dementia should focus on numerous underlying biological targets rather than just one. Likewise, a variety of compounds found in plants and plant extracts are thought to act on various molecular targets in an additive or even synergistic manner. Already, many herbal medications are used to treat dementia [71].

10.6.1 PLANTS FROM THE AMARYLLIDACEAE FAMILY

One of the most significant alkaloid-containing plant taxa is the Amaryllidoideae subfamily of the Amaryllidaceae. There are more than 800 perennial bulb species in 59 genera, which are found across the tropics and subtropics. The Amaryllidoideae subfamily's distinctive chemotaxonomic characteristic is the Amaryllidaceae alkaloids [72]. The plants from the Amaryllidaceae family that has reported medicinal activity in dementia are *Ammocharis coranica, Boophone disticha, and Crinum moorei Hook.f (Syn. Crinum imbricatum Baker), Scadoxus multiflorus, Crinum macowanii Bake, Galanthus woronowii, Galanthus alpinus, Leucojum aestivum, Lycoris radiate, Narcissus* spp. [24], *Nerine bowdenii* [73], *Ismene amancaes* (Ker Gawl.) Herb. [74].

10.6.2 PLANTS FROM THE PAPAVERACEAE FAMILY

A family of dicotyledonous flowering plants known as Papaveraceae, which belongs to the Ranunculales order, has roughly 775 species and 42 genera that are primarily found in the Northern Hemisphere [75]. The plants from the Papaveraceae family that has reported medicinal activity in dementia are *Corydalis cava, Corydalis intermedia, Corydalis solida* [24], *Argemone players* [76], *Glaucium corniculatum* [77].

10.6.3 PLANTS FROM THE ZINGIBERACEAE FAMILY

An abundant source of many bioactive phytochemicals is the Zingiberaceae family. Around 52 genera and 1,300 species of aromatic blooming perennial herbs with distinctive creeping horizontal or tuberous rhizomes make up the majority of its species [78]. The plants from the Zingiberaceae family that has reported medicinal activity in dementia are *Curcuma longa, Alpinia galangal, Alpinia hainanensis, Alpinia officinarum* [79], *Curcuma caesia* [80], *Zingiber officinale* [81], *Kaempferia parviflora*. [82].

10.6.4 PLANTS FROM THE LAMIACEAE FAMILY

The Lamiaceae family contains 236 genera and 6,900–7,200 species. Numerous beneficial medicinal plants are found in the Lamiaceae or Labiatae. The plants from the Lamiaceae family that has reported medicinal activity in dementia are *Thymus vulgaris, Salvia miltiorrhiza, Salvia lavandulifolia, Rosmarinus officinalis, Rosmarinus officinalis, Origanum vulgare, Origanum majorana, Ocimum basilicum, Mentha spicata, Melissa officinalis* [24] *Lavender Officinalis. Lavender latifolia, Lavender stoechas, Lavender angustifolia* [83], *Salvia miltiorrhiza* [84], *Dracoephalum moldavica* [85].

10.6.5 PLANTS FROM THE APIACEAE FAMILY

The approximately 3,600–3,751 plant species in the 455 genera of the Apiaceae family are frequently used as spices [86]. The plants from Apiaceae family having reported medicinal activity in dementia are *Petroselinum crispum, Ferula gummosa, Coriandrum sativum, Carum carvi, Bupleurum* species, *Angelica species, Angelica archangelica, Angelica sinensis* [24], *Smyrnium olusatrum* [87], *Pimpinella anisum* [88], *Anthriscus nemorosa* [89].

10.6.6 PLANTS FROM THE SOLANACEAE FAMILY

The Solanaceae rank as one of the most important to human beings among angiosperm families. Approximately 90 genera and 3,000–4,000 species make up the medium-sized family, with over half of them belonging to the many and diversified genus Solanum. Solanum is fascinating from an evolutionary perspective as well as for its utility to humans because this hyperdiversity in one genus is uncommon in angiosperms [90]. The plants from the Solanaceae family that have reported medicinal activity in dementia are *Nicotiana species, Acnistus arborescens,* and *Withania somnifera* [91].

10.6.7 PLANTS FROM THE FABACEAE FAMILY

The Fabaceae plant family with 770 genera and 19,500 species is the most diversified in the entire plant kingdom, ranking behind the Asteraceae and Orchidaceae as the largest angiosperm family in terms of species numbers [92]. The plants from the Fabaceae family having reported medicinal activity in dementia are *Barbieria pinnata, Cassia lucens, Clitoria ternatea, Medicago sativa* [24], *Glycyrrhiza glabra* [93], *Peltophorum pterocarpum* [94], *Sophora secundiflora Sophora tomentosa* [95], *Vigna subterranea* [96], *Astragalus mongholicus* [97], *Daniellia oliveri* [98], *Acacia auriculiformis* [99].

10.6.8 PLANTS FROM THE RUTACEAE FAMILY

The Rutaceae family has the highest number of species in the Sapindales order, mostly in (sub)tropical areas with 162 genera and about 2,085 species. The family is widely spread throughout the Americas, with 51 genera and 412–415 species, the majority of which are found in tropical America, where there are 48 genera (46 of which are indigenous to this area) and 350–400 species [100]. The plants from the Rutaceae family that has reported medicinal activity in dementia are *Toddalia asiatica* [101], *Zanthoxylum bungeanum* [102], *Melicope species* [103], and *Citrus sinensis* [104].

10.7 NUTRITIONAL CARE IN PATIENTS WITH DEMENTIA

Nutritional care refers to the support given to dementia patients living at home to ensure a sufficient intake of calories, protein, and other nutrients. There is growing evidence that combinations of foods and nutrients may work synergistically to offer benefits that are greater than those conferred by combinations of individual dietary components. Several studies have explored the impact of dietary patterns on late-life cognition. Lower cognitive deterioration and incident AD have been linked to higher adherence to the Mediterranean diet pattern [105].

Supplements and dietary elements that may have an impact on AD and cognitive decline are as follows. Omega-3 polyunsaturated fatty acids (omega-3 PUFAs) are frequently regarded as a promising non-medical alternative to enhance brain functioning and reduce the advancement of dementia. Omega-3 PUFAs are found in fish and plants [106]. Polyunsaturated fatty acids (PUFAs) are essential parts of the membranes of neuronal cells because they keep the membranes fluid during synaptic communication. Docosahexaenoic acid (DHA), eicosapentaenoic acid (EPA), and omega-3 long-chain polyunsaturated fatty acids (n–3 LC-PUFAs) enhance neuronal transmission and control neuronal membrane excitability, boosting memory and learning in healthy individuals [107]. Additionally, new research indicates that n–3 PUFA can influence innate immunity in MCI patients by causing macrophages to polarize to an intermediate M1–M2 phenotype that enhances A phagocytosis [108].

Vitamin D may play a role in the prevention and treatment of diseases like dementia and AD, according to evidence from animal and cellular research. Vitamin D is thought to have a variety of activities across the central nervous system. Although reverse causality is still a possibility, cross-sectional and case-control studies have shown that vitamin D concentrations are lower in people with dementia and cognitive impairment. Low vitamin D levels have been linked to an increased risk of cognitive deterioration and all-cause dementia, according to a small number of longitudinal studies [109]. It is thought that vitamin D lowers the amount of beta-amyloid produced in the brain. Hypercalcemia as a result of vitamin D administration is a potential side effect. No cognitive enhancement was seen when vitamin D treatment doses were increased. It is thought that excess calcium from excessive vitamin D administration has more negative impacts on cognition than positive ones [110].

1. **Curcumin:** The bioactive turmeric compound curcumin, which is derived from the powdered rhizome of *Curcuma longa* Linn, exhibits intriguing biological benefits due to its anti-inflammatory, antioxidant, and anticancer characteristics. Recent research shows that curcumin protects against brain ischemia damage and apoptosis [111]. Curcumin has been found to significantly reduce the spatial memory deficit and stimulate the function of cholinergic neurons in mice; this progress was linked with the inhibition of NF-kappa B signaling pathways and enhanced transcription by PPAR-gamma [112]. Highly absorbable curcumin decreases the buildup of amyloid and tau in persons without cognitive impairment, which may help with memory and concentration [113].
2. **Resveratrol:** It has been found to reduce MDA levels, boost SOD activity, change the expression of apoptotic proteins, and significantly improve cognitive impairment in VaD rats. The suppression of the apoptotic pathway and oxidative stress injury may be directly related to the mechanism behind its neuroprotective properties. In VaD rats, resveratrol has been found to possess anti-apoptotic characteristics as evidenced by the hippocampal expression of Bcl-2 being elevated and the hippocampal expression of Bax and caspase-3 being lowered [114].

3. **Cocoa and Cocoa-Derived Products:** It has been recognized that the cocoa bean is a significant source of flavonoids, particularly the flavanols subclass in the form of epicatechin and catechin. In addition to these useful components, chocolate also includes theobromine, caffeine, and methylxanthine, which may have an impact on neuro-cognitive function [115]. Memory and executive function have been shown to improve significantly after consumption of intermediate dosages of cocoa flavanols with a dose of 500–750 mg/day [116]. The majority of research supports cocoa flavanols' positive effects on cognitive function and neuroplasticity in young adults, indicating that consuming cocoa powder or products with high cocoa flavanol content may be a useful and reasonable preventive measure against neurodegenerative diseases and cognitive decline. Additionally, short- and medium-term impacts of daily cocoa consumption may improve verbal learning, memory, and attention in young adults, supporting academic success [117].
4. **Magnesium:** Experimental and *in-vitro* studies have demonstrated the active involvement of magnesium (Mg) in degenerative neurological disorders. Mg participates in critical pathways including the stability and control of intracellular calcium, the N-methyl-d-aspartate (NMDA)-receptor response to excitatory amino acids, and cell membrane fluidity. Additionally, several research studies have hinted that Mg may have a neuroprotective effect on synaptic function [118]. Higher magnesium consumption was linked to a lower chance of developing mild cognitive impairment and mild cognitive disorders, according to the PATH through Life Projects. According to a Japanese study, incidences of vascular dementia and all-cause dementia are lower the more magnesium is consumed [119].
5. **Microbiota and Butyrate:** The human microbiota is made up of a variety of microorganisms, including bacteria, archaea, viruses, and protozoa. The study of these microbes is one of the most active areas of biomedical research. The gut microbiota is known to generate vitamins, intestinal toxins, and intestinal neurotransmitters including GABA, acetylcholine, dopamine, or serotonin, and to affect nerve signaling, with a focus on the vagus nerve. Additionally, gut dysbiosis affects metabolic pathways important for the onset of Alzheimer's disease by impairing the synthesis of signaling proteins [120].

6. **Histamine:** A neurotransmitter that reduces tumor necrosis factor-alpha expression in the brain and functions as a neuromodulator of neuroinflammation, can be produced by *Lactobacillus, Lactococcus, Streptococcus*, and *Enterococcus* [121]. Similar to this, other bacterial taxa such as *Bacillus, Lactobacillus*, and *Bifidobacterium* are capable of synthesizing neurotransmitters such as gamma-aminobutyric acid, serotonin, norepinephrine, and acetylcholine that are involved in the regulation of memory and learning function [122]. Tryptophan metabolism-related metabolic byproducts may also encourage neuronal oxidative stress, cell death, tau phosphorylation, and tangle formation [121].
7. **Dietary-Advanced Glycation End Products (d-AGEs):** Dietary advanced glycation end products (dAGEs) are complex, heterogeneous chemicals that are created during industrial processing and home cooking by nonenzymatic glycation processes [123]. There is significant water loss and the deterioration of heat-sensitive micronutrients, including vitamin C, folates, and thiamine, when high heat is applied over an extended length of time. Additionally, those reactions contribute to the development of harmful byproducts called advanced glycation end products (AGEs) [124]. The nuclear factor-kB (NF-κB) pathway and inflammatory mediators including tumor necrosis factor (TNF), interleukin-6, and C-reactive protein are activated as a result of the interaction between RAGE receptors and AGEs. Recently, different studies reported that a raised serum level of AGEs is linked with a faster rate of cognitive decline [124].
8. **Coffee and Caffeine:** Coffee is a rich source of polyphenols. Caffeine pharmacologically acts as an adenosine A_1 and A_{2A} receptor antagonist, and these receptors are generally distributed throughout the central and peripheral nervous system [125]. An inverse relationship between coffee consumption and the occurrence of cognitive diseases (Alzheimer's disease, dementia, cognitive decline, and cognitive impairment) was found in a meta-analysis of prospective studies comprising 34,282 people. The risk was shown to be lowest at a daily intake of 1–2 cups of coffee [126].

Caffeine has well-known anti-inflammatory characteristics that include reducing the invasion of immune cells from the periphery, attenuating pro-inflammatory mediators, and inhibiting microglia activation. Higher plasma caffeine concentrations were associated with lower levels of inflammatory cytokines in the hippocampal region [127]. A recent finding suggested that caffeine has positive effects on cognitive function and dementia risk, and these effects depend on the type of caffeine source (e.g., coffee and green tea have more effects), the amount consumed (more effects with moderate amounts), and the gender of the subject, i.e., more effects are seen in female subjects [128].

A regular diet rich in sufficient polyphenols, antioxidants, and polyunsaturated fatty acids can delay the onset of chronic neurodegenerative diseases. The inflammatory system, cell signaling molecules, apoptosis, and gene expression linked to many neurodegenerative illnesses can all be impacted by diet. The nutrients in a balanced diet lessen the risk of dementia, stop motor neurons from dying, and may relieve symptoms in those with chronic degenerative disorders [129].

10.8 RECENT MEDICAL APPROACHES IN DEMENTIA

A meta-analysis on Rho-associated kinase (ROCK) and phosphodiesterase-5 (PDE-5) has shown positive results for enhancing cognitive impairment, and many factors share both of these pathways. NO/cGMP is adjusted downward as a result of ROCK's suppression of eNOS and PDE-5's suppression of NO. Additionally, they are related in several ways that can influence neuroinflammatory reactions, including MCP-1, NF-kB, and VCAM-1. *In vivo* and *in vitro* studies supported the improvement of the cGMP pathway and an improvement in mice's cognitive performance after ROCK or PDE-5 inhibition [130].

Recently, a study on Sweroside has shown that sweroside reduced scopolamine-induced anxiety and memory deficits in the zebrafish model. The mechanism was reducing brain oxidative stress and AChE activity, which ultimately improved cholinergic neurotransmission and cognitive function. Sweroside was found to be a possible anti-amnesic candidate in zebrafish for the first time in this study, adding more evidence for its potential use in the treatment of dementia-related diseases [131].

Angiopoietin-1 Mimetic Peptide (AV-001) was found to improve cognition and reduce white matter injury in middle-aged rats subjected to multiple microinfarct (MMI) models of VaD in a dose-dependent manner. Treatment of MMI with 1 μg/kg AV-001 has been found to improve axon density, remyelination, and neuroplasticity in the brain of middle-aged rats subjected to MMI [132].

Angelica purpurascen essential oil has shown beneficial effects in a zebrafish model of scopolamine-induced memory impairment by multiple pathways, including the restoration of cholinergic system function and the enhancement of the brain's oxidative state [133]. Positive modulation of hepatocyte growth factor (HGF)/MET is a crucial neurotrophic signaling mechanism, which could improve neuronal health and function and combat dementia-related neurodegeneration. Using immunocytochemistry, the most effective positive modulator of HGF/MET was discovered to be the fosgonimeton-active metabolite (forgo-AM). Enhancements in synaptogenesis and neurite outgrowth in primary hippocampal neurons treated with forgo-AM support the neurotrophic effects of positive modulators of HGF/MET. Furthermore, forgo-AM protects primary cortical neuron cultures from neurotoxic insults. Treatment with forgo-AM reversed cognitive impairments in a rat model of dementia caused by scopolamine amnesia. The metabolite forgo-AM may be therapeutically beneficial in dementia and other forms of cognitive impairment that include neurodegeneration and synaptic loss, mitochondrial malfunction, excitotoxicity, oxidative stress, cholinergic deficiencies, and neuroinflammation via positively regulating HGF/MET signaling [134].

Amitriptyline was found to increase neurogenesis and glutamate transporter-1 (GLT-1) expression in the DLB rat model, which would reduce neuronal loss and restore behavioral function. Improvements in behavioral and neurological function have been seen when GLT-1 has been raised in animal models of neurodegenerative disorders, such as Huntington's disease, Parkinson's disease, and amyotrophic lateral sclerosis [135].

Guiera senegalensis (Combretaceae) leaf hydroethanolic extract was found to ameliorate the scopolamine-induced cognitive dysfunction in zebrafish. Anti-AChE and antioxidant properties of *Guiera senegalensis* may account for its cognitive-protective effects against scopolamine-induced cognitive dysfunction [136]. Chrysin-Loaded Chitosan Nanoparticles (Chr-Chi NPs) were evaluated for neuroprotection activity in $A\beta_{1-42-}$induced neurodegenerative conditions in zebrafish. Chr-Chi NPs were found to retain memory, cognition, and synaptic connections. Chr-Chi NPs were further found to reduce aggregates of amyloid β, thus decreasing neuronal death and generation of reactive oxygen species (ROS) [137].

Amomum testaceum extract was found to reduce the malondialdehyde (MDA) levels, as well as the increased catalase and Glutathione Peroxidase levels. *Amomum testaceum* extract was also found to cause a reduction in S100B levels in brain regions associated with vascular dementia by decreasing oxidative stress [138].

For the treatment of AD, nanoparticles like liposomes and solid lipid nanoparticles are being investigated. Increasing stability, such as by adding non-natural proteins for peptide medications to make them resistant to proteolysis, and targeting the highly expressed receptors or transporters of the blood-brain barrier are two significant methods for ensuring the best possible brain selectivity. The active ingredients might even be injected directly into the nose to avoid the blood-brain barrier. Recent studies have begun focusing on liposomes as a possible pharmaceutical delivery dosage type for AD treatment [139].

Stem cell therapy has shown positive outcomes in preclinical investigations and early clinical trials for Alzheimer's disease, particularly in terms of lowering neuro-inflammation, boosting neurotransmission, accelerating neuronal development, and protein eradication, among other effects. ACh levels, phosphorylated tau, and microglial neuro-inflammation can all be reversed by a variety of stem cell types, including embryonic stem cells, induced pluripotent stem cells, umbilical cord blood/placenta stem cells, and mesenchymal stem cells (MSC). Human leukemia, bone marrow, and autologous adipose tissue are the sources of MSC [140].

The acceptance of an anti-amyloid antibody as a disease-altering therapy for Alzheimer's disease in the United States of America in 2021 was the first exceedingly contested step toward a molecular, cause-focused treatment [141]. Therapeutics that target amyloid have been the subject of numerous investigations. These include anti-A treatment combinations that address early surgical Alzheimer's disease anomalies in conjunction with other therapeutic drugs and recently found early detection biomarkers. The recent FDA approval of aducanumab, a monoclonal anti-A oligomer antibody, has raised expectations and presented new obstacles for several anti-A drugs [142].

Exosomes, a newly developed intercellular communication technique, offer a novel perspective on previously accepted treatment strategies for Alzheimer's disease. Exosomes are multicellular particles that practically every type of cell releases. By transporting miRNAs, proteins, and lipids, exosomes produced by glial cells or neurons have an impact on cell connections and consequently physiology [143]. It has been shown that microglia exosomes can transport neuroprotective substances between cells and influence synaptic activity. Microvesicles produced by microglia contribute to the upregulation of synaptic activity by increasing the synthesis of ceramide and sphingosine. Alzheimer's disease's etiology has been connected to the dysregulation of ceramide and sphingomyelin (AD). Additionally, under oxidative stress, a new glycoprotein (Synapsin-1) expressed on the surface of exosomes from people with Alzheimer's disease encourages neuritic outgrowth, which is helpful for recovery from nerve injury [144].

It is likely that low-dose radiation treatment (LD-RT), which is effective in treating both systemic amyloid deposits and chronic inflammatory disorders, can control cytokine production and amyloid burden in Alzheimer's disease. Breaking H-bonds and depolymerizing glucosamine glycans, which are extremely radiation-sensitive substances associated with amyloid fibrils, maybe the mechanism by which low-dose anti-amyloid radiation treatment works. A preclinical study found that fractionated LD-RT regimens significantly reduced amyloid plaques, approximately doubling that of hypofractionated single-dose therapy, which was linked to the regulation of pro- and anti-inflammatory cytokines and improved cognitive function [145].

Pluripotent stem cell-derived small extracellular vesicles (iPSC-sEVs) were found to provide a novelty therapeutic strategy for aged ischemic stroke and another aging-associated neurodegenerative disease [146].

10.9 CONCLUSION

In this work, we discuss the different factors that are responsible for dementia and the pathologies associated with it. Although we know that many types of dementia exist, and their pathologies are very similar to each other. Based on their pathologies, the signs and symptoms of dementia are also quite similar. Worldwide, several (semi-) synthetic medications are available for the treatment of Alzheimer's disease and some kinds of dementia. Currently, there is no cure for dementia. The main goals of pharmaceutical therapies are to slow the progression of the condition and relieve its symptoms. Some naturally occurring substances show promise as alternative therapeutic approaches. The reversible ChE inhibitor donepezil and curcumin, for instance, displayed impressive synergistic effects on cognition and oxidative stress as well as improved BBB permeability when administered together. Additionally, a transgenic mouse model of Alzheimer's disease has demonstrated that a combination supplement regimen containing several mitochondrial antioxidants, such as Acetyl-L-carnitine and lipoic acid, can improve cognitive performance in patients with age-related disorders like Alzheimer's disease and other types of dementia. However, there are still many unanswered questions in this field of study that need to be resolved by designing additional research. The scientific community requires more in-depth studies that examine plant compounds' mechanisms of action and identify their active components. Clinical investigations examining the effectiveness of the featured herbal products in the treatment of dementia will be facilitated by this research.

KEYWORDS

- **Alzheimer's disease**
- **dementia**
- **ethnopharmacology**
- **natural drugs**
- **pathophysiology**
- **pharmaceutical therapies**
- **synthetic drugs**

REFERENCES

1. Hsu, T. J., Tsai, H. T., Hwang, A. C., Chen, L. Y., & Chen, L. K. (2017). Predictors of non-pharmacological intervention effect on cognitive function and behavioral and psychological symptoms of older people with dementia. *Geriatrics & Gerontology International, 17*, 28–35.
2. Nichols, E., Steinmetz, J. D., Vollset, S. E., Fukutaki, K., Chalek, J., Abd-Allah, & Liu, X. (2022). Estimation of the global prevalence of dementia in 2019 and forecasted prevalence in 2050: An analysis for the Global Burden of Disease Study 2019. *The Lancet Public Health, 7*(2), e105–e125.
3. Brito, A., Tsang, A. C. O., Hilditch, C., Nicholson, P., Krings, T., & Brinjikji, W. (2019). Intracranial dural arteriovenous fistula as a reversible cause of dementia: Case series and literature review. *World Neurosurgery, 121*, e543–e553.
4. Jaraj, D., Wikkelsø, C., Rabiei, K., Marlow, T., Jensen, C., Östling, S., & Skoog, I. (2017). Mortality and risk of dementia in normal-pressure hydrocephalus: A population study. *Alzheimer's & Dementia, 13*(8), 850–857.
5. Cree, B. A. (2014). Acute inflammatory myelopathies. In *Handbook of Clinical Neurology* (Vol. 122, pp. 613–667).
6. Paretsky, M. (2022). The lonely path to dementia. *Neurology, 98*(13), e1406–e1408.
7. Pathak, N., Vimal, S. K., Tandon, I., Agrawal, L., Hongyi, C., & Bhattacharyya, S. (2021). Neurodegenerative disorders of Alzheimer's, Parkinsonism, amyotrophic lateral sclerosis and multiple sclerosis: An early diagnostic approach for precision treatment. *Metabolic Brain Disease*, 1–38.
8. Zotin, M. C. Z., Sveikata, L., Viswanathan, A., & Yilmaz, P. (2021). Cerebral small vessel disease and vascular cognitive impairment: From diagnosis to management. *Current Opinion in Neurology, 34*(2), 246.
9. Rosenberg, R. N., & Pascual, J. M. (Eds.). (2020). *Rosenberg's Molecular and Genetic Basis of Neurological and Psychiatric Disease: Volume 1*. Academic Press.
10. Muralidar, S., Ambi, S. V., Sekaran, S., Thirumalai, D., & Palaniappan, B. (2020). Role of tau protein in Alzheimer's disease: The prime pathological player. *International Journal of Biological Macromolecules, 163*, 1599–1617.

11. Querfurth, H., & Lee, H. K. (2021). Mammalian/mechanistic target of rapamycin (mTOR) complexes in neurodegeneration. *Molecular Neurodegeneration, 16*(1), 44.
12. Tsatsanis, A., Wong, B. X., Gunn, A. P., Ayton, S., Bush, A. I., Devos, D., & Duce, J. A. (2020). Amyloidogenic processing of Alzheimer's disease β-amyloid precursor protein induces cellular iron retention. *Molecular Psychiatry, 25*(9), 1958–1966.
13. Riphagen, J. M., Ramakers, I. H., Freeze, W. M., Pagen, L. H., Hanseeuw, B. J., Verbeek, M. M., & Jacobs, H. I. (2020). Linking APOE-ε4, blood-brain barrier dysfunction, and inflammation to Alzheimer's pathology. *Neurobiology of Aging, 85*, 96–103.
14. Rabaneda-Bueno, R., Mena-Montes, B., Torres-Castro, S., & Torres-Carrillo, N. (2021). Advances in genetics and epigenetic alterations in Alzheimer's disease: A notion for therapeutic treatment. *Genes, 12*(12), 1959.
15. Jellinger, K. A. (2020). Neuropathological assessment of the Alzheimer's spectrum. *Journal of Neural Transmission, 127*(9), 1229–1256.
16. Tiwari, S., Atluri, V., Kaushik, A., Yndart, A., & Nair, M. (2019). Alzheimer's disease: Pathogenesis, diagnostics, and therapeutics. *International Journal of Nanomedicine, 14*, 5541–5554.
17. Postuma, R. B., Berg, D., Stern, M., Poewe, W., Olanow, C. W., Oertel, W., & Deuschl, G. (2016). Abolishing the 1-year rule: How much evidence will be enough? *Movement Disorders: Official Journal of the Movement Disorder Society, 31*(11), 1623–1627.
18. Menšíková, K., Matěj, R., Colosimo, C., Rosales, R., Tučková, L., Ehrmann, J., & Kaňovský, P. (2022). Lewy body disease or diseases with Lewy bodies? *npj Parkinson's Disease, 8*(1), 3.
19. Agrawal, S., & Schneider, J. A. (2022). Vascular pathology and pathogenesis of cognitive impairment and dementia in older adults. *Cerebral Circulation-Cognition and Behavior, 3*, 100148.
20. Fotuhi, S. N., & Khalaj-Kondori, M. (2022). Imbalanced clearance of Aβ peptide causes presynaptic plaque formation. *International Journal of Neuroscience*, 1–5.
21. Trist, B. G., Hare, D. J., & Double, K. L. (2019). Oxidative stress in the aging substantia nigra and the etiology of Parkinson's disease. *Aging Cell, 18*(6), e13031.
22. Li, J. Q., Tan, L., Wang, H. F., Tan, M. S., Tan, L., Xu, W., & Yu, J. T. (2016). Risk factors for predicting progression from mild cognitive impairment to Alzheimer's disease: A systematic review and meta-analysis of cohort studies. *Journal of Neurology, 87*(5), 476–484.
23. Tisher, A., & Salardini, A. (2019). A comprehensive update on the treatment of dementia. *Seminars in Neurology, 39*(2), 167–178.
24. Tewari, D., Stankiewicz, A. M., Mocan, A., Sah, A. N., Tzvetkov, N. T., Huminiecki, L., & Atanasov, A. G. (2018). Ethnopharmacological approaches for dementia therapy and significance of natural products and herbal drugs. *Frontiers in Aging Neuroscience, 10*, 3.
25. Gellhaar, S., Sunnemark, D., Eriksson, H., Olson, L., & Galter, D. (2017). Myeloperoxidase-immunoreactive cells are significantly increased in brain areas affected by neurodegeneration in Parkinson's and Alzheimer's disease. *Cell and Tissue Research, 369*, 445–454.
26. Wright, J. R., Deen, Q. F. E., Stevenson, A., Telford-Cooke, L. L., Parker, C., Martin-Ruiz, C., & Mukaetova-Ladinska, E. B. (2022). Plasma myeloperoxidase as a potential biomarker of patient response to anti-dementia treatment in Alzheimer's. *Journal of Alzheimer's Disease, 89*, 1483–1492.

27. Perneczky, R. (2022). Dementia treatment versus prevention. *Dialogues in Clinical Neuroscience*.
28. Álvarez-Fernández, B., Bernal-López, M. R., & Gómez-Huelgas, R. (2022). Role of aripiprazole in the management of behavioral and psychological symptoms of dementia: A narrative review. *Psychogeriatrics, 22*(1), 137–144.
29. Stahl, S. M. (2017). *Prescriber's Guide: Antidepressants: Stahl's Essential Psychopharmacology*. Cambridge University Press.
30. Amariglio, R. E. (2021). Operationalizing the clinical staging scheme in the 2018 NIA–AA research framework. *Nature Reviews Neurology, 17*(7), 395–396.
31. Kverno, K. (2022). New treatment aimed at preventing Alzheimer's dementia. *Journal of Psychosocial Nursing and Mental Health Services, 60*(5), 11–14.
32. Benninghoff, J., & Perneczky, R. (2022). Anti-dementia medications and anti-Alzheimer's disease drugs: Side effects, contraindications, and interactions. In *NeuroPsychopharmacotherapy* (pp. 1–10).
33. Yin, Y. L., Liu, Y. H., Zhu, M. L., Wang, H. H., Qiu, Y., Wan, G. R., & Li, P. (2022). Floralozone improves cognitive impairment in vascular dementia rats via regulation of TRPM2 and NMDAR signaling pathway. *Physiology & Behavior, 249*, 113777.
34. Biglan, K., Munsie, L., Svensson, K. A., Ardayfio, P., Pugh, M., Sims, J., & Brys, M. (2022). Safety and efficacy of Mevidalen in Lewy body dementia: A Phase 2, randomized, placebo-controlled trial. *Movement Disorders, 37*(3), 513–524.
35. Chandran, R., Li, W., Nie, X., Voltin, J., He, L., Jamil, S., & Ergul, A. (2022). Isosorbide mononitrate and cilostazol treatment prevents temporal changes in the brain microstructure of diabetic rats following microemboli injection: Relevance to vascular cognitive impairment and dementia (VCID). *Stroke, 53*(Vol.).
36. Stummer, L., Markovic, M., & Maroney, M. (2020). Brexpiprazole in the treatment of schizophrenia and agitation in Alzheimer's disease. *Neurodegenerative Disease Management, 10*(4), 205–217.
37. Dominguez, L. J., & Barba Gallo, M. (2017). The relevance of nutrition for the concept of cognitive frailty. *Current Opinion in Clinical Nutrition and Metabolic Care, 20*(1), 61–68.
38. Vlachos, G. S., & Scarmeas, N. (2022). Dietary interventions in mild cognitive impairment and dementia. *Dialogues in Clinical Neuroscience*.
39. Aggarwal, H., Gupta, S., Sharma, P., Sharma, B. M., & Sharma, B. (2022). Neurobehavioral and neurobiochemical effect of atomoxetine and N-acetylcysteine in streptozotocin diabetes induced endothelial dysfunction and related dementia. *Physiology & Behavior, 249*, 113767.
40. Ren, Y., Wang, Q., Yang, Z., Feng, L., & Zhang, Y. (2022). MCC950 ameliorates the dementia symptom at the early age of line M83 mouse and reduces hippocampal α-synuclein accumulation. *Biochemical and Biophysical Research Communications, 611*, 23–30.
41. Dembitsky, V. M., Dzhemileva, L., Gloriozova, T., & D'yakonov, V. (2020). Natural and synthetic drugs used for the treatment of dementia. *Biochemical and Biophysical Research Communications, 524*(3), 772–783.
42. Hershey, L. A., & Coleman-Jackson, R. (2019). Pharmacological management of dementia with Lewy bodies. *Drugs & Aging, 36*, 309–319.
43. Murata, M., Odawara, T., Hasegawa, K., Iiyama, S., Nakamura, M., Tagawa, M., & Kosaka, K. (2018). Adjunct zonisamide to levodopa for DLB parkinsonism: A randomized double-blind phase 2 study. *Neurology, 90*(8), e664–e672.

44. Panza, F., Lozupone, M., Watling, M., & Imbimbo, B. P. (2019). Pharmacological management of dementia with Lewy bodies with a focus on zonisamide for treating parkinsonism. *Expert Opinion on Pharmacotherapy, 22*(3), 325–337.
45. Liu, D. D., Yuan, X., Chu, S. F., Chen, C., Ren, Q., Luo, P., & Chen, N. H. (2019). CZ-7, a new derivative of Claulansine F, ameliorates 2VO-induced vascular dementia in rats through a Nrf2-mediated antioxidant response. *Acta Pharmacologica Sinica, 40*(4), 425–440.
46. Uddin, M. S., Kabir, M. T., Rahman, M. M., Mathew, B., Shah, M. A., & Ashraf, G. M. (2020). TV 3326 for Alzheimer's dementia: A novel multimodal ChE and MAO inhibitors to mitigate Alzheimer's-like neuropathology. *Journal of Pharmacy and Pharmacology, 72*(8), 1001–1012.
47. Alzheimer's Association. (2016). Alzheimer's disease facts and figures. *Alzheimer's & Dementia, 12*(4), 459–509.
48. Kerns, J. W., Winter, J. D., Winter, K. M., Kerns, C. C., & Etz, R. S. (2018). Caregiver perspectives about using antipsychotics and other medications for symptoms of dementia. *The Gerontologist, 58*(2), e35–e45.
49. Berg-Weger, M., & Stewart, D. B. (2017). Non-pharmacologic interventions for persons with dementia. *Missouri Medicine, 114*(2), 116.
50. Miller, E., Morel, A., Redlicka, J., Miller, I., & Saluk, J. (2018). Pharmacological and non-pharmacological therapies of cognitive impairment in multiple sclerosis. *Current Neuropharmacology, 16*(4), 475–483.
51. Dyer, S. M., Harrison, S. L., Laver, K., Whitehead, C., & Crotty, M. (2018). An overview of systematic reviews of pharmacological and non-pharmacological interventions for the treatment of behavioral and psychological symptoms of dementia. *International Psychogeriatrics, 30*(3), 295–309.
52. Scuteri, D., Rombolà, L., Tridico, L., Mizoguchi, H., Watanabe, C., Sakurada, T., & Morrone, L. A. (2019). Neuropharmacological properties of the essential oil of bergamot for the clinical management of pain-related BPSDs. *Current Medicinal Chemistry, 26*(20), 3764–3774.
53. Contrada, M., Cerasa, A., Tonin, P., Bagetta, G., & Scuteri, D. (2021). Aromatherapy in stroke patients: Is it time to begin? *Frontiers in Behavioral Neuroscience, 15*, 749353.
54. Vink, A., & Hanser, S. (2018). Music-based therapeutic interventions for people with dementia: A mini-review. *Medicines, 5*(4), 109.
55. Raglio, A., Pavlic, E., & Bellandi, D. (2018). Music listening for people living with dementia. *Journal of the American Medical Directors Association, 19*(8), 722–723.
56. Van der Steen, J. T., Smaling, H. J., Van der Wouden, J. C., Bruinsma, M. S., Scholten, R. J., & Vink, A. C. (2018). Music-based therapeutic interventions for people with dementia. *Cochrane Database of Systematic Reviews, 2017(5), CD003477.*
57. Emblad, S. Y., & Mukaetova-Ladinska, E. B. (2021). Creative art therapy as a non-pharmacological intervention for dementia: A systematic review. *Journal of Alzheimer's Disease Reports, 5*(1), 353–364.
58. Wu, J., Wang, Y., & Wang, Z. (2017). The effectiveness of massage and touch on behavioral and psychological symptoms of dementia: A quantitative systematic review and meta-analysis. *Journal of Advanced Nursing, 73*(10), 2283–2295.
59. Takeda, A., Watanuki, E., & Koyama, S. (2017). Effects of inhalation aromatherapy on symptoms of sleep disturbance in the elderly with dementia. *Evidence-Based Complementary and Alternative Medicine, 2017, 1902807.*

60. Zhang, Z. Y., Liu, Z., Deng, H. H., & Chen, Q. (2018). Effects of acupuncture on vascular dementia (VD) animal models: A systematic review and meta-analysis. *BMC Complementary and Alternative Medicine, 18*(1), 1–10.
61. Brenes, G. A., Sohl, S., Wells, R. E., Befus, D., Campos, C. L., & Danhauer, S. C. (2019). The effects of yoga on patients with mild cognitive impairment and dementia: A scoping review. *The American Journal of Geriatric Psychiatry, 27*(2), 188–197.
62. Hishikawa, N., Takahashi, Y., Fukui, Y., Tokuchi, R., Furusawa, J., Takemoto, M., & Abe, K. (2019). Yoga-plus exercise mix promotes cognitive, affective, and physical functions in elderly people. *Neurological Research, 41*(11), 1001–1007.
63. Zucchella, C., Sinforiani, E., Tamburin, S., Federico, A., Mantovani, E., Bernini, S., & Bartolo, M. (2018). The multidisciplinary approach to Alzheimer's disease and dementia: A narrative review of non-pharmacological treatment. *Frontiers in Neurology, 9*, 1058.
64. Teipel, S., Babiloni, C., Hoey, J., Kaye, J., Kirste, T., & Burmeister, O. K. (2016). Information and communication technology solutions for outdoor navigation in dementia. *Alzheimer's & Dementia, 12*(6), 695–707.
65. Kamil, R. J., Bakar, D., Ehrenburg, M., Wei, E. X., Pletnikova, A., Xiao, G., & Agrawal, Y. (2021). Detection of wandering behaviors using a body-worn inertial sensor in patients with cognitive impairment: A feasibility study. *Frontiers in Neurology, 12*, 529661.
66. Ienca, M., Fabrice, J., Elger, B., Caon, M., Scoccia Pappagallo, A., Kressig, R. W., & Wangmo, T. (2017). Intelligent assistive technology for Alzheimer's disease and other dementias: A systematic review. *Journal of Alzheimer's Disease, 56*(4), 1301–1340.
67. Sobral, M., & Pestana, M. H. (2020). Virtual reality and dementia: A bibliometric analysis. *The European Journal of Psychiatry, 34*(3), 120–131.
68. Hirt, J., & Beer, T. (2020). Use and impact of virtual reality simulation in dementia care education: A scoping review. *Nurse Education Today, 84*, 104207.
69. Narasimha, S., Madathil, K. C., Agnisarman, S., Rogers, H., Welch, B., Ashok, A., & McElligott, J. (2017). Designing telemedicine systems for geriatric patients: A review of the usability studies. *Telemedicine and e-Health, 23*(6), 459–472.
70. Rosen, T., Makaroun, L. K., Conwell, Y., & Betz, M. (2019). Violence in older adults: Scope, impact, challenges, and strategies for prevention. *Health Affairs, 38*(10), 1630–1637.
71. Islam, F., Khadija, J. F., Harun-Or-Rashid, M., Rahaman, M., Nafady, M. H., Islam, M., & Mubarak, M. S. (2022). Bioactive compounds and their derivatives: An insight into prospective phytotherapeutic approaches against Alzheimer's disease. *Oxidative Medicine and Cellular Longevity, 2022*, 5100904.
72. Berkov, S., Osorio, E., Viladomat, F., & Bastida, J. (2020). Chemodiversity, chemotaxonomy and chemoecology of Amaryllidaceae alkaloids. In *The Alkaloids: Chemistry and Biology* (Vol. 83, pp. 113–185).
73. Cahlíková, L., Vaněčková, N., Šafratová, M., Breiterová, K., Blunden, G., Hulcová, D., & Opletal, L. (2019). The genus *Nerine* Herb (Amaryllidaceae): Ethnobotany, phytochemistry, and biological activity. *Molecules, 24*(23), 4238.
74. Soto-Vásquez, M. R., Rodríguez-Muñoz, C. A., Tallini, L. R., & Bastida, J. (2022). Alkaloid composition and biological activities of the Amaryllidaceae species *Ismene amancaes* (Ker Gawl.) Herb. *Plants, 11*(15), 1906.

75. Xu, Z., & Deng, M. (2017). *Identification and Control of Common Weeds* (Vol. 3). Dordrecht: Springer Netherlands.
76. Kukula-Koch, W. (2017). The elevation of LC-ESI-Q-TOF-MS response in the analysis of isoquinoline alkaloids from some *Papaveraceae* and *Berberidaceae* representatives. *Journal of Analytical Methods in Chemistry, 2017*, 8384107.
77. Bozkurt, B., Ulkar, D., Nurlu, N., Kaya, G. I., & Unver-Somer, N. (2022). Chemical profile, acetylcholinesterase, butyrylcholinesterase, and prolyl oligopeptidase inhibitory activity of *Glaucium corniculatum* subsp. *refractum*. *Brazilian Journal of Pharmaceutical Sciences, 58*(5).
78. Alolga, R. N., Wang, F., Zhang, X., Li, J., Tran, L. S. P., & Yin, X. (2022). Bioactive compounds from the *Zingiberaceae* family with known antioxidant activities for possible therapeutic uses. *Antioxidants, 11*(7), 1281.
79. de Campos Bortolucci, W., Trettel, J. R., Bernardi, D. M., Souza, M. M. Q., Lopes, A. D., Lovato, E. C. W., & Colauto, N. B. (2020). Therapeutic potential of *Zingiberaceae* in Alzheimer's disease. *Boletín Latinoamericano y del Caribe de Plantas Medicinales y Aromáticas, 19*(5), 428–465.
80. Borah, S., Sarkar, P., & Sharma, H. K. (2022). Zederone improves the fecal microbial profile in dementia-induced rat model: A first report. *CNS & Neurological Disorders-Drug Targets, 21*(4), 335–342.
81. Maqbool, I., Ali, A., Ashraf, M., ur Rehman, N., Khalid, I., Talib, S., & Hussain, A. (2022). The multi characteristics values of ginger (*Zingiber officinale*) in human nutrition and disease prevention. *GSC Biological and Pharmaceutical Sciences, 21*(2), 127–134.
82. Pham, N. K., Nguyen, H. T., & Nguyen, Q. B. (2021). A review on the ethnomedicinal uses, phytochemistry, and pharmacology of plant species belonging to *Kaempferia* L. genus (*Zingiberaceae*). *Sci. Asia, 48*, 1–24.
83. Scuteri, D., Morrone, L. A., Rombolà, L., Avato, P. R., Bilia, A. R., Corasaniti, M. T., & Bagetta, G. (2017). Aromatherapy and aromatic plants for the treatment of behavioural and psychological symptoms of dementia in patients with Alzheimer's disease: Clinical evidence and possible mechanisms. *Evidence-Based Complementary and Alternative Medicine, 2017*(6), 1–8.
84. Habtemariam, S. (2018). Molecular pharmacology of rosmarinic and salvianolic acids: Potential seeds for Alzheimer's and vascular dementia drugs. *International Journal of Molecular Sciences, 19*(2), 458.
85. Chen, S. Y., Gao, Y., Sun, J. Y., Meng, X. L., Yang, D., Fan, L. H., & Wang, P. (2020). Traditional Chinese medicine: Role in reducing β-amyloid, apoptosis, autophagy, neuroinflammation, oxidative stress, and mitochondrial dysfunction of Alzheimer's disease. *Frontiers in Pharmacology, 11*, 497.
86. Sonigra, P., & Meena, M. (2021). Metabolic profile, bioactivities, and variations in the chemical constituents of essential oils of the *Ferula* genus (*Apiaceae*). *Frontiers in Pharmacology, 11*, 608649.
87. Mustafa, A. M., Maggi, F., Papa, F., Kaya, E., Dikmen, M., & Öztürk, Y. (2016). Isofuranodiene: A neuritogenic compound isolated from wild celery (*Smyrnium olusatrum* L., *Apiaceae*). *Food Chemistry, 192*, 782–787.
88. Thiviya, P., Gamage, A., Piumali, D., Merah, O., & Madhujith, T. (2021). *Apiaceae* as an important source of antioxidants and their applications. *Cosmetics, 8*(4), 111.

89. Karakaya, S., Yılmaz, S. V., Koca, M., Demirci, B., & Sytar, O. K. S. A. N. A. (2019). Screening of non-alkaloid acetylcholinesterase inhibitors from extracts and essential oils of *Anthriscus nemorosa* (M. Bieb.) Spreng. (*Apiaceae*). *South African Journal of Botany, 125*, 261–269.
90. Ganaie, M. M., Raja, V., Reshi, Z. A., & Verma, V. (2018). Family *Solanaceae*: Taxonomy and modern trends. *Annals of Plant Science, 7*(9), 2403–2414.
91. Dembitsky, V. M., Dzhemileva, L., Gloriozova, T., & D'yakonov, V. (2020). Natural and synthetic drugs used for the treatment of dementia. *Biochemical and Biophysical Research Communications, 524*(3), 772–783.
92. Gomes, G., Silva, G., Silva, D., Oliveira, R., & Conceição, G. (2018). Botanical composition of *Fabaceae* family in the Brazilian Northeast, Maranhão, Brazil. *Asian Journal of Environment & Ecology, 6*(4), 1–10.
93. El-Saber Batiha, G., Magdy Beshbishy, A., El-Mleeh, A., Abdel-Daim, M. M., & Devkota, H. P. (2020). Traditional uses, bioactive chemical constituents, and pharmacological and toxicological activities of *Glycyrrhiza glabra* L. (*Fabaceae*). *Biomolecules, 10*(3), 352.
94. Elufioye, T. O., & Hameed, H. A. (2017). Cognitive-enhancing properties of *Morinda lucida* (*Rubiaceae*) and *Peltophorum pterocarpum* (*Fabaceae*) in scopolamine-induced amnesic mice. *African Journal of Traditional, Complementary and Alternative Medicines, 14*(3), 136–141.
95. Aly, S. H., Elissawy, A. M., Fayez, A. M., Eldahshan, O. A., Elshanawany, M. A., & Singab, A. N. B. (2021). Neuroprotective effects of *Sophora secundiflora*, *Sophora tomentosa* leaves, and formononetin on scopolamine-induced dementia. *Natural Product Research, 35*(24), 5848–5852.
96. Abaissou, H. H. N., Foyet, H. S., Wado, E. K., Nkwingwa, B. K., Kamda, J. L. D., Djomessie, L. B. K., & Bum, E. N. (2020). Cholinergic enhancing and antioxidant effect of *Vigna subterranea* (L.) Verdc. (*Fabaceae*) landrace aqueous extract on scopolamine-induced amnesia in male Swiss mice. *Pharmacognosy Research, 12*(3).
97. Dong, Q., Li, Z., Zhang, Q., Liang, H., & Xiong, L. (2022). *Astragalus mongholicus* Bunge (*Fabaceae*): Bioactive compounds and potential therapeutic mechanisms against Alzheimer's Disease. *Frontiers in Pharmacology*, 2431.
98. Beppe, G. J., Kenko Djoumessie, L. B., Keugong Wado, E., Ngatanko Abaïssou, H. H., Nkwingwa, B. K., Damo Kamda, J. L., & Foyet, H. S. (2020). Aqueous root bark extract of *Daniellia oliveri* (Hutch. & Dalz.) (*Fabaceae*) protects neurons against diazepam-induced amnesia in mice. *Evidence-Based Complementary and Alternative Medicine.*
99. Lawal, B. A., Udobre, A., Elufioye, T. O., Ahmadu, A. A., & Olanipekun, B. (2020). Novel cholinesterase inhibitory effect of α-spinasterol isolated from the leaves of *Acacia auriculiformis* A. CUNN Ex. Benth (*Fabaceae*). *Tropical Journal of Pharmaceutical Research, 19*(7), 1473–1479.
100. Groppo, M., Afonso, L. F., & Pirani, J. R. (2022). A review of systematics studies in the Citrus family (*Rutaceae*, *Sapindales*), with emphasis on American groups. *Brazilian Journal of Botany, 45*(1), 181–200.
101. Lobine, D., Pairyanen, B., Zengin, G., Yılmaz, M. A., Ouelbani, R., Bensari, S., & Mahomoodally, M. F. (2021). Chemical composition and pharmacological evaluation of *Toddalia asiatica* (*Rutaceae*) extracts and essential oil by in vitro and in silico approaches. *Chemistry & Biodiversity, 18*(4), e2000999.

102. Fan, W., Fan, L., Peng, C., Zhang, Q., Wang, L., Li, L., & Wu, C. (2019). Traditional uses, botany, phytochemistry, pharmacology, pharmacokinetics and toxicology of *Xanthium strumarium* L.: A review. *Molecules, 24*(2), 359.
103. Abdulwanis Mohamed, Z., Mohamed Eliaser, E., Mazzon, E., Rollin, P., Cheng Lian Ee, G., & Abdull Razis, A. F. (2019). Neuroprotective potential of secondary metabolites from *Melicope lunu-ankenda* (*Rutaceae*). *Molecules, 24*(17), 3109.
104. Feitosa, C. M., Cardoso, M. F. K., Oliveira, L. S. G., Figueredo, J., Melo, C. H. S., & Rashed, K. (2020). Antioxidant and anticholinergic properties of *Citrus sinensis* (L.) Osbeck (*Rutaceae*) essential oil in mice hippocampus. *Indian Journal of Natural Products and Resources, 11*(3), 199–205.
105. Mole, L., Kent, B., Abbott, R., Wood, C., & Hickson, M. (2018). The nutritional care of people living with dementia at home: A scoping review. *Health & Social Care in the Community, 26*(4), e485–e496.
106. Bischoff-Ferrari, H. A., Molino, C. D. G. R. C., Rival, S., Vellas, B., Rizzoli, R., & Kressig, R. W. (2021). DO-HEALTH: Vitamin D3-Omega-3-Home Exercise-Healthy aging and longevity trial-Design of a multinational clinical trial on healthy aging among European seniors. *Contemporary Clinical Trials, 100*, 106124.
107. Szczechowiak, K., Diniz, B. S., & Leszek, J. (2019). Diet and Alzheimer's dementia—Nutritional approach to modulate inflammation. *Pharmacology Biochemistry and Behavior, 184*, 172743.
108. Ma, Q. L., Zhu, C., Morselli, M., Su, T., Pelligrini, M., Lu, Z., & Cole, G. M. (2020). The novel omega-6 fatty acid docosapentaenoic acid positively modulates brain innate immune response for resolving neuroinflammation at early and late stages of humanized APOE-based Alzheimer's disease models. *Frontiers in Immunology*, 2364.
109. Sultan, S., Taimuri, U., Basnan, S. A., Ai-Orabi, W. K., Awadallah, A., Almowald, F., & Hazazi, A. (2020). Low vitamin D and its association with cognitive impairment and dementia. *Journal of Aging Research, 2020*, 6097820.
110. Samieri, C., Yassine, H. N., Melo van Lent, D., Lefèvre-Arbogast, S., van de Rest, O., Bowman, G. L., & Scarmeas, N. (2022). Personalized nutrition for dementia prevention. *Alzheimer's & Dementia, 18*(7), 1424–1437.
111. Pluta, R., Furmaga-Jabłońska, W., Januszewski, S., & Czuczwar, S. J. (2022). Post-ischemic brain neurodegeneration in the form of Alzheimer's disease proteinopathy: Possible therapeutic role of curcumin. *Nutrients, 14*(2), 248.
112. Liu, Z. J., Li, Z. H., Liu, L., Tang, W. X., Wang, Y., Dong, M. R., & Xiao, C. (2016). Curcumin attenuates beta-amyloid-induced neuroinflammation via activation of peroxisome proliferator-activated receptor-gamma function in a rat model of Alzheimer's disease. *Frontiers in Pharmacology, 7*, 261.
113. Small, G. W., Siddarth, P., Li, Z., Miller, K. J., Ercoli, L., Emerson, N. D., & Barrio, J. R. (2018). Memory and brain amyloid and tau effects of a bioavailable form of curcumin in non-demented adults: A double-blind, placebo-controlled 18-month trial. *The American Journal of Geriatric Psychiatry, 26*(3), 266–277.
114. Shen, D., Tian, X., Sang, W., & Song, R. (2017). Effect of melatonin and resveratrol against memory impairment and hippocampal damage in a rat model of vascular dementia. *Neuroimmunomodulation, 23*(5–6), 318–331.
115. Socci, V., Tempesta, D., Desideri, G., De Gennaro, L., & Ferrara, M. (2017). Enhancing human cognition with cocoa flavonoids. *Frontiers in Nutrition, 4*, 19.

116. Barrera-Reyes, P. K., de Lara, J. C. F., Gonzalez-Soto, M., & Tejero, M. E. (2020). Effects of cocoa-derived polyphenols on cognitive function in humans. Systematic review and analysis of methodological aspects. *Plant Foods for Human Nutrition, 75*, 1–11.
117. Martín, M. A., Goya, L., & de Pascual-Teresa, S. (2020). Effect of cocoa and cocoa products on cognitive performance in young adults. *Nutrients, 12*(12), 3691.
118. Veronese, N., Zurlo, A., Solmi, M., Luchini, C., Trevisan, C., Bano, G., & Rylander, R. (2016). Magnesium status in Alzheimer's disease: A systematic review. *American Journal of Alzheimer's Disease & Other Dementias®, 31*(3), 208–213.
119. Kirkland, A. E., Sarlo, G. L., & Holton, K. F. (2018). The role of magnesium in neurological disorders. *Nutrients, 10*(6), 730.
120. Ticinesi, A., Tana, C., Nouvenne, A., Prati, B., Lauretani, F., & Meschi, T. (2018). Gut microbiota, cognitive frailty and dementia in older individuals: A systematic review. *Clinical Interventions in Aging, 13*, 1497–1511.
121. Westfall, S., Lomis, N., Kahouli, I., Dia, S. Y., Singh, S. P., & Prakash, S. (2017). Microbiome, probiotics, and neurodegenerative diseases: Deciphering the gut-brain axis. *Cellular and Molecular Life Sciences, 74*, 3769–3787.
122. Alkasir, R., Li, J., Li, X., Jin, M., & Zhu, B. (2017). Human gut microbiota: The links with dementia development. *Protein & Cell, 8*(2), 90–102.
123. Zhang, Q., Wang, Y., & Fu, L. (2020). Dietary advanced glycation end-products: Perspectives linking food processing with health implications. *Comprehensive Reviews in Food Science and Food Safety, 19*(5), 2559–2587.
124. Abate, G., Marziano, M., Rungratanawanich, W., Memo, M., & Uberti, D. (2017). Nutrition and AGE-ing: Focusing on Alzheimer's disease. *Oxidative Medicine and Cellular Longevity, 2017, 7039816.*
125. Ran, L. S., Liu, W. H., Fang, Y. Y., Xu, S. B., Li, J., Luo, X., & Wang, W. (2021). Alcohol, coffee, and tea intake and the risk of cognitive deficits: A dose–response meta-analysis. *Epidemiology and Psychiatric Sciences, 30*, e13.
126. Barcelos, R. P., Lima, F. D., Carvalho, N. R., Bresciani, G., & Royes, L. F. (2020). Caffeine effects on systemic metabolism, oxidative-inflammatory pathways, and exercise performance. *Nutrition Research, 80*, 1–17.
127. Nordestgaard, A. T., Nordestgaard, B. G., Frikke-Schmidt, R., Rasmussen, I. J., & Bojesen, S. E. (2022). Self-reported and genetically predicted coffee consumption and smoking in dementia: A Mendelian randomization study. *Atherosclerosis, 348*, 36–43.
128. Chen, J. Q., Scheltens, P., Groot, C., & Ossenkoppele, R. (2020). Associations between caffeine consumption, cognitive decline, and dementia: A systematic review. *Journal of Alzheimer's Disease, 78*(4), 1519–1546.
129. Makkar, R., Behl, T., Bungau, S., Zengin, G., Mehta, V., Kumar, A., & Oancea, R. (2020). Nutraceuticals in neurological disorders. *International Journal of Molecular Sciences, 21*(12), 4424.
130. Lee, D. H., Lee, J. Y., Hong, D. Y., Lee, E. C., Park, S. W., Jo, Y. N., & Oh, J. S. (2022). ROCK and PDE-5 inhibitors for the treatment of dementia: Literature review and meta-analysis. *Biomedicines, 10*(6), 1348.
131. Brinza, I., Raey, M. A. E., El-Kashak, W., Eldahshan, O. A., & Hritcu, L. (2022). Sweroside ameliorated memory deficits in scopolamine-induced zebrafish (*Danio rerio*) model: Involvement of cholinergic system and brain oxidative stress. *Molecules, 27*(18), 5901.

132. Culmone, L., Powell, B., Landschoot-Ward, J., Zacharek, A., Gao, H., Findeis, E. L., & Venkat, P. (2022). Treatment with an angiopoietin-1 mimetic peptide improves cognitive outcome in rats with vascular dementia. *Frontiers in Cellular Neuroscience, 16, 869710.*
133. Boiangiu, R. S., Bagci, E., Dumitru, G., Hritcu, L., & Todirascu-Ciornea, E. (2022). *Angelica purpurascens* (Avé-Lall.) Gilli. essential oil improved brain function via cholinergic modulation and antioxidant effects in the scopolamine-induced zebrafish (*Danio rerio*) model. *Plants, 11*(8), 1096.
134. Johnston, J. L., Reda, S. M., Setti, S. E., Taylor, R. W., Berthiaume, A. A., Walker, W. E., & Church, K. J. (2022). Fosgonimeton, a novel positive modulator of the HGF/MET system, promotes neurotrophic and precognitive effects in models of dementia. *Neurotherapeutics, 20(2)*, 1–21.
135. Lin, C. L., Zheng, T. L., Tsou, S. H., Chang, H. M., Tseng, L. H., Yu, C. H., & Ho, Y. J. (2022). Amitriptyline improves cognitive and neuronal function in a rat model that mimics dementia with Lewy bodies. *Behavioral Brain Research, 435*, 114035.
136. Damo, J. L. K., Boiangiu, R. S., Brinza, I., Kenko Djoumessi, L. B., Rebe, R. N., Kamleu, B. N., & Hritcu, L. (2022). Neuroprotective potential of *Guiera senegalensis* (Combretaceae) leaf hydroethanolic extract against cholinergic system dysfunctions and oxidative stress in scopolamine-induced cognitive impairment in zebrafish (*Danio rerio*). *Plants, 11*(9), 1149.
137. Saleem, S., Banerjee, R., & Rajesh Kannan, R. (2022). Chrysin-loaded chitosan nanoparticle-mediated neuroprotection in Aβ1–42-induced neurodegenerative conditions in zebrafish. *ACS Chemical Neuroscience, 13*(13), 2017–2034.
138. Kaewkaen, P. (2022). Antioxidative effect of *Amomum testaceum* Ridl. extract for protecting against vascular dementia. *International Journal of Food Science, 2022, 1–10.*
139. Hernandez, C., & Shukla, S. (2022). Liposome-based drug delivery as a potential treatment option for Alzheimer's disease. *Neural Regeneration Research, 17*(6), 1190.
140. Athar, T., Al Balushi, K., & Khan, S. A. (2021). Recent advances on drug development and emerging therapeutic agents for Alzheimer's disease. *Molecular Biology Reports, 48*(7), 5629–5645.
141. Froelich, L., & Hausner, L. (2021). Disease-modifying treatment approaches for Alzheimer's disease. *Der Nervenarzt, 4(4)*, 203–216.
142. Jeremic, D., Jiménez-Díaz, L., & Navarro-López, J. D. (2021). Past, present, and future of therapeutic strategies against amyloid-β peptides in Alzheimer's disease: A systematic review. *Ageing Research Reviews, 72*, 101496.
143. Guo, M., Yin, Z., Chen, F., & Lei, P. (2020). Mesenchymal stem cell-derived exosome: A promising alternative in the therapy of Alzheimer's disease. *Alzheimer's Research & Therapy, 12*, 1–14.
144. Kaur, S., Verma, H., Dhiman, M., Tell, G., Gigli, G. L., Janes, F., & Mantha, A. K. (2021). Brain exosomes: Friend or foe in Alzheimer's disease? *Molecular Neurobiology, 58(12), 6610–6624.*
145. Ceyzeriat, K., Tournier, B. B., Millet, P., Frisoni, G. B., Garibotto, V., & Zilli, T. (2020). Low-dose radiation therapy: A new treatment strategy for Alzheimer's disease? *Journal of Alzheimer's Disease, 74*(2), 411–419.
146. Niu, X., Xia, Y., Luo, L., Chen, Y., Yuan, J., Zhang, J., & Wang, Y. (2023). iPSC-sEVs alleviate microglia senescence to protect against ischemic stroke in aged mice. *Materials Today Bio, 19*, 100600.

CHAPTER 11

Role of Diet, Micronutrients, and Macronutrients in Managing the Alzheimer's Disease

ANURADHA MISHRA,[1] SUNAYNA CHOUDHARY,[2] VINOD KUMAR GAUTTAM,[3] and KAVITA MUNJAL[4*]

[1]*Department of Food Technology, M.M.I.C.T. & B.M., Maharishi Markandeshwar (Deemed to be University), Mullana, Ambala, Haryana, India*

[2]*Department of Pharmacognosy, M.M. College of Pharmacy, Maharishi Markandeshwar (Deemed to be University), Mullana, Ambala, Haryana, India*

[3]*Department of Pharmacognosy, Shiva Institute of Pharmacy, Bilaspur, Himachal Pradesh, India*

[4]*Department of Pharmacy, Amity Institute of Pharmacy, Amity University, Noida, Uttar Pradesh, India*

*Corresponding author.

ABSTRACT

Alzheimer's disease (AD) is an age-associated neurodegenerative syndrome that mainly impacts cognitive and memory functions and is accompanied by behavioral disorders such as apathy, aggressiveness, and depression. It severely impacts the lives of not only the demented patients but also people related to them (caregivers, family members, colleagues, and friends). Currently, no proven methods exist to prevent or cure the disease. Dietary and lifestyle modifications contribute a significant role in slowing AD symptom progression. The reports published in several scientific studies

Neuro-Nutraceuticals and Drug Discovery and Delivery in Alzheimer's Disease, Volume 1: Targeting Key Pathological Pathways. Varinder Singh, Amit Kumar, Parul Sood (Eds.)

indicate that dietary supplementation of antioxidants, polyphenols, poly- and mono-unsaturated fatty acids, proteins, vitamins, and minerals is beneficial in managing AD. It is also proposed that the reduction in the intake of coffee and fructose and an increase in vitamin and certain minerals consumption may decrease the risk of AD. Epidemiological studies generally report the potential neuronal protective effects of various micronutrients. The disease is difficult to cure completely, so early detection and prevention are important perspectives to manage AD. Numerous studies have confirmed the usage of medicinal plants as an alternative approach to developing new therapeutics for AD. A balanced diet rich in micronutrients, along with regular exercise and mental activity, can help prevent the onset and progression of dementia. This chapter aims to describe the significance of phytochemicals, diet, and nutrition in the management of the progression/development of AD.

11.1 INTRODUCTION

The most common type of dementia, which affects adults over 65 worldwide, is Alzheimer's disease (AD). Clinically, most individuals with AD also experience signs of a mental condition in addition to their complete dementia, which includes memory loss, cognitive impairment, and behavioral and personality abnormalities [1]. Although these symptoms can be momentarily alleviated with careful attention and medication, there is no known way to prevent or treat AD [2].

According to estimates, 6.5 million Americans aged 65 and older suffer from AD. By 2060, this number may rise to 13.8 million if no medical improvements are discovered to prevent, slow down, or cure AD. According to official death certificates, 1,21,499 fatalities in 2019, the most recent year for which data are available, were attributable to AD. The disease was ranked as the sixth-leading cause of death in the US in 2019 and the seventh-leading cause of death in 2020 and 2021 when COVID-19 entered the top 10 causes of death [3].

Dementia prevalence in South Asia was estimated to be 1.9% in 2005; it is expected to rise to 3.6 million by 2020 and 7.5 million by 2040. According to several epidemiological studies, dementia prevalence in India ranges from 2 per 1,000 to 35 per 1,000 people [4].

Pharmacological treatment for AD focuses solely on symptom relief because the genesis of the condition is still poorly understood. Due to the strong correlation between illness burden and age at onset, it is expected that as the population ages and life expectancy increases, disease burden will also increase. Along with age, lifestyle choices are known to impact the likelihood of developing AD. There are additional risk factors for dementia, including high blood pressure, obesity, diabetes, and physical inactivity in osteoarthritis, according to a recent study published in the Lancet Commission [5, 6]. Hearing loss, smoking, depression, illiteracy, and infrequent social interaction [2, 7–9]. In fact, within 360 days of receiving their original COVID-19 diagnosis, patients with the condition were found to be considerably more likely to receive a new diagnosis of AD [10–12].

Since dementia has no known treatment, there is an urgent but unmet need for accessible prevention measures. Because early behavioral intervention may arrest the progression of the disease and future memory loss, it is imperative to research the effects of lifestyle factors, such as eating habits, on memory impairment. After repeated attempts and their unfortunate failure in pharmacotherapy, the research trend has changed away from using synthetic origin molecules against AD in favor of using plants in diet or medication form that are potentially clinically interesting for the treatment of AD and have positive effects on cognitive disorders and strong acetylcholinesterase (AChE) inhibitory, anti-inflammatory, and antioxidant activities [13]. In this regard, polyunsaturated fatty acids (PUFA), B vitamins, different minerals, and antioxidants spark the most interest [14–16]. Following specific diets, such as the Mediterranean diet, the DASH diet, and the MIND diet, may help prevent AD, which has recently drawn a lot of attention due to its positive effects on overall diet composition, for the delay of dementia and AD, according to some studies [17, 18].

11.2 HISTORICAL BACKGROUND

Commonly dementia is AD, which is a slowly progressive neurodegenerative disease. Dementia has existed in humanity long before it was named. In 2000 B.C., the ancient Egyptians were previously aware that memory deteriorates over time [19]. According to Pythagoras, the Greek mathematician and physician (570–495 B.C.), there are six stages of life: infancy (birth to age six), adolescence (age seven to 21), adulthood (age 22 to 49), middle age (age 50 to 62), senescence (age 63 to 79), and old age (age 80 and over). It was believed that senescence and old age were phases of declining mental and physical abilities. Both the Greek physicians Plato (428–347 B.C.) and Hippocrates (460–370 B.C.) believed that dementia is mostly brought on by aging because mental capacity inevitably declines with age. Hippocrates believed that cognitive disorder results from brain damage. Instead, the Roman philosopher, politician, and jurist Marcus Tullius Cicero (106–43 B.C.) observed that, except for people with weak wills, aging does not usually cause a reduction in mental capacity. In a brief statement, he said that dementia is not necessarily a sign of aging (Cicero, 1923).

Around the second century, Aretheus, a physician in ancient Turkey, classified dementia into two categories: dementia, an irreversible chronic condition, and delirium, a reversible acute impairment of cognitive function. Doctor Thomas Willis (1621–1675) is credited with creating the term "neurology" and the medical specialty that uses it. He initially provided a scientific description of vascular dementia in his book, "De Anima Brutorum." [20] In the Modern Era, dementia as recognition was first acquired as a medical word in 1797 by French physician Philippe Pinel (1745–1826). Dementia, according to Pinel's follower Jean Etienne Dominique Esquirol (1772–1840), is characterized by cognitive, intellectual, and willpower impairments brought on by brain disorders, the loss of joyous enjoyment, and the plight of the wealthy. Along with Alois Alzheimer, Swiss-born Otto Ludwig Binswanger researched neurosyphilis, one of the causes of dementia (1864–1915). In the academic world, he described numerous varieties of vascular dementia in 1894. German doctor Emil Kraepelin distinguished between senile dementia and presenile dementia in 1910. After Alois Alzheimer, he was the first person to use the term "AD" [21]. AD was named after the German scientist Alois Alzheimer. He observed symptoms like memory loss, unusual behavior, and brain shrinkage in a patient known as "Auguste D." in 1906 [22]. The name AD was coined by Dr. Alzheimer's colleague Emil Kraepelin in the medical book 1910 [22]. Alzheimer's biopsy of her brain after her death in 1906 showed broad cortical atrophy and "specific alterations in cortical cell clusters." At a German psychiatric conference that year, Alzheimer made a presentation on "Auguste D," claiming that these cortical lesions were to blame for her symptoms. The following year, he submitted a research article, and AD was first mentioned in a psychiatric textbook in 1910. In the U.S., the clinical diagnostic standards for AD were standardized in 1984. They were updated in 2011 and 2018 to highlight the importance of biomarkers in diagnosing AD and to generate distinct diagnoses for the preclinical, mild cognitive impairment (MCI), and dementia stages of the disease. The US Congress, as part of the National Institutes of Health (NIH), founded the National Institute on Aging (NIA) in 1974.

11.3 CAUSES AND RISK FACTORS OF AD

Figure 11.1 illustrates the various risk factors for AD, which include advancing age, hereditary variables, brain traumas, vascular-related disease, infections, and environmental factors (heavy metals, trace metals, and others). Even though the causes of AD are still largely unclear, there is mounting evidence that various risk and protective variables play a part in the disease's progression. The development of AD surely involves a compound interaction of factors, including the type of lifestyle, which may initiate or hasten the neurodegenerative process, similar to other chronic diseases [23].

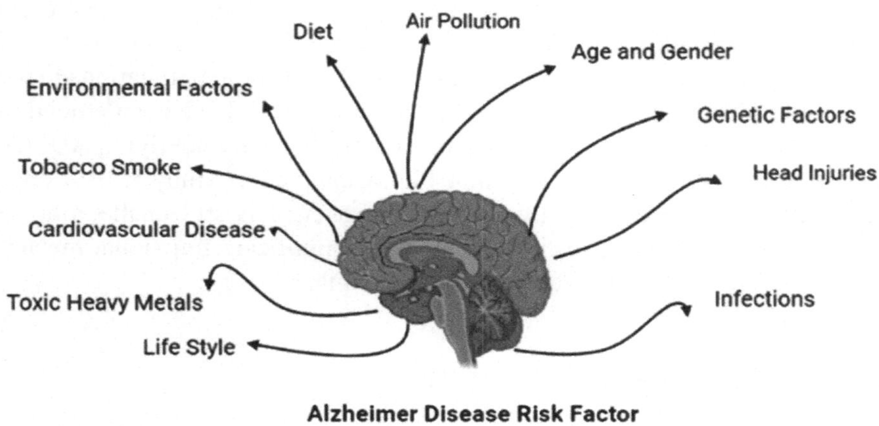

FIGURE 11.1 Risk factors for Alzheimer's disease.

11.4 RISK FACTORS

11.4.1 AGING

Age is still the biggest risk factor for Alzheimer's and is a major component in the progression of the illness. The rate of global population aging is unparalleled and unmatched in human history [24]. The percentage of older people increased throughout the 20th century, and this tendency has persisted into the 21st [24]. For the first time, by 2050, there will be more senior people than younger people on the planet. The number of individuals in the world who are 60 or older is expected to increase by 56% between 2015 and 2030, and by 2050, the number of people in this age group is expected to more than quadruple. Aging is the main risk factor for AD. The occurrences of AD start after 65 years of age, and younger people rarely contract this illness [25]. Aging is a critical and irreversible process that influences several organs and cell systems, shrinking and thinning the brain, eradicating synapses, and enlarging some ventricles [26].

11.4.2 GENETICS

Over the years, genetic factors have been uncovered, and it has been determined that they significantly contribute to the onset of AD. The majority of cases of EOAD are inherited in an autosomal dominant manner, and mutations in the key genes apolipoprotein E (ApoE), Amyloid precursor protein (APP), and presenilin-1 (PSEN-1) are associated with AD. Around 70% of AD cases are attributed to genetic causes [24, 25]. Although mutations in the Amyloid precursor protein (APP), PSEN1, and PSEN2 have been crucial in the current understanding of the pathogenic mechanism underlying AD, the results from GWAS and the Macular Photocoagulation Study (MPS) once again highlight the complexity of AD. However, it is still challenging to translate genetic discoveries into biologically significant functional mechanisms for disease causation and therapy planning.

11.4.3 ENVIRONMENTAL FACTORS

The recognition of modifiable environmental risk variables can have a significant impact on AD and related dementia prevention and therapy. Numerous chemicals in the environment have long been known to be neurotoxic. Air pollution, heavy metals, infections, and many other harmful environmental factors can be a source of oxidative stress and inflammation, which raises the likelihood of developing AD. Here, we list the most significant environmental elements and their connections to AD.

11.4.4 AIR POLLUTION

By introducing some chemical, physical, or biological contaminants into the surrounding atmosphere, air pollution alters the composition of the original atmosphere. It has lately been shown to be linked to AD as well as respiratory and cardiovascular illnesses. National Ambient Air Quality Standards (NAAQSs) in the USA have identified six air pollutants, for example ozone

(O_3), particulate matter (PM), nitrogen oxides (NOx), carbon monoxide (CO), sulfur dioxide (SO_2), and lead, which are threats to human health. The highest levels of air pollution can harm the frontal cortex area, as well as the olfactory mucosa and bulb, similar to what is seen in AD, according to some studies on cellular and animal models [27]. Cigarette smoke was discovered to be related to an increased incidence of dementia in a sectional study of around 6,000 people in different regions of China [28].

11.4.5 TOXIC HEAVY METALS

Given the broad exposure of the population, the effects of some heavy metals like lead, cadmium, and manganese on the environment are of particular interest. Even at modest levels of such exposure found in the normal population, lead and cadmium are remarkable metals for their neurotoxic effects. Although manganese is a crucial trace element needed for many physiological processes, including the health of neurons, it is hazardous when present in low or excessive amounts. It is essential to comprehend how these heavy metals contribute to the genesis of AD and associated dementias [29].

11.5 ROLE OF DIET IN AD

11.5.1 DASH DIET

The Dietary Approaches to Stop Hypertension (DASH) diet, recommended by the National Heart, Lung, and Blood Institute (NHLBI, USA), is a dietary pattern first designed to control hypertension for a healthy heart. The DASH diet contains minerals like calcium, potassium, proteins, and fiber. It discourages using processed meats, full-fat dairy products, oils, sugary drinks, desserts, excessive salt, saturated fats, and cholesterol [30]. This diet has been demonstrated to reduce the risk of cardiovascular disease and modify the pathogenic processes (oxidative stress, inflammation, and insulin resistance) related to AD. Elevated levels of antioxidant capacity and decreased inflammation have been linked to diets rich in fruits, vegetables, and vegetable oils, vitamins C and E, beta-carotene, and flavonoids. DASH and MD share many dietary components but vary in the frequency with which low-fat dairy products are consumed, as shown in Table 11.1 [31, 32]. The outcomes of these dietary intervention studies suggest that dietary patterns may lessen the risk of dementia or AD due to their impact on inflammatory pathways and oxidative stress [33].

TABLE 11.1 Different Dietary Patterns to Prevent AD [32]

Diets	Measures of Consumption	
	Moderate-to-High	**Low**
Dietary approaches to stop hypertension (DASH)	• Foods made with whole grains • Green vegetables • Fruits • Milk and milk products (average to high intake) • Chicken (two times a week) • Seafood (once or twice a week) • Beans and other legumes (twice weekly)	• Saturated fats • Salt, Drinks with added sugar, Processed meat
Mediterranean diet (MD)	• Eat a serving or two of whole-grain cereal with each major meal. • Eat two servings of vegetables with every major meal. • Eat some fruit with every big meal (two to four servings). • Infused with olive oil. • Nuts and seeds (twice daily). • Low-calorie diaries (two entries each day). • Herbs and spices. • Garlic/onions (every day). • Chicken or duck eggs (twice or four times a week). • Two servings of white meat every week. • Seafood/fish (2x/week). • Avocado (3 times a week). • Beans (2x/week). • (Red) wine.	• Incorporated salt. • Consuming red meat on a weekly basis (less than two servings). • Tinned beef (once every seven days). • Sugary treats (once every two weeks).
Mediterranean-DASH intervention for neurodegenerative delay (MIND)	• Eat a lot of leafy green veggies. • A handful of nuts (one every five days). • Fruit (about twice a week). • Kidney beans (about three times a week). • Three servings of whole grains each day. • Fish (once a week). • Chickens (2 times a week). • Infused with olives and olive oil (primary oil used). • One glass of wine (red) every day.	• Consumption of red meat (once every four days). • Margarines, including butter and stick varieties. • Cheese (1 s/week). • Desserts (about once a week). • Processed food (once every several weeks).

11.5.2 Mediterranean Diet (MD)

In recent years, MD has earned widespread attention for its positive impact on several illnesses, including neurodegenerative disorders (NDs). Although the Greeks and Romans initially introduced MD, it wasn't until Castelvetro made the connection to health in 1634. In the early 1960s, Professor Ancel Keys studied the dietary patterns and eating habits of people in Mediterranean nations. High intake of olive oil, green vegetables, whole grain cereals, polyphenolic substances, fruits, chickpeas, legumes, fatty acids (mono- and polyunsaturated fatty acids), and nuts; medium consumption of fish, meat, and red wine; and low use of saturated fats constitute the Mediterranean diet [34]. Most of the phytoconstituents found in the MD are flavonoids which showed beneficial and protective effects against common pathways, including inflammation, oxidative stress, and signaling cascades in cells, which are involved in the progression of AD [35, 36].

Using antioxidants to prevent oxidative stress (OS) has been researched as one of the most effective preventative measures against neurodegenerative disorders, including AD. The antioxidant ability of polyphenolic compounds, a primary component in MD, has been the subject of substantial research and study against a wide range of NDs [36]. These antioxidants neutralize free radicals, block pro-apoptotic pathways, and boost protective signaling cascades during OS. The antioxidant properties of olive oil (a key ingredient in MD) and it's phenolic constituents hydroxytyrosol and oleuropein have protective effects against OS through various mechanisms, including preventing the oxidation of low-density lipids; limiting the generation of short-chain malondialdehyde, aldehydes, 4-hydroxynonenal-lysine adducts, and peroxides; metals chelation; and inhibiting free radicals [35, 37]. F2-isoprostane (a by-product of arachidonic acid peroxidation) levels were shown to be considerably reduced in a randomized cross-over trial when participants had a phenolic-enriched meal that included olive oil [38].

Another compound named resveratrol (3,5,4-trihydroxy-trans-stilbene) is one of the most researched natural compounds due to its biological and medicinal significance [39]. It is found in grapes and red wine. Resveratrol has been shown to have a substantial neuroprotective effect against OS produced by Aβ, stroke, streptozotocin, and MPTP, among other neurodegenerative diseases, in a wide range of research investigations [35]. According to Zini et al., resveratrol's antioxidant effect is manifested in the following distinct ways: (i) competing for coenzyme Q and inhibiting the site of ROS generation (through complex 1-III in the mitochondrial respiratory chain); (ii) inhibiting $O_2^{\bullet-}$ radicals and lipid peroxidation in the mitochondria; and

(iii) preserving the levels of antioxidant enzymes [40] The hydroxyl and gallate group in epigallocatechin-3-gallate provides the beverage with its antioxidant properties by scavenging free radicals and chelating metals [41]. It also suppresses ROS by regulating the nuclear factor erythroid 2-related factor 2 (Nrf2) cascade and expressions of enzymes, including glutathione S-transferase, glutathione peroxidase, glutamate cysteine ligase, heme oxygenase-1. Carotenoids exert significant antioxidant potential through direct and indirect pathways. β-carotene, lycopene, and lutein exhibited antioxidant activity by direct physical quenching and indirectly by interacting with various signaling pathways at the cellular level [42, 43]. Furthermore, flavonoids like naringenin, quercetin, and kaempferol in the MD also showed antioxidant properties by scavenging ROS or inhibiting enzymes or components involved in free radical formation. It also reduces their synthesis through chelation and augments the production of antioxidant genes [35, 36].

11.5.3 MIND DIET

The MIND diet (Mediterranean-DASH Intervention for Neurodegenerative Delay) was developed by a group of researchers from Rush University and Harvard Public Health School in the USA [30]. Greens, veggies, fruits, berries, whole grains, nuts, legumes, olive oil, lean proteins, and red wine are a few examples of the 10 brain-healthy foods that make up the MIND diet, with decreased intake of red meats, saturated fats, cheese, pastries, sweets, and processed food [32, 33]. Fish intake is reduced on the MIND and DASH diets compared to the MD, with both plans recommending no more than one serving of fish per week. The results of the prospective Rotterdam trial, which investigated the function of fish intake in preventing AD, are consistent with this low level of fish consumption [44, 45]. The n–3 fatty acids from fish consumption decrease amyloid-β formation, oxidative stress, and inflammation [46]. Several clinical studies (Table 11.2) found a statistically significant correlation between these dietary patterns and a reduced risk of cognitive impairment in older adults. The MIND diet also contains berries which exhibited substantial improvement in cognitive function because of antioxidant and anti-inflammatory activities in neuronal toxicity cellular models [47, 48]. *In vivo* investigations of animals fed with high berries diet showed the reduction of age-related neuronal loss and enhanced motor coordination, cognitive function, and hippocampal plasticity [49–51].

TABLE 11.2 Summary of the Clinical Trials Examining the Effect of Dietary Patterns in Preventing Cognitive Decline and AD

Different Diets	Study Design	Study Population	Duration of Treatment	Results	References
DASH	Cohort	Older American women	6 years	DASH diet followers had higher mean cognitive scores, but there is no correlation between diet and cognitive decline or improvement throughout the follow-up period.	[52]
DASH	RCT (ENCORE)	Obese and sedentary individuals	4 months	Those who followed the DASH diet saw marginal gains in psychomotor speed.	[53]
MD	Cohort	Elderly Americans	4 years	A significantly reduced chance of developing AD was seen in those with higher MD adherence.	[54]
MD	Cohort	Elderly Americans	5.4 years	Increases in both physical activity and adherence to a Mediterranean diet have been linked to a lower incidence of AD.	[55]
MD	Cohort	Elderly Americans	3.8 years	The chance of developing AD is inversely proportional to one's Modified Rankin Scale score. The chance of acquiring AD was reduced by 34% in the top tertile.	[56]
MD	Cohort	Elderly Americans	4.3 years	MD adherence causes 48% less risk of developing AD.	[57]
MD	Cohort	Elderly Americans	4.4 years	AD patients with better adherence to the MD had a decreased risk of dying.	[58]
MD	Cross-sectional	Older Americans	NA	Greater adherence to the MD was connected to reduced AD risk.	[59]
MD	Cross-sectional	Elderly Greeks	NA	Maintaining a regimen of MD has been linked to improved cognitive function and a reduced risk of developing dementia.	[60]
MD	Cross-sectional (AIBL) study	Elderly Australians	NA	When subjects with AD and MCI were maintained on MD, they exhibited a decreased risk of transitioning to AD.	[61]
MD	RCT (MedLey)	Elderly Australians	6 months	There is no proof that MD involvement improves memory or cognitive skills in healthy elderly people.	[62]
MD	RCT (NU-AGE)	European populations	1 year	Groups showed significant cognitive improvement.	[63]

TABLE 11.2 *(Continued)*

Different Diets	Study Design	Study Population	Duration of Treatment	Results	References
MD	RCT (PREDIMED)	Individuals at a high cardiovascular (CV) risk	4.1 years	Improved cognitive function.	[64]
MD	RCT (PREDIMED)	Individuals with heart problems	6.5 years	In comparison to a low-fat diet, dietary supplementation with MD seems to increase cognitive performance.	[65]
MD DASH	Cohort	Elderly American women	9.1 years	No link between MED and DASH scores.	[66]
MD DASH MIND	Cohort	Older Americans	4.5 years	High-MD and high-DASH adherents had a 54% and 39% decreased chance of acquiring AD, respectively.	[66]
MD MIND	Cross-sectional	Elderly population	NA	Higher levels of adherence to the MD and MIND diet enhance cognitive performance.	[67]

11.6 ROLE OF VITAMINS IN AD

Generally speaking, vitamins are regarded as organic substances that are necessary for the growth and regular operation of the body. Vitamins cannot be manufactured by the body; they must therefore be received from the diet. Importantly, vitamins frequently serve as enzymatic cofactors or antioxidants. In general, vitamins have a special benefit for neurodegenerative illnesses. Therefore, it is crucial to learn more about these vitamins and how important they are for both preventing and treating AD.

11.6.1 AD AND VITAMIN D

Vitamin D seems to be able to affect the central nervous system in addition to its numerous other roles. Vitamin D receptors have been found in several important brain areas that are neuron-rich [68]. It has also been displayed that the brain includes enzymes that facilitate the local union of calcitriol. According to some experimental investigations, the vitamin's multifarious mechanisms of action through modulating anti-inflammatory, vasculoprotective, and neuroprotective processes may be able to prevent the development of dementia. Scientists advise achieving blood vitamin D concentrations of at least 30 ng/mL to prevent dementia [69]. This can be done by getting sun exposure as much as possible, eating enough vitamin D-rich food items, or taking dietary supplements containing at least 800 IU of vitamin D daily [68]. One clinical trial revealed that increasing vitamin D levels can have a particularly beneficial impact on the mental capacities that regulate thought and activity [70]. Such 'executive functions' are frequently found impaired in AD patients who are still in the preclinical stages of this disease.

11.6.2 AD AND VITAMIN B-COMPLEX

Thiamine (B1), riboflavin (B2), niacin (B3), pyridoxine (B6), folate (B9), and cobalamin are all members of the B-vitamin class (B12). It is commonly accepted that the B-complex vitamins, especially folate, B12, and B6, can stop AD and aging cognitive decline. Increased generality of gastritis and other digestion-related problems that hinder absorption cause vitamin B12 deficiency, which affects more than 20% of people 65 years of age and older, to become increasingly common as people age [71, 72]. Thiamine and niacin deficits are the root causes of two uncommon neurologic disorders. Pellagra is a condition marked by symptoms of dementia, diarrhea, and dermatitis that can be treated with niacin supplementation and is known to be brought on by niacin insufficiency [73]. According to some reports, vitamin B6 can prevent oxidative stress in AD [74].

11.6.3 ROLE OF MINERALS IN AD

In human bodies, metals like iron, copper, and zinc are found naturally. These metals must be present in our bodies and brains at minute levels to maintain correct function. They are implicated in a wide range of functions, including the generation and management of numerous significant molecules in the body, the flow of oxygen, and the production of energy. A connection between naturally occurring metals and the onset or continuation of AD is likely to exist (Figure 11.2). However, it is not yet clear from the evidence if this connection contributes to AD.

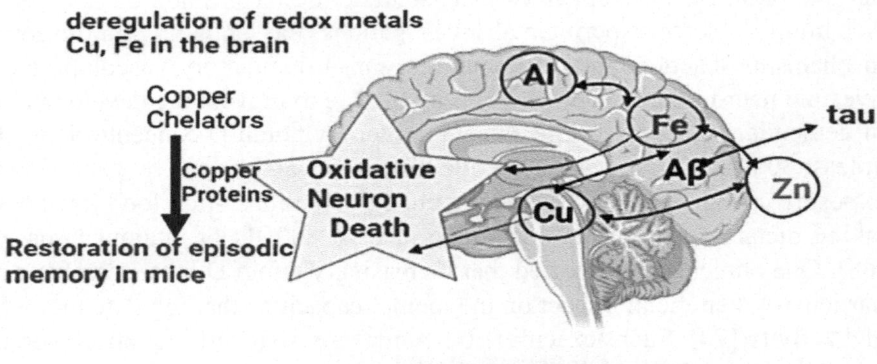

FIGURE 11.2 Deregulation of redox metals in the brain.

Source: Adapted from Ref. [161]

11.6.4 AD AND ZINC

One of the body's important micronutrients and the second-most prevalent micronutrient in the human body's nervous system is zinc [75, 76]. Growth and development, wound healing, immunological control, catalytic processes, and substance synthesis all involve zinc. In the brain, zinc controls both excitatory and inhibitory neurotransmitters [77, 78]. Zinc treatment was reported to postpone hippocampal-dependent memory problems in AD mice models and to diminish both A and tau pathology in the hippocampus [79]. In AD, a zinc shortage can cause a decline in learning capacity and memory. One study found that supplementing with zinc (3 mg/kg) improved learning and memory [24].

11.6.5 AD AND IRON

One of the vital trace metals, iron is abundantly distributed throughout the human body. Iron influences lipid peroxidation, cell differentiation, growth and development, transport of materials, growth, and development, and gene expression. AD is likelier to have abnormal heme levels and disturbed iron homeostasis [80]. Many neurodegenerative diseases are characterized by iron accumulation in the brain. Post-mortem studies have discovered a considerably greater concentration of ferritin and hemosiderin collection in the brain tissues of patients with critical AD [81]. Iron deficiency in the fetal brain tissue may result from inadequate iron consumption during pregnancy, raising the risk of neurological abnormalities. Age-related brain tissue-amyloid protein deposition and plaque can lead to iron accumulation in the brain tissue, which in turn encourages more iron deposition [81].

11.6.6 AD AND SELENIUM

In recent years, it has become increasingly obvious how crucial Selenium is to biology and health [82]. Its cellular functions, which are crucial for life, include a wide variety of enzymatic and non-enzymatic activities that affect hormones, signal transduction, and transcription factors, and participate in antioxidant and redox control [82]. By utilizing selenomethionine, selenium can interact with metals and enhance the body's antioxidant capacity. In mice with AD, chondroitin sulfate selenium has been demonstrated to enhance memory and spatial learning deficits, lessen synaptic edema in hippocampal neurons, and safeguard mitochondrial integrity.

11.6.7 AD AND SILICON

One of the most prevalent micronutrients in the body is silicon. It is separated into crystalline silicon, which is found as silicon dioxide or silicate, and amorphous silicon. The immune system, bone mineralization, immune system modulation, and Tau phosphorylation are all affected by silicon [83, 84]. Recent research has demonstrated silicon's positive effects on human health. In the human body, soluble silicic acid is a beneficial form of silicon. Human health is directly correlated with the soluble silicic acid absorption, distribution, and metabolic properties in the human body. Soluble silicic acid's special capacity for cross-linking and its opposition to poisonous aluminum may offer protection from AD. A study shows that beer, which contains silicon and hops in abundance, is crucial in preventing brain diseases as silicon lowers the risk of AD. This is essentially connected to beer's capacity to control oxidation, inflammation, and cholinesterase activity [85].

11.6.8 AD AND MANGANESE

One of the vital micronutrients in the body is manganese. It participates in processes that are mostly connected to the alkylation of manganese, such as oxidation-reduction, lipid formation, and protein breakdown. Studies have demonstrated how manganese helps in AD diagnosis. Assessing the degree of pathogenic Tau build-up can be done using manganese-enhanced magnetic resonance imaging [86]. A new approach to the therapeutic therapy of AD may be found in the use of manganese-chelating compounds in the treatment of neurodegenerative illnesses like AD. A viable method for stopping or reducing AD may be effectively regulating manganese neurotoxicity. When prion proteins exhibit abnormal conformation in healthy cells, they can develop into pathogenic prion proteins that bind to micronutrients like manganese, copper, and zinc and cause AD [87].

11.6.9 AD AND ARSENIC

The body needs arsenic as a micronutrient. It is frequently encountered in nature as ash, black, and yellow arsenic. Although highly dangerous, arsenic has some advantages in tiny doses. Protein synthesis, material metabolism, and biotransformation are all affected by arsenic. In clinical research, inductively coupled plasma mass spectrometry was used to assess the amounts of arsenic in the nails and hair of 40 AD patients. Compared to controls, AD had greater arsenic levels. This suggests that higher arsenic levels are common in AD patients [88]. Arsenic in drinking water has been linked to irregular circadian rhythm, abnormal motility, and amyloid protein buildup in the frontal cortex and hippocampus in AD mice, according to animal research.

This was discovered to be connected to the mice's arsenic-induced lipid peroxidation [88]. Gallic acid (100 mg/kg) was observed to attenuate the behavioral abnormalities and memory changes caused by sodium arsenite in male rats with AD, demonstrating the neuroprotective action of gallic acid.

11.7 ROLE OF MACRONUTRIENTS IN AD

Clinical interest is growing in the use of polyunsaturated fatty acids (PUFAs), specifically eicosapentaenoic (EPA) and docosahexaenoic (DHA) acids, for the prevention of cognitive decline. These fatty acids show neuroprotective action, including enhancing neuroplasticity in neuronal cell membranes, stimulation of synapse formation, regulation of intracellular signaling pathways, and reducing inflammation response [89]. The 'Washington Hamilton Heights, Inwood, Columbia Aging Project' (WHICAP) research recommends the consumption of PUFAs, particularly DHA, EPA, and omega-3 fatty acids, for controlling the inflammation occurring in patients with AD [90]. The study indicates that increased consumption of omega-3s and length of unsaturated fatty acids lowers the chance of getting AD. On the other hand, increased use of monounsaturated fatty acids (MUFAs) and fat content increases the risk of AD [90, 91].

People with mild AD who took omega-3 and alpha-lipoic acid supplements for one year showed less cognitive decline. However, the research has its limitations due to the small sample size [90]. Omega-3 PUFA (800 mg DHA and 225 mg EPA) intake for three years in older patients with memory complaints did not corroborate the impact of intake on learning and memory in the Multidomain Alzheimer Preventive Trial [92]. Therefore, those who lack these nutrients, particularly in the early stages before cognitive damage sets in, should be studied to determine the effects of PUFA supplementation on dementia [92].

Moreover, EPA, DHA, and n–3 PUFA have been widely documented for their protective benefits against neuroinflammation in AD. Some of the ways in which n–3 PUFAs have been demonstrated to be anti-inflammatory include blocking the activity of the transcription factor NF-κB, decreasing the generation of NO, and boosting microglial phagocytic activity through the M2 pathway [93]. DHA also aids in the production of resolvins, which have anti-inflammatory effects and prevent a rise in cytokines and nitric oxide [94]. DHA is the neuroprotection D1 precursor, suppressing the production of cytokines, nuclear factor kappa B (NF-κB), caspase 3, and cyclo-oxygenase-2 [95, 96]. DHA restricts Aβ from fibrillating by preventing the production of Aβ oligomers and β-sheets [97]. It also increases the nonamyloidogenic processing of amyloid precursor protein and protects neurons from Aβ-induced damage in cultured PC12 cells via upregulating the PI3/AKT neuronal survival pathway [98].

11.8 ROLE OF PHYTOCHEMICALS IN AD

11.8.1 AB AND B-SECRETASE INHIBITORS

β-Secretase inhibition forms a suitable therapeutic approach for treating AD patients. Various plant extracts and their phytoconstituents (given in Table 11.3) also showed a beneficial effect against Aβ and β-secretase activity [99]. Compounds isolated from *Curcuma longa*, like calebin-A, curcumin, and demethoxycurcumin, protected PC12 cells from Aβ-induced damage [100, 101]. Ginsenoside Rg3 from *P. ginseng* lowered Aβ concentration (IC_{50}, under 25 μmol/L) in SK-N-SH cells transfected with β-APP [102]. Single oral doses of other ginsenosides like Rg1 and Re also exhibited significant reductions in the amount of Aβ detected in the brains of animals. Ginsenoside Rg1 from Sanchi ginseng (*Panax notoginseng*) also showed a neuroprotective effect in PC12 cells (*in vitro*) by inhibiting β-secretase activity against $A\beta_{25-35}$ [103].

Berberine, an isoquinoline alkaloid isolated from *Coptidis rhizoma*, effectively reduced the levels of $A\beta_{40}$ and $A\beta_{42}$ (IC_{50} = 5 μmol/L) [117]. Berberine has also ameliorated Aβ pathology, gliosis, and cognitive impairment in a transgenic mouse model of AD [118]. It has inhibited the Aβ-stimulated production of interleukin-6, lowered the activity of beta-site APP cleaving enzyme-1 (BACE-1), and downregulated the expression of cyclooxygenase-2 [119–121].

Salvia miltiorrhiza (commonly known as Danshen) is a well-known plant in traditional Chinese medicine. Salvianolic acid B (SalB, 10 mg/kg, p.o.) isolated from the plant was found to significantly reverse the memory impairments induced by scopolamine (1 mg/kg, i.p.) and $A\beta_{25-35}$ (10 nmol/5 mL, i.c.v.) injection [112]. The aqueous/ethanol extracts of the root of *Salvia miltiorrhiza* reversed $A\beta_{25-35}$-induced cytotoxicity. Danshensu and SalB protected the PC-12 cells by blocking $A\beta_{25-35}$-induced Ca^{2+} uptake, lactate dehydrogenase expression, and cell death through apoptosis [122]. Cryptotanshinone (CTS, concentration: 10 μM) not only improves cognitive ability

TABLE 11.3 Plants and Phytoconstituents with Aβ and β-Secretase Inhibitory Activity

Plants	Phytoconstituents	Type of Extract	References
Callistemon lanceolatus (Myritaceae)	4′,5-Dihydroxy-6,8-dimethyl-7-methoxyflavanone, Eucalyptin, Sideroxylin, and Quercetin	Methanol extract	[104]
Curcuma longa (Zingiberaceae)	Curcumin	–	[105]
Eleutherococcus senticosus (Araliaceae)	Eleutheroside B, Eleutheroside E and Isofraxidin	Methanol extract	[106]
Elsholtzia rugulosa (Lamiaceae)	Luteolin	Ethanol extract	[107]
Eragrostis ferruginea (Poaceae)	7-Demethyl-ageconyflavone A, Tricin, 4-Ketopinoresinol	Methanol extract	[108]
Magnolia officinalis (Magnoliaceae)	Magnolol, Honokiol, and 4-*O*-Methylhonokiol	Ethanol extract	[109]
Plumbago genus (Plumbaginaceae)	Plumbagin	–	[110]
Pueraria lobate (Fabaceae)	Genistein, Biochanin A, Sissotrin, Puerol B, 2-(*α*, *α*-Dimethylallyl) coumestrol	Ethyl acetate-soluble extract	[111]
Salvia miltiorrhiza (Lamiaceae)	Salvianolic acid B and Danshensu	Aqueous and ethanol extracts	[112]
Salvia officinalis (Lamiaceae)	Rosmarinic acid	Hydroalcoholic extract	[113]
Schisandra chinensis (Schisandraceae)	Schisantherin A and Schisandrin B-C	Hexane extract	[114]
Withania somnifera (Solanaceae)	Withanamide A and C	–	[115, 116]

in AD transgenic mice and promotes APP metabolism in rat cortical neuronal cells, but also decreases the levels of $A\beta_{42}$ by 45% [123].

Camelia sinensis (Green tea) infusion (0.03 mg/ml) inhibited BACE 1 activity by 27% after 5 min incubation and 38% inhibition after 60 min incubation time [124]. Epigallocatechin gallate (EGCG) reduces the intracellular generation of both $A\beta_{1-40}$ and $A\beta_{1-42}$ peptides [125] and Aβ generation and deposition in cell cultures [125, 126]. Two compounds present in *Magnolia officinalis* – honokiol and magnolol – significantly decreased the Aβ-induced cell death [109]. Silybin (Silibinin), a flavonoid derived from milk thistle

(*Silybum marianum*), inhibited memory impairment in an $A\beta_{25-35}$ model of AD [127]. Tenuigenin, isolated from *Polygala tenuifolia*, limited the production of Aβ and C99 in SH-SY5Y APP695 cells [128]. Additionally, it blocked BACE1's proteolytic activity (beta-secretase). Another compound, Tenuifolin, prevented the beta-site APP cleaving enzyme, which caused a decrease in Aβ secretion from the transfected cells [129].

Flavonoids such as quercetin, luteolin, myricetin, kaempferol, apigenin, morin; flavones like kuwanon A, morusin, kuwanon C, norartocarpetin, 2,3-dihydroamentoflavone, 2,3-dihydro-6-methylginkgetin, bilobetin, ginkgetin, amentoflavone-7,7″-dimethyl ether, amentoflavone, and sequoiaflavone, sotetsuflavone, podocarpusflavone A, podocarpusflavone B, isoginkgetin, also exhibited β-secretase-inhibitory activity [130, 131]. Additionally, furanocoumarins (5-geranyloxy-8-methoxypsoralen) are found to be the most active for drug development for AD because of their lower IC_{50} value and high lipophilicity [131, 132]. Other phytoconstituents/compounds that reduce the Aβ levels in various experimental studies are vanillic acid, vanillin, tramiprosate (also known as homotaurine, from red algae *Grateloupia livida*), vitamin C, D_3 and E, docosahexaenoic acid (from fish and algae), melatonin, resveratrol (from *Vitis vinifera*) and nicotine (from *Nicotiana tabacum*) [105, 133, 134].

11.8.2 Γ-SECRETASE INHIBITORS

γ-Secretase is involved in the generation of Aβ peptides ($A\beta_{40}$ and $A\beta_{42}$) by cleaving APP in the final step. Despite potential action, interference in the metabolism of nonamyloid substrates and Notch processing leads to adverse effects and neurotoxicity, which is the main obstacle to developing γ-secretase inhibitors [135]. Because of these difficulties, only a small number of plant extracts and active compounds have been screened for γ-secretase inhibitory activity. The compound SPI-014 (identified as 24-O-acetylhydroshengmanol (Δ-16,17)-enol ether-3-O-β-D-xylopyranoside) from the alcoholic extract of *Actaea racemosa* (Syn: *Cimicifuga racemosa*, Family – Ranunculaceae) inhibits the formation of $A\beta_{42}$ (IC_{50} = 0.1 μM). Furthermore, it increases the concentration of $A\beta_{37}$ and $A\beta_{39}$ (smaller fragments) in the brain and does not affect Notch signaling. These findings show that SPI-014 has the potential to act as a lead molecule for developing new therapeutics. The main issue with SPI-014 is its low penetration in the brain due to the BBB, but recently, the structure has been optimized to increase its bioavailability in the brain [136]. SPI-1865 (semisynthetic derivatives of SPI-014) was found to be effective and has been selected for further preclinical trials [137]. The aqueous extract of kino and stem bark of *Pterocarpus erinaceus* (Fabaceae) also shows γ-secretase inhibitory activity without inhibiting γ-secretase-dependent Notch intracellular domain release. *Malus domestica* (Apple, Family – Rosaceae) reduces Aβ production by reducing γ-secretase expression.

11.8.3 TAU INHIBITORS

Tau proteins are responsible for the stabilization of the microtubules in the neurons. Hyperphosphorylation of tau proteins develops neurofibrillary tangles, which disrupt normal neuronal function. Due to its rich chemical diversification, many plants/phytoconstituents have been explored as new AD therapeutics (Table 11.4) for clearing tau aggregation [1].

11.9 ROLE OF LIFESTYLE MODIFICATIONS AND ALTERNATIVE THERAPIES TO TREAT AD

Sedentary behavior is one of the risk factors for many diseases in the twenty-first century [153]. A physical workout is any skeletal muscle action of the body that involves the use of energy. People who are physically active are generally healthy and free of various ailments. Recent research showed that relative declines of 10% per decade in the prevalence of some adjustable risk variables might cut the incidence of AD by 8.3% globally by 2050 [156, 157].

According to a different study, exercise depletes energy and raises the AMP/ATP ratio, which prompts the cell's AMPK protein kinase to become active. Another potentially beneficial non-pharmacologic strategy for slowing down the aging process of the brain is calorie restriction (CR), which enhances metabolic health [158]. CR works by counteracting the negative effects of ROS and oxidative damage. In light of this, CR may be thought of as a viable nutritional interposition for the prevention of several age-related chronic diseases in addition to physical workouts and exercise. Patients may also benefit from keeping track of their food and exercise-related behaviors, feelings, and thoughts [159, 160]. Once they have achieved their lifestyle goals, patients may find it helpful to use cognitive rewards to help them cope with the frustration of limited weight loss

TABLE 11.4 Plants and Phytoconstituents with Tau Inhibitory Activity

Plants	Phytoconstituents	Type of Extract	References
Allium sativum (Alliaceae)	*S*-allyl-cysteine, and diallyl-disulfide	Aged garlic extract	[138]
Anemarrhena asphodeloides (Asparagaceae)	Saponin B	–	[139]
Camellia sinensis (Theaceae)	EGCG and (–)-epicatechin-3-gallate	–	[140]
Centella asiatica (Apiaceae)	Asiatic acid	–	[141]
Cinnamonium zeylanicum (Lauraceae)	Cinnamaldehyde	Aqueous extract	[142]
Cnidium monnieri (Apiaceae)	Osthole	–	[143]
Cocos nucifera (Arecaceae)	Estrone, 17-β-estradiol and β-sitosterol	Juice of young coconut	[144]
Curcuma longa (Zingiberaceae)	Curcumin	Standardized turmeric extract (contains 82% curcuminoids by weight)	[145, 146]
Hibiscus sabdariffa (Malvaceae)	Gossypetin	–	[147, 148]
*Ilex latifolia (*Aquifoliaceae)	The primary component of bitter Chinese tea called "*Kudingcha*"	Ethanol extract	[149]
Maclura pomifera (Moraceae)	Morin	–	[150]
Myrica cerifera (Myricaceae)	(+)-aR,11S-myricanol, Myricetin, Myricitrin	Aqueous extract of Bayberry	[151]
Olive oil from fruits of *Olea europaea* (Oleaceae)	Oleocanthal, oleuropein, oleuropein aglycone and hydroxytyrosol	–	[152]
Panax ginseng (Araliaceae)	Ginsenoside Rb1, ginsenoside Rd	–	[153]
Red wine, grapes, berries, peanuts	Resveratrol	–	[154]

and to boost their confidence in body weight management and leading a healthy lifestyle. Clinicians may also employ positive reinforcement, and they should always thank their patients for their accomplishments and never blame them when they fail.

11.10 REFLECTION POINTS FOR FUTURE RESEARCH

AD is one of the complex diseases of the CNS that needs extra care along with medications. The life of a person with AD is very difficult and challenging as memory and recall of situations become hard for the patients, making things worse. The current chapter briefly discusses the role of a balanced diet and lifestyle in the development as well as the management of AD and associated symptoms. Nutrients and lifestyle contribute not only to the management of metabolic diseases but also play a key role in CNS-related disorders. As explained, the contribution of macro- and micro-nutrients in the prevention of the disease reflects their role during the ongoing treatment of the disease with some allopathic medicines. The role and mechanism of dietary minerals and vitamins in the prevention or treatment need to be explored and supported by a greater number of clinical studies. Allopathic medicines alone are not capable enough to manage the disease. Therefore, herbs or other time-tested traditional diets should be examined scientifically for benefits in the management of AD and related diseases.

11.11 CONCLUSION

AD is a disease of the CNS in which short-term or long-term memory loss is a prominent and characteristic symptom. Although modern science has developed a lot, there is still no permanent and successful treatment available for AD. Researchers have tried to explore the role of a balanced diet and traditional herbs in the treatment of AD. Some of the herbs are even documented for their success in pre-clinical studies using established animal models of AD. The published reports on macro- and micro-nutrients are encouraging and provide evidence of their contribution to slowing the progression of memory loss. This chapter includes consolidated data on herbs and dietary nutrients that have shown promising results in the management of AD or other CNS-related disorders. The chapter also provides insight into a balanced diet, its composition, and essential nutrients that can help delay memory loss or conditions like dementia. Traditional systems of medicine are time-tested healthcare systems that have been in place since time immemorial. Such systems support the role of natural ingredients in managing a variety of diseases and can also serve as a guide to developing medicines for the treatment of AD and other CNS-related complications. Therefore, medical practitioners need to focus on a holistic approach to treatment, including a balanced diet.

KEYWORDS

- **Alzheimer's disease (AD)**
- **dementia**
- **lifestyle modifications**
- **macronutrients**
- **Mediterranean diet**
- **micronutrients**

REFERENCES

1. Malik, J., Munjal, K., & Deshmukh, R. (2015). Attenuating effect of standardized lyophilized *Cinnamomum zeylanicum* bark extract against streptozotocin-induced experimental dementia of Alzheimer's type. *Journal of Basic & Clinical Physiology & Pharmacology, 26*(3), 275–285.
2. Li, X., Feng, X., Sun, X., Hou, N., Han, F., & Liu, Y. (2022). Global, regional, and national burden of Alzheimer's disease and other dementias, 1990–2019. *Alzheimer's & Dementia, 14*, 937486.
3. 2022 Alzheimer's disease facts and figures. (2022). *Alzheimer's & Dementia: The Journal of the Alzheimer's Association, 18*(4), 700–789.
4. Choudhary, A., Ranjan, J., & Asthana, H. (2021). Prevalence of dementia in India: A systematic review and meta-analysis. *Journal of Clinical Neuroscience, 65*(2), 152–158.
5. Haye, A., Ansari, M., Saini, A., Ahmed, Z., Munjal, K., Shamsi, Y., & Sharma, M. (2022). Polyherbal formulation improves glucose-lipid metabolism and prevents hepatotoxicity in streptozotocin-induced diabetic rats: Plausible role of IRS-PI3K-Akt-GLUT2 signaling. *Pharmacognosy Magazine, 18*, 52.
6. Sonali, V., Sumeet, G., Rina, D., Kavita, M., Meenakshi, D., Dinesh Kumar, M., Gurudev, G., & Anshu, G. (2023). Unraveling the approaches to treat osteoarthritis: A focus on the potential of medicinal plants. *Pharmacognosy Research, 15*(1), 13–25.
7. Stefaniak, O., Dobrzyńska, M., Drzymała-Czyż, S., & Przysławski, J. (2022). Diet in the prevention of Alzheimer's disease: Current knowledge and future research requirements. *Nutrients, 14*(21), 4654.
8. Munjal, K., Ahmad, S., Gupta, A., Haye, A., Amin, S., & Mir, S. (2020). Polyphenol-enriched fractions and the compounds isolated from *Garcinia indica* fruits ameliorate obesity through the suppression of digestive enzymes and oxidative stress. *Pharmacognosy Magazine, 16*(70), 236–245.
9. Sharma, A., Gupta, D. S., Sharma, S., Dhanawat, M., & Munjal, K. (2021). Combination effect of *Spirulina fusiformis* with rutin or chlorogenic acid in lipopolysaccharide-induced septic cardiac inflammation in an experimental diabetic rat model. *Pharmacognosy Magazine, 17*, 257.

10. Kciuk, M., Mujwar, S., Rani, I., Munjal, K., Gielecińska, A., Kontek, R., & Shah, K. (2022). Computational bioprospecting of guggulsterone against ADP ribose phosphatase of SARS-CoV-2. *Molecules, 27*, 8287.
11. Munjal, K., Kumar, G., Gauttam, V., Arora, A., & Sawale, J. (2022). Scope and limitations of digital learning in developing countries: A real-time survey. *Annals of Phytomedicine: An International Journal*, COVID-19 Special.
12. Wang, L., Davis, P. B., Volkow, N. D., Berger, N. A., Kaelber, D. C., & Xu, R. (2022). Association of COVID-19 with new-onset Alzheimer's disease. *Journal of Alzheimer's Disease, 89*(2), 411–414.
13. Omar, S. H., Scott, C. J., Hamlin, A. S., & Obied, H. K. (2017). The protective role of plant biophenols in mechanisms of Alzheimer's disease. *The Journal of Nutritional Biochemistry, 47*, 1–20.
14. Baker, L. D., Manson, J. E., Rapp, S. R., Sesso, H. D., Gaussoin, S. A., Shumaker, S. A., & Espeland, M. A. (2022). Effects of cocoa extract and a multivitamin on cognitive function: A randomized clinical trial. *Alzheimer's & Dementia: The Journal of the Alzheimer's Association, 19*(4), 1308–1319.
15. Purushothaman, S., Ragavi, A., Basavaraju, P., Moorthi, P., & Anand, A. (2020). The role of trace elements in Alzheimer's disease. *Journal of Clinical Neuroscience, 21*(2), 107–111.
16. Tomata, Y., Larsson, S. C., & Hägg, S. (2020). Polyunsaturated fatty acids and risk of Alzheimer's disease: A Mendelian randomization study. *European Journal of Nutrition, 59*(4), 1763–1766.
17. Dutta, R. (2019). Role of MIND diet in preventing dementia and Alzheimer's disease. *Current Alzheimer Research, 4*(3), 1–8.
18. Agarwal, P., Wang, Y., Aggarwal, N. T., Cherian, L. J., James, B. D., Dhana, K., Leurgans, S. E., Bennett, D. A., & Schneider, J. A. (2021). MIND and Mediterranean diet association with Alzheimer's disease pathology. *Journal of Alzheimer's Disease, 17*(S10), e055679.
19. Yang, H. D., Kim, D. H., Lee, S. B., & Young, L. D. (2016). History of Alzheimer's disease. *Dementia and Neurocognitive Disorders, 15*(4), 115–121.
20. Román, G. (2003). Vascular dementia: A historical background. *International Psychogeriatrics, 15*(Suppl 1), 11–13.
21. L., S. B. (2002). Historical sketch of dementia concept. *Dementia and Neurocognitive Disorders, 1*(2).
22. Yang, H. D., Kim, D. H., Lee, S. B., & Young, L. D. (2016). History of Alzheimer's Disease. *Dementia and Neurocognitive Disorders, 15*, 115–121.
23. Gustaw-Rothenberg, K. (2009). Dietary patterns associated with Alzheimer's disease: Population-based study. *International Journal of Environmental Research and Public Health, 6*(4), 1335–1340.
24. Morris, M. C., S. J., & Tangney, C. C. (2006). Thoughts on B vitamins and dementia. *Journal of Alzheimer's Disease, 9*(4), 429–433.
25. Guerreiro, R., & Bras, J. (2015). The age factor in Alzheimer's disease. *Genome Medicine, 7*, 106.
26. Breijyeh, Z., & Karaman, R. (2020). Comprehensive review on Alzheimer's disease: Causes and treatment. *Molecules, 25*(24).

27. Croze, M. L., & Zimmer, L. (2018). Ozone atmospheric pollution and Alzheimer's disease: From epidemiological facts to molecular mechanisms. *Journal of Alzheimer's Disease, 62*(2), 503–522.
28. Brayne, C., McCracken, C., & Matthews, F. E. (2006). Cohort profile: The Medical Research Council Cognitive Function and Ageing Study (CFAS). *International Journal of Epidemiology, 35*(5), 1140–1145.
29. De Benedictis, C. A., Vilella, A., & Grabrucker, A. M. (2019). The role of trace metals in Alzheimer's disease. In T. Wisniewski (Ed.), *Alzheimer's Disease* (pp. 1–16). Codon Publications.
30. van den Brink, A. C., Brouwer-Brolsma, E. M., Berendsen, A. A. M., & van de Rest, O. (2019). The Mediterranean, dietary approaches to stop hypertension (DASH), and Mediterranean-dash intervention for neurodegenerative delay (MIND) diets are associated with less cognitive decline and a lower risk of Alzheimer's disease—A review. *Advances in Nutrition, 10*(6), 1040–1065.
31. Hu, N., Yu, J. T., Tan, L., Wang, Y. L., Sun, L., & Tan, L. (2013). Nutrition and the risk of Alzheimer's disease. *BioMed Research International, 2013*, 524820.
32. Cremonini, A. L., Caffa, I., Cea, M., Nencioni, A., Odetti, P., & Monacelli, F. (2019). Nutrients in the prevention of Alzheimer's disease. *Oxidative Medicine and Cellular Longevity, 2019*, 9874159.
33. Samadi, M., Moradi, S., Moradinazar, M., Mostafai, R., & Pasdar, Y. (2019). Dietary pattern in relation to the risk of Alzheimer's disease: A systematic review. *Neurological Sciences, 40*(10), 2031–2043.
34. Gauttam, V., Munjal, K., Mujwar, S., Sawale, J., Rohilla, M., & Gupta, S. (2022). Comparative study of developed formulation and market formulation for antidiabetic potential in alloxan-induced diabetic Wistar rats. *Journal of Young Pharmacists, 14*, 387–393.
35. Malik, J., & Choudhary, S. (2018). The molecular basis for protective effect of Mediterranean diet in neurodegenerative disorders. In *Role of the Mediterranean Diet in the Brain and Neurodegenerative Diseases* (pp. 53–76). Elsevier.
36. Stefaniak, O., Dobrzyńska, M., Drzymała-Czyż, S., & Przysławski, J. (2022). Diet in the prevention of Alzheimer's disease: Current knowledge and future research requirements. *Nutrients, 14*(21), 4564.
37. Omar, S. H., Scott, C. J., Hamlin, A. S., & Obied, H. K. (2018). Olive biophenols reduce Alzheimer's pathology in SH-SY5Y cells and APPswe mice. *International Journal of Molecular Sciences, 20*(1), 125.
38. Visioli, F., Caruso, D., Galli, C., Viappiani, S., Galli, G., & Sala, A. (2000). Olive oils rich in natural catecholic phenols decrease isoprostane excretion in humans. *Biochemical and Biophysical Research Communications, 278*(3), 797–799.
39. Pangeni, R., Sahni, J. K., Ali, J., Sharma, S., & Baboota, S. (2014). Resveratrol: Review on therapeutic potential and recent advances in drug delivery. *Expert Opinion on Drug Delivery, 11*(8), 1285–1298.
40. Zini, R., Morin, C., Bertelli, A., Bertelli, A. A., & Tillement, J. P. (2002). Resveratrol-induced limitation of dysfunction of mitochondria isolated from rat brain in an anoxia-reoxygenation model. *Life Sciences, 71*(26), 3091–3108.
41. Pietta, P. G. (2000). Flavonoids as antioxidants. *Journal of Natural Products, 63*(7), 1035–1042.

42. Ben-Dor, A., Steiner, M., Gheber, L., Danilenko, M., Dubi, N., Linnewiel, K., Zick, A., Sharoni, Y., & Levy, J. (2005). Carotenoids activate the antioxidant response element transcription system. *Molecular Cancer Therapeutics, 4*(1), 177–186.
43. Stahl, W., & Sies, H. (2003). Antioxidant activity of carotenoids. *Molecular Aspects of Medicine, 24*(6), 345–351.
44. Larrieu, S., Letenneur, L., Helmer, C., Dartigues, J., & Barberger-Gateau, P. (2004). Nutritional factors and risk of incident dementia in the PAQUID longitudinal cohort. *Journal of Nutrition, Health & Aging, 8*(3), 150–154.
45. Kalmijn, S., Launer, L. J., Ott, A., Witteman, J. C., Hofman, A., & Breteler, M. M. (1997). Dietary fat intake and the risk of incident dementia in the Rotterdam Study. *Annals of Neurology, 42*(5), 776–782.
46. Morris, M. C., Evans, D. A., Bienias, J. L., Tangney, C. C., Bennett, D. A., Wilson, R. S., Aggarwal, N., & Schneider, J. (2003). Consumption of fish and n-3 fatty acids and risk of incident Alzheimer's disease. *Archives of Neurology, 60*(7), 940–946.
47. Cásedas, G., Les, F., Gómez-Serranillos, M. P., Smith, C., & López, V. (2017). Anthocyanin profile, antioxidant activity, and enzyme inhibiting properties of blueberry and cranberry juices: A comparative study. *Food & Function, 8*(11), 4187–4193.
48. Tavares, L., Figueira, I., McDougall, G. J., Vieira, H. L., Stewart, D., Alves, P. M., Ferreira, R. B., & Santos, C. N. (2013). Neuroprotective effects of digested polyphenols from wild blackberry species. *European Journal of Nutrition, 52*(1), 225–236.
49. Shukitt-Hale, B., Cheng, V., & Joseph, J. A. (2009). Effects of blackberries on motor and cognitive function in aged rats. *Nutritional Neuroscience, 12*(3), 135–140.
50. Malin, D. H., Lee, D. R., Goyarzu, P., Chang, Y. H., Ennis, L. J., Beckett, E., Shukitt-Hale, B., & Joseph, J. A. (2011). A short-term blueberry-enriched diet prevents and reverses object recognition memory loss in aging rats. *Nutrition, 27*(3), 338–342.
51. Casadesus, G., Shukitt-Hale, B., Stellwagen, H. M., Zhu, X., Lee, H. G., Smith, M. A., & Joseph, J. A. (2004). Modulation of hippocampal plasticity and cognitive behavior by short-term blueberry supplementation in aged rats. *Nutritional Neuroscience, 7*(5–6), 309–316.
52. Berendsen, A. A., Kang, J. H., van de Rest, O., Feskens, E. J., de Groot, L. C., & Grodstein, F. (2017). The dietary approaches to stop hypertension diet, cognitive function, and cognitive decline in American older women. *Journal of the American Medical Directors Association, 18*(5), 427–432.
53. Smith, P. J., Blumenthal, J. A., Babyak, M. A., Craighead, L., Welsh-Bohmer, K. A., Browndyke, J. N., Strauman, T. A., & Sherwood, A. (2010). Effects of the dietary approaches to stop hypertension diet, exercise, and caloric restriction on neurocognition in overweight adults with high blood pressure. *Hypertension, 55*(6), 1331–1338.
54. Scarmeas, N., Stern, Y., Tang, M. X., Mayeux, R., & Luchsinger, J. A. (2006). Mediterranean diet and risk for Alzheimer's disease. *Annals of Neurology: Official Journal of the American Neurological Association and the Child Neurology Society, 59*(6), 912–921.
55. Scarmeas, N., Luchsinger, J. A., Schupf, N., Brickman, A. M., Cosentino, S., Tang, M. X., & Stern, Y. (2009). Physical activity, diet, and risk of Alzheimer disease. *JAMA, 302*(6), 627–637.
56. Gu, Y., Luchsinger, J. A., Stern, Y., & Scarmeas, N. (2010). Mediterranean diet, inflammatory and metabolic biomarkers, and risk of Alzheimer's disease. *Journal of Alzheimer's Disease, 22*(2), 483–492.

57. Scarmeas, N., Stern, Y., Mayeux, R., Manly, J. J., Schupf, N., & Luchsinger, J. A. (2009). Mediterranean diet and mild cognitive impairment. *Archives of Neurology, 66*(2), 216–225.
58. Scarmeas, N., Luchsinger, J. A., Mayeux, R., & Stern, Y. (2007). Mediterranean diet and Alzheimer disease mortality. *Neurology, 69*(11), 1084–1093.
59. Scarmeas, N., Stern, Y., Mayeux, R., & Luchsinger, J. A. (2006). Mediterranean diet, Alzheimer's disease, and vascular mediation. *Archives of Neurology, 63*(12), 1709–1717.
60. Anastasiou, C. A., Yannakoulia, M., Kosmidis, M. H., Dardiotis, E., Hadjigeorgiou, G. M., Sakka, P., Arampatzi, X., Bougea, A., Labropoulos, I., & Scarmeas, N. (2017). Mediterranean diet and cognitive health: Initial results from the Hellenic Longitudinal Investigation of Ageing and Diet. *PLoS One, 12*(8), e0182048.
61. Gardener, S., Gu, Y., Rainey-Smith, S. R., Keogh, J. B., Clifton, P. M., Mathieson, S., Taddei, K., Mondal, A., Ward, V. K., & Scarmeas, N. (2012). Adherence to a Mediterranean diet and Alzheimer's disease risk in an Australian population. *Translational Psychiatry, 2*(10), e164.
62. Knight, A., Bryan, J., Wilson, C., Hodgson, J. M., Davis, C. R., & Murphy, K. J. (2016). The Mediterranean diet and cognitive function among healthy older adults in a 6-month randomized controlled trial: The MedLey Study. *Nutrients, 8*(9), 579.
63. Marseglia, A., Xu, W., Fratiglioni, L., Fabbri, C., Berendsen, A. A., Bialecka-Debek, A., Jennings, A., Gillings, R., Meunier, N., & Caumon, E. (2018). Effect of the NU-AGE diet on cognitive functioning in older adults: A randomized controlled trial. *Frontiers in Physiology, 9, 349.*
64. Valls-Pedret, C., Sala-Vila, A., Serra-Mir, M., Corella, D., De la Torre, R., Martínez-González, M. Á., Martínez-Lapiscina, E. H., Fitó, M., Pérez-Heras, A., & Salas-Salvadó, J. (2015). Mediterranean diet and age-related cognitive decline: A randomized clinical trial. *JAMA Internal Medicine, 175*(7), 1094–1103.
65. Martínez-Lapiscina, E. H., Clavero, P., Toledo, E., Estruch, R., Salas-Salvadó, J., San Julián, B., Sanchez-Tainta, A., Ros, E., Valls-Pedret, C., & Martínez-Gonzalez, M. Á. (2013). Mediterranean diet improves cognition: The PREDIMED-NAVARRA randomized trial. *Journal of Neurology, Neurosurgery & Psychiatry, 84*(12), 1318–1325.
66. Haring, B., Wu, C., Coker, L. H., Seth, A., Snetselaar, L., Manson, J. E., Rossouw, J. E., & Wassertheil-Smoller, S. (2016). Hypertension, dietary sodium, and cognitive decline: Results from the Women's Health Initiative Memory Study. *American Journal of Hypertension, 29*(2), 202–216.
67. McEvoy, C. T., Guyer, H., Langa, K. M., & Yaffe, K. (2017). Neuroprotective diets are associated with better cognitive function: The Health and Retirement Study. *Journal of the American Geriatrics Society, 65*(8), 1857–1862.
68. Eyles, D. W., Smith, S., Kinobe, R., Hewison, M., & McGrath, J. J. (2005). Distribution of the vitamin D receptor and 1 alpha-hydroxylase in human brain. *Journal of Chemical Neuroanatomy, 29*(1), 21–30.
69. Lu'o'ng, K. V., & Nguyen, L. T. (2013). The role of vitamin D in Alzheimer's disease: Possible genetic and cell signaling mechanisms. *American Journal of Alzheimer's Disease & Other Dementias, 28*(2), 126–136.
70. Mizwicki, M. T., Menegaz, D., Zhang, J., Barrientos-Durán, A., Tse, S., Cashman, J. R., Griffin, P. R., & Fiala, M. (2012). Genomic and nongenomic signaling induced by 1α,25(OH)2-vitamin D3 promotes the recovery of amyloid-β phagocytosis by Alzheimer's disease macrophages. *Journal of Alzheimer's Disease, 29*(1), 51–62.

71. Munjal, K., Sharma, S., Sharma, S., Kumar, D., Choudhary, A., Berwal, R., & Kumar, A. (2021). Comparison of serum 25-hydroxyvitamin D levels after a single oral dose of vitamin D3 formulations in mild vitamin D3 deficiency. *RSC Advances, 12*(4), 163–167.
72. Morris, M. S., Jacques, P. F., Rosenberg, I. H., & Selhub, J. (2002). Elevated serum methylmalonic acid concentrations are common among elderly Americans. *Journal of Nutrition, 132*(9), 2799–2803.
73. Morris, M. C., Schneider, J. A., & Tangney, C. C. (2006). Thoughts on B-vitamins and dementia. *Journal of Alzheimer's Disease, 9*(4), 429–433.
74. Pal, T., Bhimaneni, S., Sharma, A., & Flora, S. J. S. (2020). Design, synthesis, biological evaluation, and molecular docking study of novel pyridoxine-triazoles as anti-Alzheimer's agents. *RSC Advances, 10*(44), 26006–26021.
75. Xie, Z., Wu, H., & Zhao, J. (2020). Multifunctional roles of zinc in Alzheimer's disease. *Neurotoxicology, 80*, 112–123.
76. Khalighinejad, P., Parrott, D., & Sherry, A. D. (2020). Imaging tissue physiology in vivo by use of metal ion-responsive MRI contrast agents. *Pharmaceuticals (Basel), 13*(10), 268.
77. Narayanan, S. E., Rehuman, N. A., Harilal, S., Vincent, A., Rajamma, R. G., Behl, T., Uddin, M. S., Ashraf, G. M., & Mathew, B. (2020). Molecular mechanism of zinc neurotoxicity in Alzheimer's disease. *Environmental Science and Pollution Research International, 27*(35), 43542–43552.
78. Lippi, S. L. P., Kakalec, P. A., Smith, M. L., & Flinn, J. M. (2020). Wheel-running behavior is negatively impacted by zinc administration in a novel dual transgenic mouse model of AD. *Frontiers in Neuroscience, 14*, 854.
79. Corona, C., Masciopinto, F., Silvestri, E., Viscovo, A. D., Lattanzio, R., Sorda, R. L., Ciavardelli, D., Goglia, F., Piantelli, M., Canzoniero, L. M., & Sensi, S. L. (2010). Dietary zinc supplementation of 3xTg-AD mice increases BDNF levels and prevents cognitive deficits as well as mitochondrial dysfunction. *Cell Death & Disease, 1*(10), e91.
80. Ashraf, A., Ashton, N. J., Chatterjee, P., Goozee, K., Shen, K., Fripp, J., Ames, D., Rowe, C., Masters, C. L., Villemagne, V., Hye, A., Martins, R. N., & So, P. W. (2020). Plasma transferrin and hemopexin are associated with altered Aβ uptake and cognitive decline in Alzheimer's disease pathology. *Alzheimer's Research & Therapy, 12*(1), 72.
81. van der Weerd, L., Lefering, A., Webb, A., Egli, R., & Bossoni, L. (2020). Effects of Alzheimer's disease and formalin fixation on the different mineralized-iron forms in the human brain. *Scientific Reports, 10*(1), 16440.
82. Loef, M., Schrauzer, G. N., & Walach, H. (2011). Selenium and Alzheimer's disease: A systematic review. *Journal of Alzheimer's Disease, 26*(1), 81–104.
83. Deepak, K., Pandey, S., Kumar, S., Kumar, A., Rai, D. K., Munjal, K., Rani, M., & Narayan, S. (2020). Change in bone mineral density in premenopausal women with rheumatoid arthritis managed with or without prednisolone. *The Journal of Rheumatology, 47*(2), 201–210.
84. Lu, Q., Chen, C., Xiong, Y., Li, G., Zhang, X., Zhang, Y., Wang, D., Zhu, Z., Li, X., Qing, G., Sun, T., & Liang, X. (2020). High-efficiency phosphopeptide and glycopeptide simultaneous enrichment by hydrogen bond-based bifunctional smart polymer. *Analytical Chemistry, 92*(9), 6269–6277.
85. Tedesco, E., Benetti, F., & Pezzani, R. (2020). In vitro evaluation of different organic matrices used to modulate silicon bioavailability. *FASEB Journal, 34*(9), 12229–12238.

86. Bowman, A. B., Kwakye, G. F., Herrero Hernández, E., & Aschner, M. (2011). Role of manganese in neurodegenerative diseases. *Journal of Trace Elements in Medicine and Biology, 25*(4), 191–203.
87. Martins, A. C., Jr., Morcillo, P., Ijomone, O. M., Venkataramani, V., Harrison, F. E., Lee, E., Bowman, A. B., & Aschner, M. (2019). New insights on the role of manganese in Alzheimer's disease and Parkinson's disease. *International Journal of Environmental Research and Public Health, 16*(19), 3511.
88. Tyler, C. R., & Allan, A. M. (2014). The effects of arsenic exposure on neurological and cognitive dysfunction in human and rodent studies: A review. *Current Environmental Health Reports, 1*(2), 132–147.
89. Zhang, Y., Chen, J., Qiu, J., Li, Y., Wang, J., & Jiao, J. (2015). Intakes of fish and polyunsaturated fatty acids and mild-to-severe cognitive impairment risks: A dose-response meta-analysis of 21 cohort studies. *The American Journal of Clinical Nutrition, 103*(2), 330–340.
90. Simonetto, M., Infante, M., Sacco, R. L., Rundek, T., & Della-Morte, D. (2019). A novel anti-inflammatory role of omega-3 PUFAs in prevention and treatment of atherosclerosis and vascular cognitive impairment and dementia. *Nutrients, 11*(10), 2279.
91. Gustafson, D. R., Bäckman, K., Scarmeas, N., Stern, Y., Manly, J. J., Mayeux, R., & Gu, Y. (2020). Dietary fatty acids and risk of Alzheimer's disease and related dementias: Observations from the Washington heights-Hamilton heights-in wood Columbia aging project (WHICAP). *Alzheimer's & Dementia, 16*(12), 1638–1649.
92. Andrieu, S., Guyonnet, S., Coley, N., Cantet, C., Bonnefoy, M., Bordes, S., Bories, L., Cufi, M. N., Dantoine, T., & Dartigues, J. F. (2017). Effect of long-term omega-3 polyunsaturated fatty acid supplementation with or without multidomain intervention on cognitive function in elderly adults with memory complaints (MAPT): A randomized, placebo-controlled trial. *The Lancet Neurology, 16*(5), 377–389.
93. Laye, S. (2010). Polyunsaturated fatty acids, neuroinflammation, and well-being. *Prostaglandins, Leukotrienes and Essential Fatty Acids (PLEFA), 82*(4–6), 295–303.
94. Delpech, J. C., Madore, C., Joffre, C., Aubert, A., Kang, J. X., Nadjar, A., & Layé, S. (2015). Transgenic increase in the n-3/n-6 fatty acid ratio protects against cognitive deficits induced by an immune challenge through the decrease of neuroinflammation. *Neuropsychopharmacology, 40*(3), 525–536.
95. Bazan, N. G. (2006). Cell survival matters Docosahexaenoic acid signaling, neuroprotection, and photoreceptors. *Trends in Neurosciences, 29*(5), 263–271.
96. Bazan, N. (2013). The docosanoid neuroprotectin D1 induces homeostatic regulation of neuroinflammation and cell survival. *Prostaglandins, Leukotrienes and Essential Fatty Acids, 88*(1), 127–129.
97. Hossain, S., Hashimoto, M., Katakura, M., Miwa, K., Shimada, T., & Shido, O. (2009). Mechanism of docosahexaenoic acid-induced inhibition of in vitro Aβ1–42 fibrillation and Aβ1–42-induced toxicity in SH-SY5Y cells. *Journal of Neurochemistry, 111*(2), 568–579.
98. Eckert, G. P., Chang, S., Eckmann, J., Copanaki, E., Hagl, S., Hener, U., Müller, W. E., & Kögel, D. (2011). Liposome-incorporated DHA increases neuronal survival by enhancing non-amyloidogenic APP processing. *Biochimica et Biophysica Acta (BBA)–Biomembranes, 1808*(1), 236–243.

99. Kumar, N. S., & Nisha, N. (2014). Phytomedicines as potential inhibitors of β amyloid aggregation: Significance to Alzheimer's disease. *Chinese Journal of Natural Medicines, 12*(11), 801–818.
100. Satyavert, Gupta, S., Choudhury, H., Jacob, S., Nair, A. B., Dhanawat, M., & Munjal, K. (2021). Pharmacokinetics and tissue distribution of hydrazinocurcumin in rats. *Pharmacological Reports, 73*(6), 1734–1743.
101. Park, S. Y., & Kim, D. S. (2002). Discovery of natural products from *Curcuma longa* that protect cells from beta-amyloid insult: A drug discovery effort against Alzheimer's disease. *Journal of Natural Products, 65*(9), 1227–1231.
102. Yang, L., Hao, J., Zhang, J., Xia, W., Dong, X., Hu, X., Kong, F., & Cui, X. (2009). Ginsenoside Rg3 promotes beta-amyloid peptide degradation by enhancing the gene expression of neprilysin. *The Journal of Pharmacy and Pharmacology, 61*(13), 375–380.
103. Wang, Y. H., & Du, G. H. (2009). Ginsenoside Rg1 inhibits beta-secretase activity in vitro and protects against Abeta-induced cytotoxicity in PC12 cells. *Journal of Asian Natural Products Research, 11*(7), 604–612.
104. Park, S. Y., Lim, J. Y., Jeong, W., Hong, S. S., Yang, Y. T., Hwang, B. Y., & Lee, D. (2010). C-methyl flavonoids isolated from *Callistemon lanceolatus* protect PC12 cells against Abeta-induced toxicity. *Planta Medica, 76*(9), 863–868.
105. Anand, A., Patience, A. A., Sharma, N., & Khurana, N. (2017). The present and future of pharmacotherapy of Alzheimer's disease: A comprehensive review. *European Journal of Pharmacology, 815*, 364–375.
106. Bai, Y., Tohda, C., Zhu, S., Hattori, M., & Komatsu, K. (2011). Active components from *Siberian ginseng* (*Eleutherococcus senticosus*) for protection of amyloid β (25–35)-induced neuritic atrophy in cultured rat cortical neurons. *Journal of Natural Medicines, 65*(3–4), 417–423.
107. Liu, R., Meng, F., Zhang, L., Liu, A., Qin, H., Lan, X., Li, L., & Du, G. (2011). Luteolin isolated from the medicinal plant *Elsholtzia rugulosa* (Labiatae) prevents copper-mediated toxicity in β-amyloid precursor protein Swedish mutation overexpressing SH-SY5Y cells. *Molecules, 16*(3), 2084–2096.
108. Na, C. S., Hong, S. S., Choi, Y. H., Lee, Y. H., Hong, S. H., Lim, J. Y., Kang, B. H., Park, S. Y., & Lee, D. (2010). Neuroprotective effects of constituents of *Eragrostis ferruginea* against Aβ-induced toxicity in PC12 cells. *Archives of Pharmacal Research, 33*(7), 999–1003.
109. Hoi, C. P., Ho, Y. P., Baum, L., & Chow, A. H. (2010). Neuroprotective effect of honokiol and magnolol, compounds from *Magnolia officinalis*, on beta-amyloid-induced toxicity in PC12 cells. *Phytotherapy Research, 24*(10), 1538–1542.
110. Nakhate, K. T., Bharne, A. P., Verma, V. S., Aru, D. N., & Kokare, D. M. (2018). Plumbagin ameliorates memory dysfunction in streptozotocin-induced Alzheimer's disease via activation of the Nrf2/ARE pathway and inhibition of β-secretase. *Biomedicine & Pharmacotherapy, 101*, 379–390.
111. Choi, Y. H., Hong, S. S., Shin, Y. S., Hwang, B. Y., Park, S. Y., & Lee, D. (2010). Phenolic compounds from *Pueraria lobata* protect PC12 cells against Aβ-induced toxicity. *Archives of Pharmacal Research, 33*(10), 1651–1654.
112. Kim, D. H., Park, S. J., Kim, J. M., Jeon, S. J., Kim, D. H., Cho, Y. W., Son, K. H., Lee, H. J., Moon, J. H., Cheong, J. H., Ko, K. H., & Ryu, J. H. (2011). Cognitive dysfunctions induced by a cholinergic blockade and Aβ 25–35 peptide are attenuated by salvianolic acid B. *Neuropharmacology, 61*(8), 1432–1440.

113. Sallam, A., Mira, A., Ashour, A., & Shimizu, K. (2016). Acetylcholine esterase inhibitors and melanin synthesis inhibitors from *Salvia officinalis*. *Phytomedicine, 23*(10), 1005–1011.
114. Song, J. X., Lin, X., Wong, R. N. S., Sze, S. C. W., Tong, Y., Shaw, P. C., & Zhang, Y. B. (2011). Protective effects of dibenzocyclooctadiene lignans from *Schisandra chinensis* against beta-amyloid and homocysteine neurotoxicity in PC12 cells. *Phytotherapy Research, 25*(3), 435–443.
115. Roy, A. J. S. J. H. M. (2017). A review on medicinal plants for Alzheimer's disease. *SciFed Journal of Herbal Medicine, 1*(2), 1–6.
116. Jayaprakasam, B., Padmanabhan, K., & Nair, M. G. (2010). Withanamides in *Withania somnifera* fruit protect PC-12 cells from beta-amyloid responsible for Alzheimer's disease. *Phytotherapy Research, 24*(6), 859–863.
117. Asai, M., Iwata, N., Yoshikawa, A., Aizaki, Y., Ishiura, S., Saido, T. C., & Maruyama, K. (2007). Berberine alters the processing of Alzheimer's amyloid precursor protein to decrease Abeta secretion. *Biochemical and Biophysical Research Communications, 352*(2), 498–502.
118. Durairajan, S. S., Liu, L. F., Lu, J. H., Chen, L. L., Yuan, Q., Chung, S. K., Huang, L., Li, X. S., Huang, J. D., & Li, M. (2012). Berberine ameliorates β-amyloid pathology, gliosis, and cognitive impairment in an Alzheimer's disease transgenic mouse model. *Neurobiology of Aging, 33*(12), 2903–2919.
119. Jia, L., Liu, J., Song, Z., Pan, X., Chen, L., Cui, X., & Wang, M. (2012). Berberine suppresses amyloid-beta-induced inflammatory response in microglia by inhibiting nuclear factor-kappaB and mitogen-activated protein kinase signaling pathways. *The Journal of Pharmacy and Pharmacology, 64*(10), 1510–1521.
120. Panahi, N., Mahmoudian, M., Mortazavi, P., & Hashjin, G. S. (2013). Effects of berberine on β-secretase activity in a rabbit model of Alzheimer's disease. *Archives of Medical Research, 9*(1), 146–150.
121. Jung, H. A., Min, B. S., Yokozawa, T., Lee, J. H., Kim, Y. S., & Choi, J. S. (2009). Anti-Alzheimer and antioxidant activities of *Coptidis Rhizoma* alkaloids. *Biological and Pharmaceutical Bulletin, 32*(8), 1433–1438.
122. Durairajan, S. S., Yuan, Q., Xie, L., Chan, W. S., Kum, W. F., Koo, I., Liu, C., Song, Y., Huang, J. D., Klein, W. L., & Li, M. (2008). Salvianolic acid B inhibits Abeta fibril formation disaggregates preformed fibrils and protects against Abeta-induced cytotoxicity. *Neurochemistry International, 52*(4–5), 741–750.
123. Mei, Z., Zhang, F., Tao, L., Zheng, W., Cao, Y., Wang, Z., Tang, S., Le, K., Chen, S., Pi, R., & Liu, P. (2009). Cryptotanshinone, a compound from *Salvia miltiorrhiza*, modulates amyloid precursor protein metabolism and attenuates beta-amyloid deposition through upregulating alpha-secretase in vivo and in vitro. *Neuroscience Letters, 452*(2), 90–95.
124. Okello, E. J., Savelev, S. U., & Perry, E. K. (2004). In vitro anti-beta-secretase and dual anti-cholinesterase activities of *Camellia sinensis* L. (tea) relevant to the treatment of dementia. *Phytotherapy Research, 18*(8), 624–627.
125. Lin, C. L., Chen, T. F., Chiu, M. J., Way, T. D., & Lin, J. K. (2009). Epigallocatechin gallate (EGCG) suppresses β-amyloid-induced neurotoxicity by inhibiting c-Abl/FE65 nuclear translocation and GSK 3β activation. *Neurobiology of Aging, 30*, 81–92.
126. Rezai-Zadeh, K., Shytle, D., Sun, N., Mori, T., Hou, H., Jeanniton, D., Ehrhart, J., Townsend, K., Zeng, J., Morgan, D., Hardy, J., Town, T., & Tan, J. (2005). Green tea epigallocatechin-3-gallate (EGCG) modulates amyloid precursor protein cleavage and

reduces cerebral amyloidosis in Alzheimer's transgenic mice. *Journal of Neuroscience, 25*(38), 8807–8814.

127. Lu, P., Mamiya, T., Lu, L. L., Mouri, A., Zou, L., Nagai, T., Hiramatsu, M., Ikejima, T., & Nabeshima, T. (2009). Silibinin prevents amyloid beta peptide-induced memory impairment and oxidative stress in mice. *British Journal of Pharmacology, 157*(7), 1270–1277.
128. Jia, H., Jiang, Y., Ruan, Y., Zhang, Y., Ma, X., Zhang, J., Beyreuther, K., Tu, P., & Zhang, D. (2004). Tenuigenin treatment decreases secretion of the Alzheimer's disease amyloid beta-protein in cultured cells. *Neuroscience Letters, 367*(1), 123–128.
129. Lv, J., Jia, H., Jiang, Y., Ruan, Y., Liu, Z., Yue, W., Beyreuther, K., Tu, P., & Zhang, D. (2009). Tenuifolin, an extract derived from tenuigenin, inhibits amyloid-beta secretion in vitro. *Acta Physiologica (Oxford, England), 196*(4), 419–425.
130. Munjal, K., Uniyal, R., Kumar, A., Arora, A., Gupta, A., Haye, A., & Gauttam, V. (2020). Development of validated HPTLC method for quantification of luteolin in *Eclipta alba* and its formulation. *Journal of Pharmacological and Toxicological Methods, 2685–2695.*
131. Malik, J. (2017). Phytomedicine: A possible tool for Alzheimer's disease therapeutics. In T. Farooqui & A. A. Farooqui (Eds.), *Neuroprotective Effects of Phytochemicals in Neurological Disorders* (pp. 167–198). John Wiley & Sons.
132. Munjal, K., Amin, S., Mir, S. R., Gauttam, V., & Gupta, S. (2022). Furanocoumarins and lectins as food toxins. In *Food Toxins* (pp. 67–80).
133. Andrade, S., Ramalho, M. J., Loureiro, J. A., & Pereira, M. D. C. (2019). Natural compounds for Alzheimer's disease therapy: A systematic review of preclinical and clinical studies. *International Journal of Molecular Sciences, 20*(9), 2313.
134. Munjal, K., Gauttam, V., Gupta, S., Gupta, A., Abidin, L., Jhawat, V., & Altaf, A. (2022). Traditional uses and phytochemistry of *Cinnamomum* species: A mini-review. *Research Journal of Pharmacy and Technology, 15*, 5363–5367.
135. Tyagi, S., Singh, U., Kalra, T., & Munjal, K. (2010). Applications of metabolomics: A systematic study of the unique chemical fingerprints: An overview. In *Metabolomics Applications*.
136. He, Q., Liu, J., Liang, J., Liu, X., Li, W., Liu, Z., Ding, Z., & Tuo, D. (2018). Towards improvements for penetrating the blood-brain barrier: Recent progress from a material and pharmaceutical perspective. *Cells, 7*(4).
137. Findeis, M. A., Schroeder, F. C., Creaser, S. P., McKee, T. D., & Xia, W. (2015). Natural product and natural product-derived gamma-secretase modulators from *Actaea racemosa* extracts. *Medicines (Basel, Switzerland), 2*(3), 127–140.
138. Chauhan, N. B. (2006). Effect of aged garlic extract on APP processing and tau phosphorylation in Alzheimer's transgenic model Tg2576. *Journal of Ethnopharmacology, 108*(3), 385–394.
139. Zhong, L., Tan, J., Ouyang, S., & Xu, J. P. (2006). Effects of saponin B from *Anemarrhena asphodeloides* Bunge on tau hyperphosphorylation induced by beta-amyloid peptide (25–35) in rats. *Nan Fang Yi Ke Da Xue Xue Bao = Journal of Southern Medical University, 26*(8), 1106–1109.
140. Bulic, B., Pickhardt, M., & Mandelkow, E. (2013). Progress and developments in tau aggregation inhibitors for Alzheimer's disease. *Journal of Medicinal Chemistry, 56*(11), 4135–4155.

141. Rather, M. A., Thenmozhi, A. J., Manivasagam, T., Saravanababu, C., Guillemin, G. J., & Essa, M. M. (2019). Asiatic acid attenuates aluminum chloride-induced tau pathology, oxidative stress, and apoptosis via AKT/GSK-3β signaling pathway in Wistar rats. *Neurotoxicity Research, 35*(4), 955–968.
142. Peterson, D. W., George, R. C., Scaramozzino, F., LaPointe, N. E., Anderson, R. A., Graves, D. J., & Lew, J. (2009). Cinnamon extract inhibits tau aggregation associated with Alzheimer's disease in vitro. *Journal of Alzheimer's Disease, 17*(3), 585–597.
143. Yao, Y., Wang, Y., Kong, L., Chen, Y., & Yang, J. (2019). Osthole decreases tau protein phosphorylation via PI3K/AKT/GSK-3β signaling pathway in Alzheimer's disease. *Life Sciences, 217*, 16–24.
144. Radenahmad, N., Saleh, F., Sawangjaroen, K., Vongvatcharanon, U., Subhadhirasakul, P., Rundorn, W., Withyachumnarnkul, B., & Connor, J. R. (2011). Young coconut juice, a potential therapeutic agent that could significantly reduce some pathologies associated with Alzheimer's disease: Novel findings. *The British Journal of Nutrition, 105*(5), 738–746.
145. Shytle, R. D., Tan, J., Bickford, P. C., Rezai-Zadeh, K., Hou, L., Zeng, J., Sanberg, P. R., Sanberg, C. D., Alberte, R. S., Fink, R. C., & Roschek, B., Jr. (2012). Optimized turmeric extract reduces beta-amyloid and phosphorylated tau protein burden in Alzheimer's transgenic mice. *Current Alzheimer Research, 9*(4), 500–506.
146. Tang, M., & Taghibiglou, C. (2017). The mechanisms of action of curcumin in Alzheimer's disease. *Journal of Alzheimer's Disease, 58*(4), 1003–1016.
147. Seung, T. W., Park, S. K., Kang, J. Y., Kim, J. M., Park, S. H., Kwon, B. S., Lee, C. J., Kang, J. E., Kim, D. O., Lee, U., & Heo, H. J. (2018). Ethyl acetate fraction from *Hibiscus sabdariffa* L. attenuates diabetes-associated cognitive impairment in mice. *Food Research International, 105*, 589–598.
148. Calcul, L., Zhang, B., Jinwal, U. K., Dickey, C. A., & Baker, B. J. (2012). Natural products as a rich source of tau-targeting drugs for Alzheimer's disease. *Future Medicinal Chemistry, 4*(13), 1751–1761.
149. Kim, J. Y., Lee, H. K., Jang, J. Y., Yoo, J. K., & Seong, Y. H. (2015). *Ilex latifolia* prevents amyloid β protein (25–35)-induced memory impairment by inhibiting apoptosis and tau phosphorylation in mice. *Journal of Medicinal Food, 18*(12), 1317–1326.
150. Gong, E. J., Park, H. R., Kim, M. E., Piao, S., Lee, E., Jo, D. G., Chung, H. Y., Ha, N. C., Mattson, M. P., & Lee, J. (2011). Morin attenuates tau hyperphosphorylation by inhibiting GSK3β. *Neurobiology of Disease, 44*(2), 223–230.
151. Jones, J. R., Lebar, M. D., Jinwal, U. K., Abisambra, J. F., Koren, J. III, Blair, L., O'Leary, J. C., Davey, Z., Trotter, J., Johnson, A. G., Weeber, E., Eckman, C. B., Baker, B. J., & Dickey, C. A. (2011). The diarylheptanoid (+)-aR,11S-myricanol, and two flavones from bayberry (*Myrica cerifera*) destabilize the microtubule-associated protein tau. *Journal of Natural Products, 74*(1), 38–44.
152. Li, W., Sperry, J. B., Crowe, A., Trojanowski, J. Q., Smith, A. B. III, & Lee, V. M. Y. (2009). Inhibition of tau fibrillization by oleocanthal via reaction with the amino groups of tau. *Journal of Neurochemistry, 110*(4), 1339–1351.
153. Li, L., Liu, J., Yan, X., Qin, K., Shi, M., Lin, T., Zhu, Y., Kang, T., & Zhao, G. (2011). Protective effects of ginsenoside Rd against okadaic acid-induced neurotoxicity in vivo and in vitro. *Journal of Ethnopharmacology, 138*(1), 135–141.

154. Shati, A. A., & Alfaifi, M. Y. (2019). Trans-resveratrol inhibits tau phosphorylation in the brains of control and cadmium chloride-treated rats by activating PP2A and PI3K/Akt induced-inhibition of GSK3β. *Neurochemical Research, 44*(2), 357–373.
155. Blair, S. N. (2009). Physical inactivity: The biggest public health problem of the 21st century. *British Journal of Sports Medicine, 43*(1), 1–2.
156. Norton, S., Matthews, F. E., Barnes, D. E., Yaffe, K., & Brayne, C. (2014). Potential for primary prevention of Alzheimer's disease: An analysis of population-based data. *Lancet Neurology, 13*(8), 788–794.
157. Luck, T., & Riedel-Heller, S. G. (2016). Prevention of Alzheimer's dementia in Germany: A projection of the possible potential of reducing selected risk factors. *Nervenarzt, 87*(11), 1194–1200.
158. Wahl, D., Solon-Biet, S. M., Cogger, V. C., Fontana, L., Simpson, S. J., Le Couteur, D. G., & Ribeiro, R. V. (2019). Aging, lifestyle, and dementia. *Neurobiology of Disease, 130*, 104481.
159. Bhatti, G. K., Reddy, A. P., Reddy, P. H., & Bhatti, J. S. (2019). Lifestyle modifications and nutritional interventions in aging-associated cognitive decline and Alzheimer's disease. *Frontiers in Aging Neuroscience, 11*, 369.
160. Alkefai, N., Mir, S. R., Amin, S., Ahamad, J., Munjal, K., & Gauttam, V. (2022). NMR in analysis of food toxins. In *Food Toxins* (pp. 131–139).
161. Liu Y, Nguyen M, Robert A, Meunier B. Metal Ions in Alzheimer's Disease: A Key Role or Not? *Acc Chem Res.* 2019 Jul 16; *52*(7):2026-2035. doi: 10.1021/acs.accounts.9b00248. Epub 2019 Jul 5. PMID: 31274278.

Index

L

M

N

O

P

T

Y

Z